ALTERNATIVE HEALING AND YOUR HEALTH

THE DIAGRAM GROUP

Editors Moira Johnson, Susan Bosanko
Indexer Maureen Cartwright

Art director Richard Hummerstone
Design assistance Point Three
Artists James Dallas
Brian Hewson
Lee Lawrence
Paul McCauley
Kathleen McDougall
Philip Patenall
Micky Pledge
Jane Robertson
Graham Rosewarne
Dino Skeete

Other Diagram Group titles also published by Ballantine Books:

PREDICTING YOUR FUTURE
WHO ARE YOU?
WHO WERE YOU?
YOUR MIND OVER MATTER

Published in the United States by Ballantine Books, a division of Random House, Inc., New York, and simultaneously in Canada by Random House of Canada Limited, Toronto.

Library of Congress Catalog Card Number: 90-93516

ISBN: 0-345-36692-1

Manufactured in the United States of America

First Edition: June 1991

10 9 8 7 6 5 4 3 2 1

ALTERNATIVE HEALING AND YOUR HEALTH

by J. Maya Pilkington
and the Diagram Group

BALLANTINE BOOKS · NEW YORK

Foreword

Alternative Healing and Your Health is yet another in the fine series of books by Maya Pilkington and the Diagram Group in which a diversity of fascinating knowledge and ideas is collected together and presented concisely so that you can dip into the pages either for a brief encounter or a detailed exploration of the whole magical world of healing.

This book of **Alternative Healing and Your Health** is a compulsive read for anyone who has a natural human interest in good health and longevity. From the mystique of ancient worlds, through the myriad strands of primitive medical systems, to the mysteries of modern discoveries, every page is an adventure in itself.

The connections that link mankind's search for health and healing across the centuries and around the world will keep you enthralled, especially when some of what was called the medicine man's mumbo-jumbo has turned out to have an indisputable scientific basis. The attractive visual presentation and the wealth of detailed examples in **Alternative Healing and Your Health** help you to uncover your own outlook.

Alternative Healing and Your Health leads you through six aspects of medicine that are different facets of the same concern with human well-being. Three approaches applied from outside the body, which often require the cooperation of the patient are: healing through stimulating the body's energy streams; healing by touch; and healing by harnessing natural phenomena such as hot springs, mineral waters and sunlight. Treatment by changing the diet, by taking remedies or by surgery are methods applied to the inside of the body while outwardly the patient remains relatively passive. On the other hand, there are medical rituals and faith healing whose success often depends on the attitude of the patient.

In **Alternative Healing and Your Health** some fundamental concerns are explored concerning human life and the nature of ill-health and disease, and the relationship between tribal medicines, the world's major medical systems and the growing number of alternative approaches. **Alternative Healing and Your Health** also presents some unusual approaches to diagnosis and brings you up to date on the newest and most avant-garde ideas.

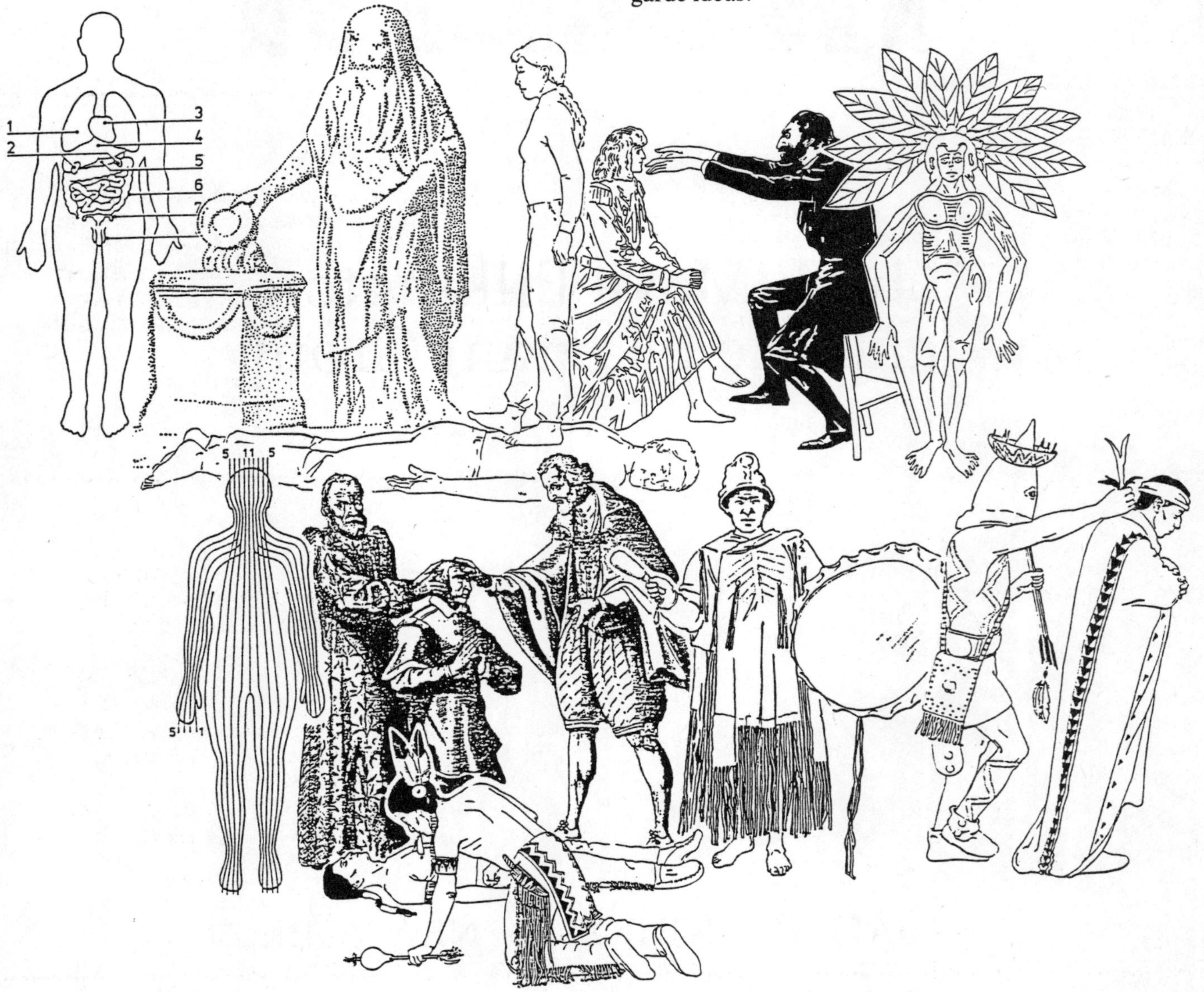

Alternative Healing and Your Health presents you with an unusually refreshing approach to medical care around the world and through time, explaining and describing a plethora of fascinating treatments that have been used to cure human ills since man walked upright.

There are details of what to expect from a shaman and how to consult a witchdoctor. Remedies for minor ills and possible solutions to major plagues are explored; surprisingly, much of what is taken for granted as modern medicine was in common use centuries ago. But medicine was not always a serious business. Primitive rituals sometimes included humor in their routine prescriptions, and some of the methods themselves will bring a smile to the modern mind.

The horrors of a Cesarean delivery without painkillers, and infections without a known antidote will give you goosepimples, yet many weird treatments were very successful, and the courage of patients and doctors who worked these primitive miracles of healing can only be admired. Many of their successes may leave you wondering if the Western medicine chest is overfull.

Alternative Healing and Your Health will stretch your imagination as you pore through the wonders of medical endeavors practiced by our forebears. The challenge to understanding will be even greater as alternative medicines are seen to be founded both on primitive beliefs and on the most up-to-date scientific research.

The author does not make recommendations but leaves you to make up your own mind. **Alternative Healing and Your Health** is not a reference book for the would-be patient but a compendium of insights into the world of healing.

Modern understanding of how the body and its immune system works is slowly dawning. Researchers are uncovering the facts about biochemical mysteries that ancient peoples could only guess at. Yet their intuitive healing has much to teach us, as we enter an era during which allopathic concepts of health-care are likely to be overturned in favor of holistic approaches. Many theories of health and disease are presented in this book and, as always, we leave you to make up your own mind as you enjoy the journey through the world of **Alternative Healing and Your Health**.

HEALTH WARNING

Ordinary people are capable of harming themselves because they are ignorant about methods or ignorant about themselves. The power to heal lies in knowledge of both. Any particular treatment will not be suitable for all people or all cases of the same disease.

None of the methods outlined in this book should be attempted by amateurs. If you have ill-health, chronic complaints or any other disturbance, you should consult a properly qualified and experienced practitioner, whether orthodox, alternative, primitive or religious.

To find a qualified practitioner, consult the registers held by official associations and institutes, addresses for which can be found in main reference libraries and telephone listings. Any genuine practitioner will offer proof of training and experience.

DRUGS AND MEDICINES — CAUTION!

The notes below apply to anything that can be taken, injected or applied, whether of herbal or laboratory origin.

1 It is possible for anyone to become dependent upon any mind-altering substance.

2 The effect of a drug or medicine depends on dose, expectations, the mental and physical condition of the consumer, the setting in which it is taken and the manner by which it is taken.

3 Processed, concentrated or synthesized substances are often more potent and have more side-effects than their natural plant equivalents.

4 Frequent or long-term use of any substance will increase the difficulties on withdrawal, which will produce the very opposite of the effect the drug or medicine was designed to have. For example, withdrawal from long-term use of tranquilizers will cause great agitation and anxiety. Withdrawal from an addiction will, temporarily, produce a very bad trip, for example, the well-documented DTs (*delirium tremens*) of alcoholic withdrawal.

5 Mixing drugs or medicines with each other or with other substances, such as alcohol, is often harmful, and even lethal.

Contents

SECTION ONE
UNIVERSAL ENERGY

8 Opener
10 Five life-forces
12 In sickness and in health
14 The balance of life
16 The human body
18 Science and magic
20 The creative cycle
22 Parts and wholes
24 Energy states
26 Handling pain
28 Magical healing methods

SECTION TWO
CREATIVE TOUCH

30 Opener
32 The way of the Orient: Acupuncture 1
34 Acupuncture 2
36 The meridians
38 The balancing touch
40 Techniques of manipulation
42 The laying-on of hands
44 A loving touch
46 Any old bones
48 Handwork
50 It's all in the sole 1
52 It's all in the sole 2

SECTION THREE
RITUAL TRANSFORMATION

54 Opener
56 The way of the Vedas
58 Ritual is magic
60 Magical rituals
62 Magic charms
64 What's in a name?
66 Portents and familiars
68 The magic circle
70 Alchemy
72 The imagery of alchemy

SECTION FOUR
NATURE AND NURTURE

74 Opener
76 The way of mother earth
78 Fertility
80 Childbirth
82 What's in a diet?
84 Good red blood
86 Sweat it out
88 Nectar of the gods
90 New life for old
92 Water of life
94 Inheritance or environment?

SECTION FIVE
RELAXING INTO FAITH

96 Opener
98 The way of the believer
100 The tree of life
102 Hidden patterns
104 Shamanism
106 A little black box
108 The mystical senses
110 A healthy charge
112 Suggestive healing
114 A pinch of optimism
116 The sounding board
118 Rainbow health

SECTION SIX
ADAPTIVE POTIONS

120 Opener
122 The primitive pharmacopoeia
124 Folklore remedies
126 Old wives' tales
128 Drugs for all occasions
130 Mystical excursions
132 Which potions?
134 Homeopathic remedies
136 Flower remedies
138 Natural remedies
140 An alphabet of vitamins

SECTION SEVEN
HOW ARE YOU?

142 Opener
144 Diagnostic alternatives 1
146 Diagnostic alternatives 2
148 Divining the diagnosis
150 How fit are you?
152 The best of both worlds

154 Glossary
158 Index

Section one

UNIVERSAL ENERGY

What keeps us alive and healthy, and is death the ultimate state of ill-health? Is there a life-force, an emotional body chemistry or an electricity that powers the thousands of reactions that take place within our skins every day? And does this same life energy bring about aging?

Is health affected by psychology, morality or spirituality? Does the body include the mind, and can a person be healthy who commits evil acts?

What causes an illness? Is a person responsible for his total well-being, so if he falls ill, is it his fault? Can we help ourselves to get better, or will ill-health get the better of us regardless of how positive we are?

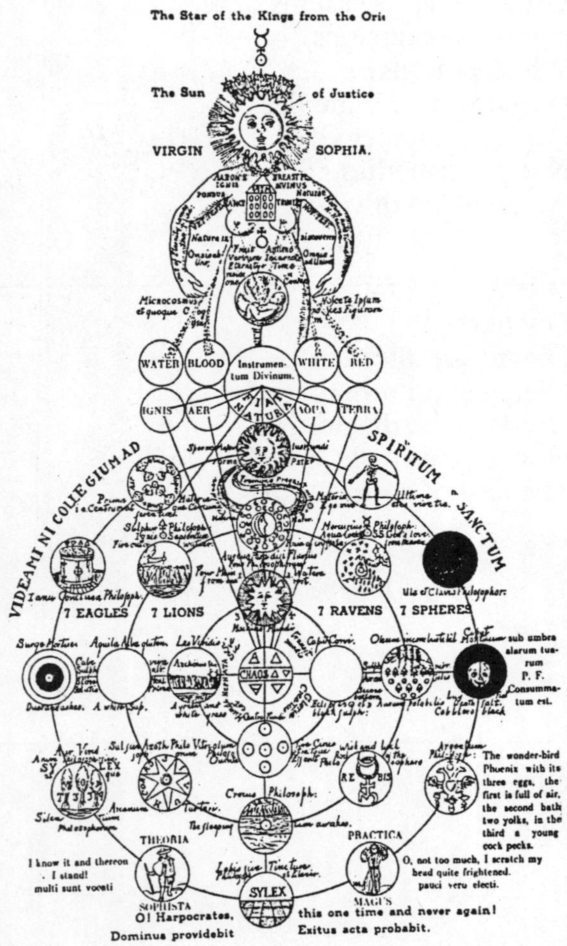

Creation: A Rosicrucian diagram of the female as the origin and provider of life forces, 19th century engraving.

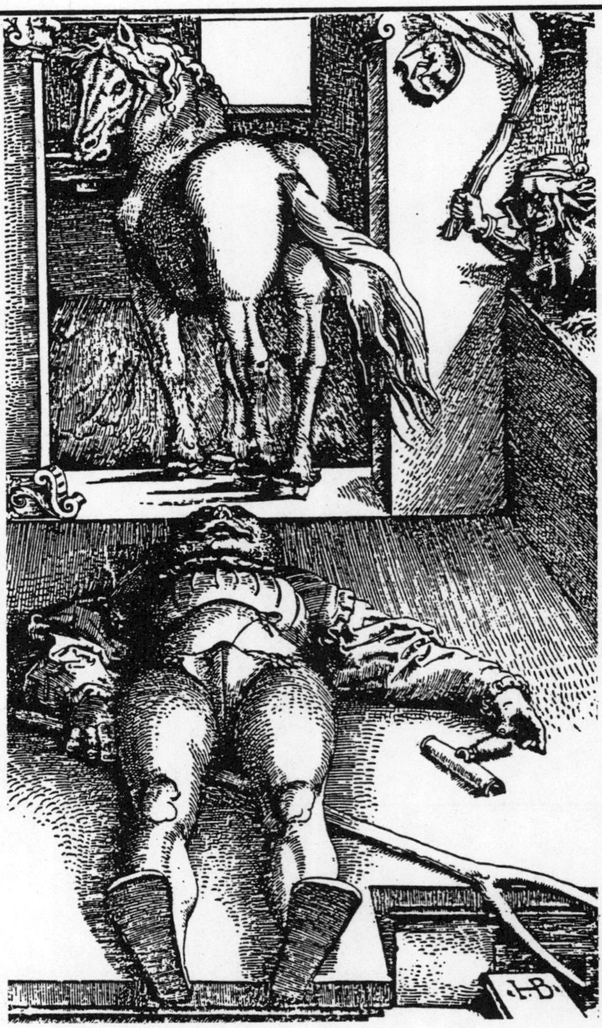

Illness: Medieval superstition believed health could be influenced by external forces such as witchcraft. "The Bewitched Groom", a German 16th century woodcut.

Are different aspects of this life energy in a continually changing state of balance? Is sickness a loss of balance, and if so what are the things that need to be in balance? Can these energies be used to heal personal ills and the ills of other people? Is the energy of a group more powerful than individual energies, and are rhythms and cycles important?

All these questions are explored in this section, which introduces the idea of a universal human life energy that can be affected by different approaches to healing.

Looking at the wide spectrum of healing methods, ranging from modern Western medicine and the many alternatives to the most primitive of ancient practices, they are seen to be based on very different philosophies and yet, in practice, often there is little to choose between what we call science and what our ancestors called magic.

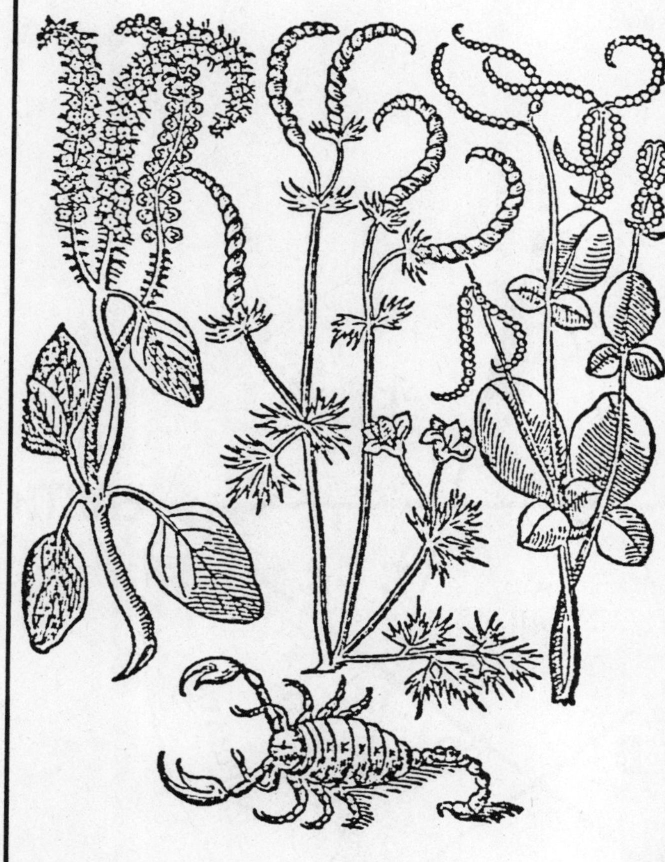

Sympathetic medicine: The idea that "like cures like". A herb believed to be a remedy for scorpion stings because its flowers curl in a similar way to a scorpion's tail. Woodcut from the Italian physicist Giambattista della Porta's *Phytognomonica* (1588).

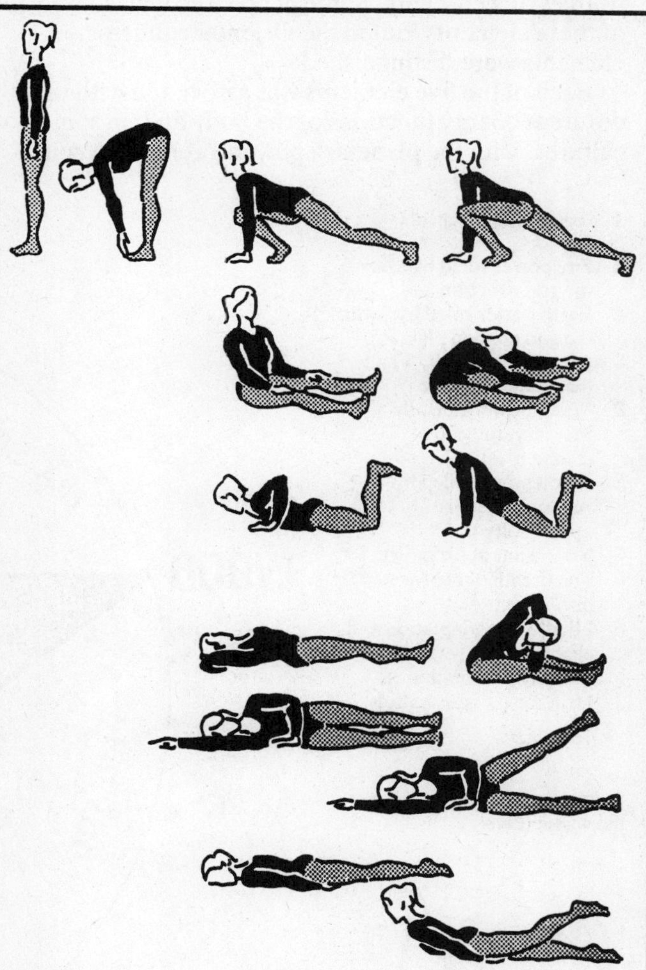

Preventive medicine: Exercise sequence designed to maintain a healthy, fit body. A 20th century instructional illustration for a program prepared by the US President's Council on Physical Fitness.

Five life-forces

In very early tribal civilizations, people were injured, became sick and inherited diseases, just as happens today. While they did not have hospitals, wonder drugs, miracle technology, replacement surgery, cloning, screening and other facilities available to them, they did have many effective practices and some powerful beliefs to sustain them.

Primitive healing methods were regarded as magical, since they could not be understood. Magic to primitive people was not a deception, nor a sleight of hand, but a genuine source of awesome wonder. Magic was a resource to be called upon when needed; its potency depended upon the power of the universal energy or life energy it was acting upon.

The five elements

Manifestations of universal energy, such as water, air, fire and earth, were regarded by primitive peoples as the sources of well-being. Some people recognized only four of these elements, but in the Oriental cultures five elements were distinguished.

Each of the five elements was associated with the different energy functions of the body and, in some cultures, with the planetary powers (gods) that ruled them. Sickness was said to be caused by too much or too little energy at work in one element, which would immediately affect all the others, thus pushing the whole person off balance. Modern holistic, alternative therapies have developed from these early ideas in which the human body-mind was regarded as a balanced, interactive whole. Needless to say, while primitive people firmly believed the spirits controlled these powers, modern practitioners tend to believe we can affect our own destiny.

The pentagram of health

The pentagram is a very old symbol of magical powers and was worn by the select membership of the Pythagorean Society founded by Pythagoras in Ancient Greece. Pythagoras was of the opinion that the universe could be explained and understood mathematically, a point of view that is becoming increasingly evident through modern research. The pentagram, containing a series of dynamic triangles, demonstrates the interdependence of the parts in maintaining a balanced whole.

The balanced pentagram
(*right*)

- **A** Fire power ruled by Mars, the god of action
- **B** Earth power ruled by Saturn, the god of good planning
- **C** Air power ruled by Venus, the goddess of love
- **D** Water power ruled by Mercury, the god of communication
- **E** Wood power ruled by Jupiter, the god of opportunity
- F Nourishment for growth
- G The breath of life for inspiration
- H Fluidity for adaptation and change
- I Fertility for creation
- J Heat for transformation

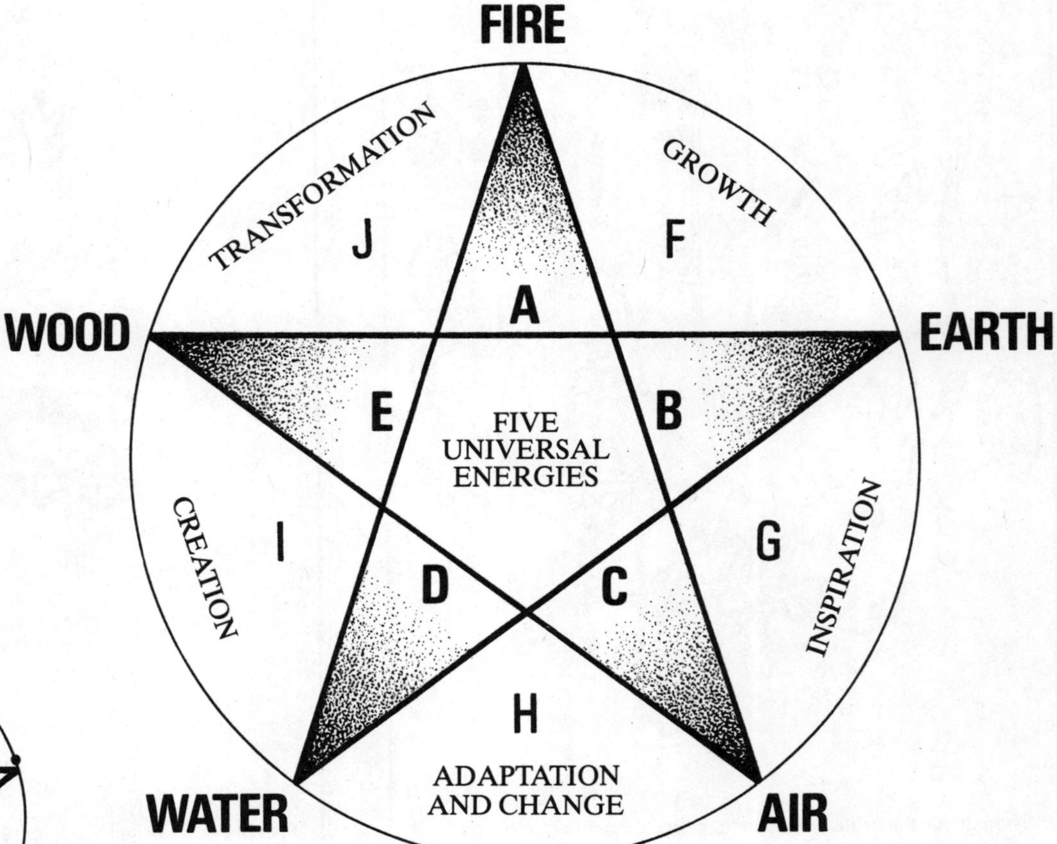

A small irregularity unbalances the whole (*below*)

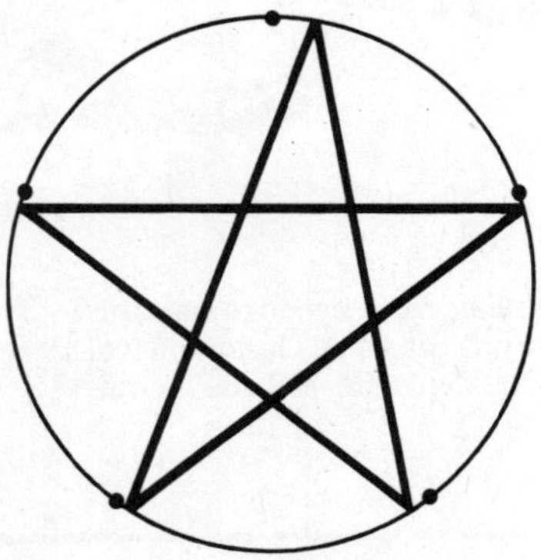

Chaos and order

Called the Butterfly Effect, the line between a balanced order and chaos is very, very much finer than we ever imagined, as the new science of chaology is discovering. For example, meteorologist Edward Lorenz of the Massachusetts Institute of Technology gave a talk on the subject of chaos entitled: "Does the flap of a butterfly's wings in Brazil set off a tornado in Texas?"

The paradox is that even random chaos can be predicted because chaos itself is self-organizing, which appears to reflect the way of all living processes. Reacting molecules make wonderfully ordered shapes and patterns; one organization of these patterns is the fractal, a word coined by Benoit Mandelbrot of the IBM computer research laboratories in the USA. Fractals are shapes which divide and subdivide into replicas of themselves and are all around us in the natural world. Cabbages, onions, cauliflowers, trees, river systems, molecular activity in living cells and the human nervous system are all examples of fractals.

When unpredictability is plotted by the use of complex mathematics, a computer picture of the graph has three wing-shapes and has been nick-named "the Strange Attractor." It is a fractal: regardless of how many times each part of each wing is enlarged it will be found to consist of smaller and smaller replicas of the original three-winged shape.

Many scientists claim that chaology, this new area of scientific enquiry made visible by the use of computer graphics, will revolutionize all our previous ideas about life and living things. Inevitably this will affect medical practice and perhaps take us full circle back to the instincts of early peoples who found magic in life and the universal energy.

What links us with our primitive ancestors?

Homo sapiens is the Latin name for the genus mankind. *Homo* means "having the same" or "similar"; *sapiens* means "wisdom"; thus our genus name implies we have much knowledge and wisdom in common with others in the present and in the past, perhaps through our collective unconscious as suggested in the early 20th century by the Swiss psychologist Dr Carl Jung.

If there is a common wisdom between us and our primitive ancestors, perhaps it lies in the correspondence between the intuitive beliefs of antiquity and our modern understanding of chaology. Tiny irregularities can result in chaos, albeit predictable chaos. Perhaps these tiny irregularities are what lead eventually to immune deficiencies, aging processes and degenerative diseases.

Keeping a balance between the energies at work in the body is the job of prevention. Correcting imbalances is the job of healers. This was the view of ancient peoples; perhaps it will become the view of modern *homo sapiens*.

No two snowflakes are alike, yet every one is a variation of a delicate six-sided star pattern

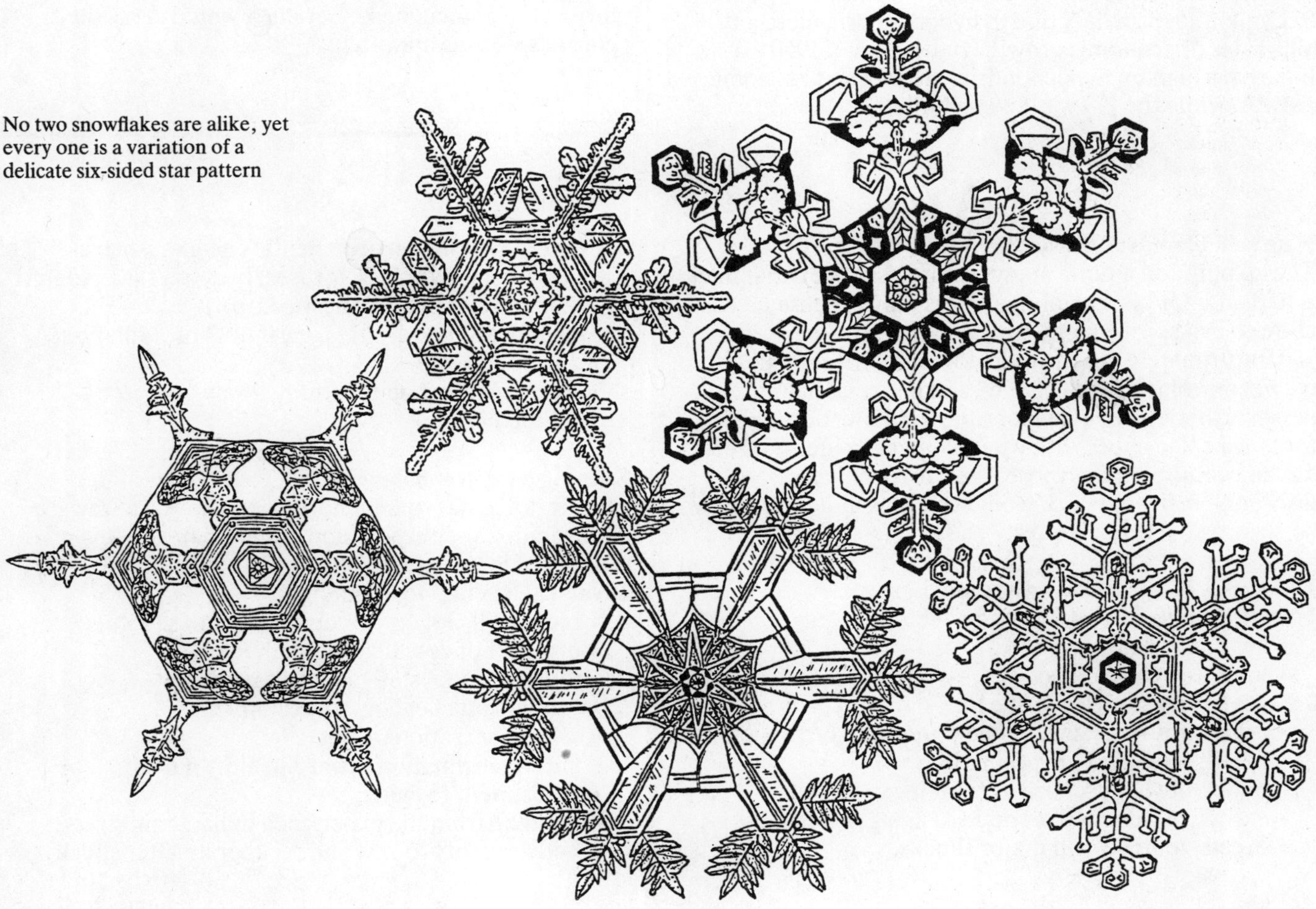

In sickness and in health

The World Health Organization has defined health as "a state of complete physical, mental and social well-being." This is a fixed, utopian view which does not allow for social variations. Health is probably better defined as a dynamic rather than a static state; for example, you are healthy if you can function properly in your social role and sick if you cannot. This definition does not equate health with a particular age or level of strength or stamina.

Ill-health could similarly be defined as an inability to function in your social role, which may be due to physical or psychological disorders. Another point of view would argue that a physical abnormality, such as the inability to walk, is not necessarily a mark of ill-health; many people function very well in wheelchairs . . . some better than those who can walk.

Attitudes to health

National attitudes to health vary. For example, the Japanese are extremely sensitive about the body. The tiniest imperfection, such as one nostril being slightly larger than the other, jeopardizes a girl's chances of marriage. On the other hand, a propensity to slight illness or a generally weak body indicates that a person is *shinkeishitsu*, i.e. different from others because he or she is so very sensitive.

In the 1960s several psychological studies indicated a strong tendency toward hypochondria among the Japanese, and in a study of 11 different countries by R.Lynn in 1968 anxiety due to hypochondria matched high rates of economic growth. In the period 1950–65 Japan was high on hypochondrial anxiety and economic growth, while the US was low on both.

EXORCIZING PLAGUE SPIRITS BY MAGICAL MEANS

Across all cultures it was believed that when a disease struck a community it was caused by the visitation of evil spirits. It was common practice to expel evil spirits by embodying them in objects or people, who would then draw the plague spirits away from the community.

The East Indian island of Ceram

When sickness struck a village, a small boat was loaded with rice, tobacco and eggs, etc., and launched with the words: "O all ye sicknesses, ye smallpoxes, agues, measles . . . who have visited us so long and wasted us so sorely . . . we have furnished you with provender sufficient for the voyage . . . Depart . . . never come near us again . . ." The exhortation continued as the boat drifted out to sea. If the sickness attacked again, it was considered to be a different sickness that needed another boat and another exhortation.

Scapegoating

The use of animals or people as scapegoats for the ills of whole communities is commonplace. Even today, civilized nations like to blame their leaders for all manner of social and economic ills!

In 1857 the Aymara Indians of Peru and Bolivia suffered a devastating plague. They attempted to rid themselves of the evil by loading the clothes of plague victims onto a llama, sprinkling them with brandy. They turned the animal loose, hoping it would carry the plague spirits away with it.

Who is to blame for disease?

The assumption among many cultures has been that man is to blame for his own ill-health, usually because he has allowed evil spirits to enter his body.

Unfortunately this attitude does not differentiate between evolutionary "blame" and personal blame. A person cannot be held responsible for being born, only for how he/she copes with what happens in life. If disease has an evolutionary purpose, the causes of human disorders, many of which would count as ill-health, could be classified in three groups.

The causes of human disorders and illness

1 **Constitutional defects**, due to:
- genetic mishaps;
- inherited conditions.

2 **Degenerative disorders**, due to:
- poor nurturing, such as bad parenting, or lack of health screening or vaccination;
- unhealthy habits, such as smoking;
- excessive wear and tear due to aging or occupation;
- excessive stress and major shocks.

3 **Failure to master environmental enemies**, such as:
- predators, parasites, viruses, bacteria (an epidemic is imperfect evolutionary control);
- chemicals, floods, fires, earthquakes, radiation;
- food deficiencies;
- encroachment on territory;
- accidents.

Keeping a natural balance

The life-force has some built-in mechanisms to thwart the evolutionary purpose and maintain health, even in the face of handicaps.

1 **Natural healing**, for example:
- blood will clot on contact with air to seal cuts;
- broken bones will knit together;
- the immune system will fight invaders.

2 **Developmental healing**, for example:
- self-preservation instinct;
- natural inclination toward healthy habits;
- adjustment to aging;
- learning from the experience of handling stress;
- body's ability to rest and recuperate after shock.

On the day of Atonement the Jewish high priest used to confess the sins of the Children of Israel, transferring them by touch to a goat, which was then banished to the wilderness.

The sufferings of deliberately tortured animals and people were said to draw away the evil. Dogs have been intoxicated and stoned to death and people banished with their bones broken to prevent them from returning with the plague.

Finally, the scapegoat may be a divine animal or person. In Ancient Egypt, divine bulls would be ritually slaughtered. The Albanians of the eastern Caucasus used to keep sacred slaves, one of whom would be killed by having a sacred spear thrust into his side. From the way he fell, forecasts were made of future well-being and everyone in the community would trample on the body, leaving their sicknesses with it.

Regicide was a regular practice among the Khazars of southern Russia; their kings would be put to death when a calamity hit the kingdom or even at the height of their powers so that the people might continue to live in prosperity and health.

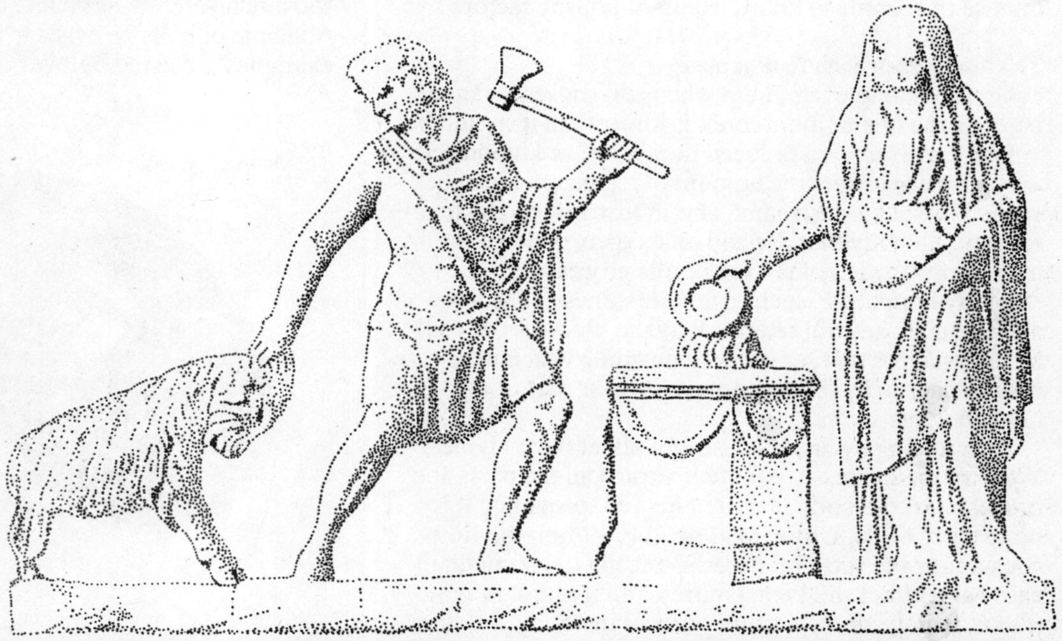

A literal Roman scapegoat is dragged to the altar of sacrifice where a priestess officiates

3 Controlling environmental enemies, for example:
- the building of new, specific immunities;
- traveling distances to satisfy dietary needs;
- adaptation, e.g. a lizard will drop its tail when being chased and grow a new one later;
- resolving territorial differences by social systems.

Medical systems
Three kinds of medical approaches have evolved to assist the life-force to cure or control ill-health. All approaches overlap to some extent.

1 Local folklore traditions
These include the use of local herbs, insects and mineral sources; for example, in parts of India, it was noticed that certain species of termites make their nests by stapling leaves together, so the termite was used to stitch large wounds together.

Sometimes sorcery and rituals were developed by one tribe or even one family, and often a particular local person became the accepted healer or medicine-man.

2 Some regional religious or cultural systems
- Chinese traditional medicine
- Kanpo (Japanese version of Chinese medicine)
- Ayurveda (Hindu medicine)
- Unani (Islamic medicine)
- Shamanism (Arctic Asian medicine)
- Allopathy (Western/European medicine)

3 A worldwide cosmopolitan medical system
This has developed in the 20th century from allopathic beginnings in Europe. Cosmopolitan medicine is based on "Western" medicine and embraces some practices from folklore and regional systems, such as the use of leeches, certain drugs such as opium and practices such as acupuncture anesthesia.

The World Health Organization, while training local and regional "barefoot" doctors in hygiene and midwifery, is encouraging the use of successful local and regional remedies, thus adding these to the great body of cosmopolitan medicine.

The balance of life

Each medical system that has evolved over the centuries has balance as one of its most fundamental principles. When the parts or the processes of the human body are in an active state of balance with one another, then the body is healthy. When any one part or process is off-balance, this throws the whole body-system off-balance and sickness is the result.

Western medicine, and those other systems that have adopted Western approaches at the expense of their own, tend to disregard the full implications of the principle of balance and use a linear method of tracing disease that omits to take account of holistic factors.

The linear approach to diagnosis

Take 'for example' a patient who is diagnosed as anemic because the hemoglobin count is lower than it should be. A low count means a reduced number of red blood cells which in turn lowers the amount of oxygen that can be carried in the bloodstream. This in turn affects the many parts of the body that depend on oxygen, which is a major constitutent of the metabolic process.

Many symptoms, such as breathlessness, may arise and there are several reasons why the blood count could be low, such as diet, or internal bleeding which in its turn may be caused by damage to a particular part of the intestine, and so on.

This tracing by linear cause and effect that is typical of Western medicine can eventually trace all the parts and processes of the body that are affected, providing it is done thoroughly. Unfortunately, this is often too time-consuming and too expensive. Basically the immediate cause and effect will be diagnosed and treated. Any minor damage done to other parts of the body and their functions by the protracted lack of oxygen will be ignored. Any major damage is often regarded as a separate diagnosis, although Western doctors are not ignorant of interconnections.

The holistic approach to diagnosis

Medical systems other than Western medicine, such as Chinese, Japanese, Indian, Arabic, Tibetan and other traditions, have tended to base their diagnoses upon a holistic view, assuming that any disturbance in one part of the body will affect the balance of all other parts.

The pulse diagnosis used in traditional Chinese Acupuncture is a measure of the balance of the 12 meridians or energy pathways that connect all organs of the body. Needling is then used to re-balance what has been thrown off-balance. Acupuncture is discussed further at the beginning of **Section Two**.

Tibetan pulsing seeks a balance similar to that of the acupuncture but uses pressure points and sound to bring about a balance in the energy system.

Some of these medical systems have modernized their approaches by combining the scientific Western methods with their own holistic traditions, and have often gained by it. Some Western doctors are reciprocating by beginning to take into account the principles of balance, some of which are described on this page.

YIN-YANG

The principle of the balance of opposites is as old as the universe and the oriental philosophy of yin and yang is one way in which this principle has been thoroughly explored.

The words yin and yang originate from Old Chinese, yin meaning heaven, the force of expansion, and yang meaning earth, the force of contraction. Yin and yang are antagonistic opposites, yet complementary. Together they make the whole, because one is continuous from the other. Too much yin swings the balance to yang, and too much yang swings back to yin. The yin-yang principle of balance exists in every aspect of life. Some examples are listed below.

The yin-yang symbol

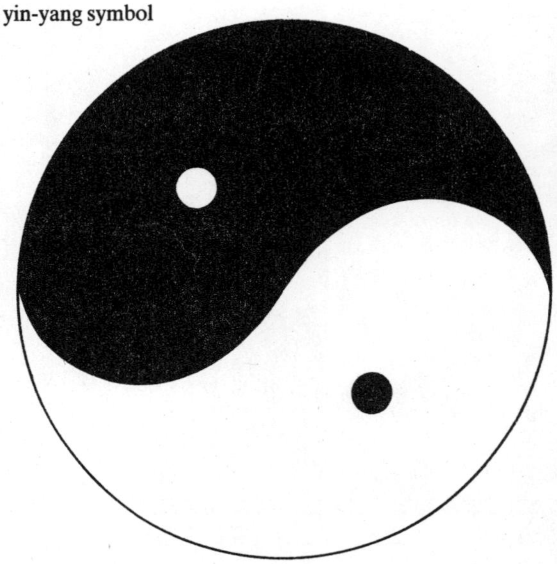

YIN qualities	YANG qualities
heaven above, expansion	earth below, contraction
feminine, growth	masculine, initiation
dissipating force	binding force
sweet, e.g. sugar	bitter, e.g. salt
acid, e.g. vinegar	alkali, e.g. soap
cold climate, short time	hot climate, long time
low pressure	high pressure
inebriating, e.g. alcohol, some drugs	sobering, e.g. ginseng, soy sauce
night time, dark, winter	day time, light, summer
inert, passive	dynamic, active
dry, lack of fluids	wet, too much fluid
sympathetic nervous system	parasympathetic nervous system
positive ions	negative ions
hypo- i.e. below normal	hyper- i.e. above normal
hypoglycemia, i.e. low blood sugar	hyperglycemia, i.e. high blood sugar
low blood pressure, depression, coma	high blood pressure, fevers, convulsion

The yin-yang of disease

About AD 200, Chang Chung-Ching a doctor, wrote in his treatise the *Shan Han Lun*, that while some diseases are yin and some are yang, the progress of an illness advances in six stages. The first three stages are yang, while the person still has enough energy to help himself, and the second three stages are yin, during which the patient becomes weaker and unable to help himself.

The six stages of an illness

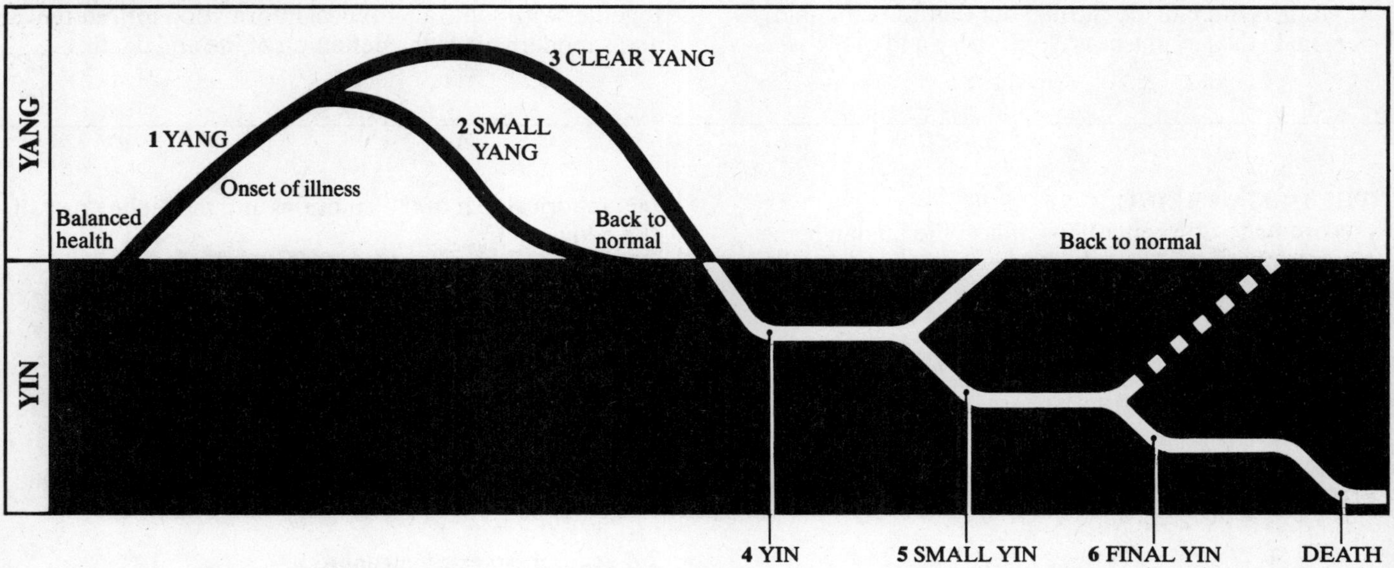

1 YANG The beginning of any illness is a yang disease. The yang is felt on the surface of the body: a strong superficial pulse, some pains, chills, fever, coughs, headache or stiffness. At this stage the patient can cure himself by wrapping up to induce sweating. Rapid changes can take place, a rapid cure or a change toward a deeper, yin state.

2 SMALL YANG This is the normal route if care is taken and the illness is mild. There may be sickness, constipation and a yellow tongue, but fever will reduce and normal balance be regained.

3 CLEAR YANG If care is not taken and the general health is not good anyway, the first stage may move directly into this severe yang stage: strong deep pulse, pain in stomach, constipation, hard abdomen, vomiting, dizziness, bitter taste in mouth, thirst, fast heartbeat, loss of appetite. If the treatment is correct, the disease will change for the better. If not it will quickly change into a yin disease.

4 YIN This is the first stage of any yin disease and the fourth stage of an illness. The yin level is in the stomach, which is soft and aches. There is no appetite, constipation may change to diarrhea and there may be vomiting. The feet become cold and the deep pulse becomes weak. Proper treatment at this stage will return the patient to normal.

5 SMALL YIN At this stage the heart becomes weak and the patient cannot sit up. Earlier symptoms continue and all pulses weaken. There is loss of weight. At this stage, people with a yang constitution may die suddenly because they change quickly and the illness affects the heart and liver. People with a yin constitution may get better or may remain ill but last for months or even years, slowly deteriorating.

6 FINAL YIN This is the most serious stage when all the organs deteriorate. Appetite is gone and the head may be hot while the feet are cold. There is usually loss of fluid. (In hospitals run on Western principles, there is often a drip to feed the patient with sugar and salt dissolved in water and there may be a catheter from the bladder.) The old texts contained lists of herbal teas that were used at each stage.

THE TRI-DOSAS

The three humors (principles of body-functions) of Ayurveda, the ancient Indian system of medicine are known as the dosas. Physical health is maintained when the three dosas work in harmony. When upset, they become illnesses.

Vatta dosa is concerned with the functions of movement, elimination and the nervous system.

Pitta dosa is concerned with functions of heat, digestion and metabolism.

Kapha dosa is concerned with the functions of structure of the body, strength and tissue resistance to disease.

REFERENCE: There is more information about systems of balance in **Section Two: The balancing touch** (pp.38–39).

The human body

Looking at the range of medicine from ancient folk remedies to the most sophisticated of modern bio-technology, the question of human identity arises. Just what are consultants, doctors, alternative practitioners, shamans, para-medics and a host of primitive medicine men treating?

It is clear that more than only the physical body is involved, but what are the other parts of a person? Mention is often made throughout this book of mind, personality, consciousness, spirit, aura and other aspects of the living human being. It may be that none of these actually exist as separable entities. It may be that only some of them exist at all. To enjoy delving into the many methods of healing, whether rational or magical, it is best to keep an open mind about the human body.

For information only, and not to prove anything is right or wrong, or real or imaginary, some of the ancient, philosophical ideas about human life are presented here, together with some anatomical information for reference and a modern, working definition of life and death.

THE HUMAN BEING
According to different philosophies, the human being consists of many interlocked systems. Two main viewpoints are given here.

1 A broadly modern viewpoint
Of the eight parts listed, some people would omit, for example, part D, according to personal belief.
A BODY The biological body.
B MIND The thinking, conscious part of the body.
C HEART (or stomach or solar plexus) The metaphorical seat of the emotions and the feeling part of the body.
D SOUL The part of a body that survives death.
E SPIRIT The life-force, life energy or electrical impulses that keep the system going.
F INTELLIGENCE The ability to understand; the natural instincts and know-how of the body.
G INTUITION Immediate understanding without reason.
H MORALITY Inherent principles of right and wrong, good and evil.

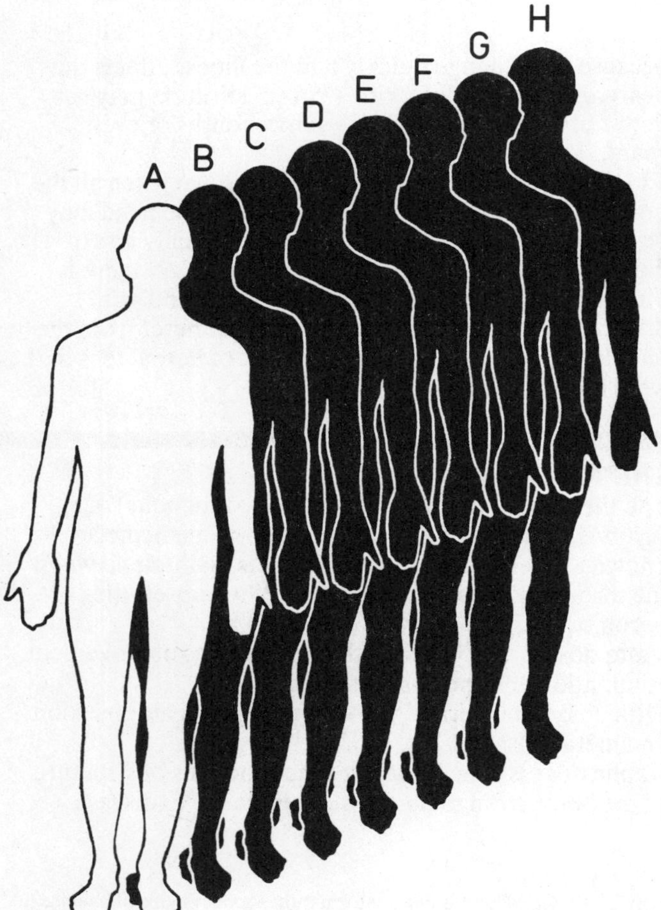

2 A general esoteric viewpoint
These ideas come from Eastern religions. The living person is seen as having seven parts.

Immortal INDIVIDUALITY

SPIRIT Carries the karmic imprint from previous lives
1. Atman The original divine cosmic principle.
2. Buddhi A state of nirvana or bliss.
3. Manas An individual's cosmic intelligence.

Perishable PERSONALITY

SOUL
4. Ego The psyche or personal, body consciousness.
5. Astral body Free-floating consciousness.
6. Etheric body The life-giving force that also forms the aura which pulsates around the body.
MATTER
7. The physical body of flesh, bones, tissues, etc., which includes mind, heart, intelligence, morality, intuition, skills, memories, thoughts.

The life force
This is known by many names, for example:
Oriental ch'i energy
Ancient Hindu prana (breath)
The Alchemist's ether
Mesmer's animal magnetism
Radiesthetist's etheric force
Wilhelm Reich's orgone energy or vegetative streamings
Alexander Lowen's bio-energy
Western medicine's psychosomatic phenomena
Primitive communities often gave the life force the name of an animal.

SOME HUMAN ANATOMY

When treating a patient, Western medicine tends to pinpoint areas of the body anatomy, while Eastern medicines tend to pinpoint a particular system.

The skeleton and muscles

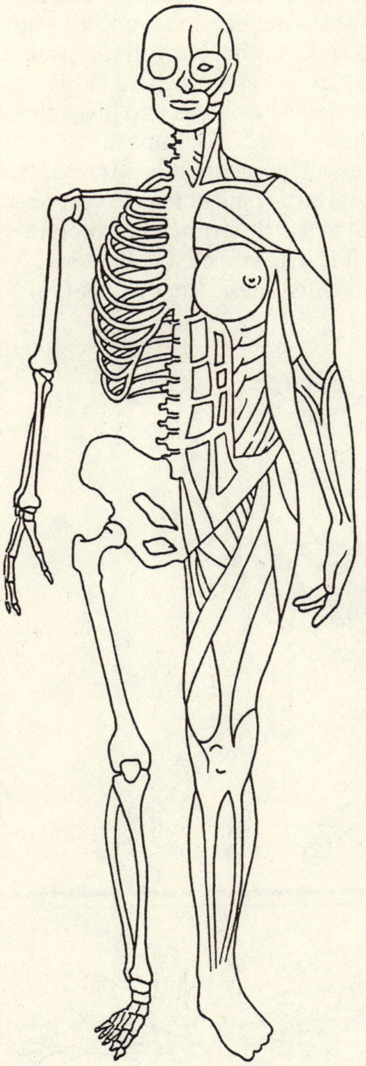

Some major organs

1 Lungs
2 Kidneys
3 Heart
4 Liver
5 Stomach
6 Intestines
7 Reproductive organs (female)
8 Reproductive organs (male)

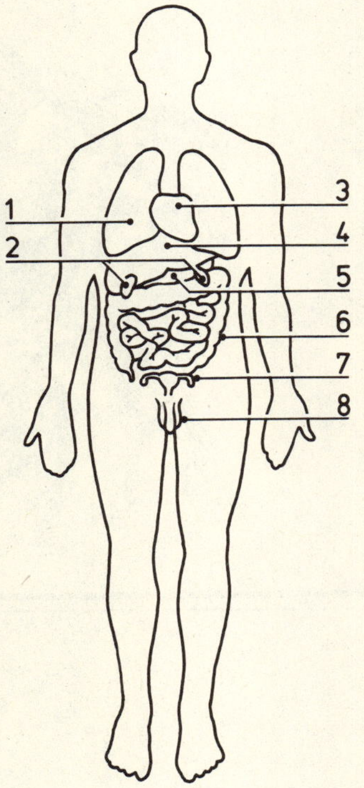

The central nervous system

The brain and spinal cord receive, interpret and send information via the peripheral nervous system (PNS) that reaches all parts of the body.

The PNS has two parts, the somatic system that serves parts of the body under voluntary control, such as the walking musles, and the autonomic system that controls unconscious activities such as heart beat and digestion.

The autonomic system has two sub-systems acting in opposition to each other and keeping a balance. During stress the sympathetic system dominates and during relaxation the parasympathetic system is in control.

LIFE AND DEATH

A new human body begins to be formed when a sperm from a man fertilizes an egg from a woman to produce a morula, which is the name given to a fertilized egg during its first eight days.

The morula contains 23 double strings of deoxyribonucleic acid (DNA), one from each parent. These strings, or chromosomes, contain all the genetic material required to build an entirely new human body.

By the ninth day the morula has acquired a fluid sac and has become implanted in the wall of the womb as the blastocyst. By the 16th day, three layers of differentiated cells have grown, which will become the organs of the body, and it is known as an embryo. At 20 days there are swellings recognizable as head, heart and stomach and by day 34, there are eyes, a nose, arms and legs.

So when did the embryo become alive and can it be called a human being? Does the embryo have a mind, a soul or a spirit?

What happens at death?

Although there are theories, philosophies and beliefs about what happens after earthly life, the only certainty concerns the symptoms of physical death. Medically there are two kinds of death, clinical and brain.

Clinical death

The most reliable indicators of death are the absence of clinically detectable signs of life. For example, the heart and the breathing stop for an extended period of time, the blood pressure drops so low it is undetectable, the pupils of the eyes dilate and the body temperature drops. Although resuscitation can often take place when only one symptom occurs, the period during which this may be possible is 30 minutes at the maximum.

Brain death

The electrical activity of the brain can be traced on the print-out of an electroencephalograph machine, known as an EEG. Death has occurred when the electrical activity of the brain has completely ceased.

It takes time to set up an EEG so brain death is only usually detectable in an intensive care unit where the EEG would have been working already. When the readings are flat the brain has ceased to be active and the person is declared dead. Very low brain activity in cases can give a flat reading, in cases such as hypothermia or a drug overdose, so clinical indications are always sought as well.

Science and magic

Magic is the art of influencing events by occult or other inexplicable means. The validity of magic is in its being. Pacific Trobriand Islanders would explain that the importance of a magic spell is in its use by the right person at the right time for the right purpose. Magical occurrences cannot be proved, they simply ARE.

Science is the art of proving how events occur by observation, experiment or logical thought. From these activities a body of scientific knowledge is built up systematically. Scientists will only accept "magical" occurrences if they can be validated scientifically.

The illusions of magic
Since magic is a mystery, and we all love to be surprised, we are vulnerable to trickery. The modern entertainer who delights us with his magical routines uses our own illusions to deceive us. He distracts, tempts and persuades us. He suggests what he wants us to believe and, because we believe, we are convinced, despite the logic that tells us it is only a trick.

His counterpart might seem to be the primitive witchdoctor, the difference being that death was the penalty when his magic failed to produce results. Yet many witchdoctors and medicine men had a high degree of success and lived to ripe old ages.

The imperfections of science
An old story of the scientist and the flea is often told to demonstrate the fallibility of scientific experiment. It should also remind us of our common tendency to misinterpret what we see.

The scientist and the flea
A scientist has been researching the behavior of a large flea for some time. He has already conditioned the flea to jump over a match-box on the command "jump." Watching the flea jump, he wonders what gives the flea the ability to respond to his command.

He theorizes that it must be the front of the flea's three pairs of legs. So the scientist tears off the flea's front legs and gives the command to jump. The flea jumps, so the scientist adjusts his theory. It must be the middle pair of legs that enables the flea to respond... but no, without its middle pair of legs, the flea still jumps as before. The scientist is very excited by now and in his enthusiasm he tears off the flea's back legs and gives the command to jump. This time the flea does not move.

What can have happened? The scientist is puzzled. It is obvious the flea needed its back pair of legs to respond to the command... so what is the difference between the back legs and the other pairs? The scientist concludes that removing the back legs must make the flea deaf!

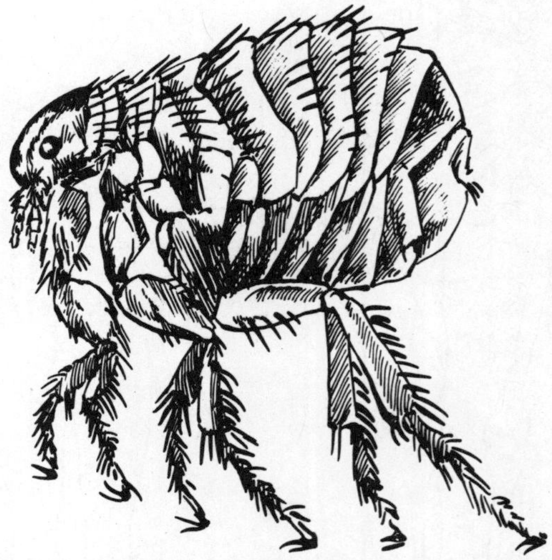

TWO KINDS OF MAGIC
There are two kinds of magic that recur throughout all primitive forms of healing. Magic can be positive or negative.

1 Sympathetic magic: things that are similar have similar effects.

Make-believe, for example, is a form of sympathetic magic used among the Dyaks of Borneo. Two wizards would attend a woman having a difficult labor. One would help by using physical manipulation based on a knowledge of anatomy while the other would use sympathetic magic by lying down and imitating the birth process.

Homeopathic medicine is a form of sympathetic magic. The tinctures are taken to induce the illness that is being treated, thus stimulating the body to respond by attacking the disease.

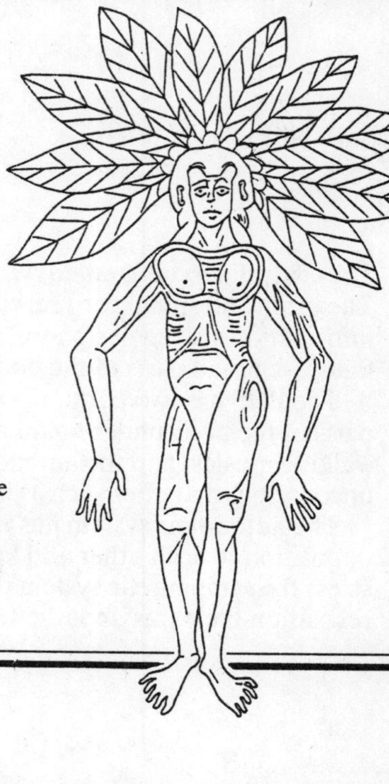

A mandrake root, said to have healing properties because it resembles the human figure as in this 15th century medical treatise drawing

Science in healing

The Western world tends to dismiss what cannot be scientifically proved. Consequently, most of Western medical practice is based on scientific principles, and magical methods of healing are dismissed as dangerous nonsense. Our fear of magic is often expressed as contempt for anything unscientific.

It is typical of our illogical human natures that many of us who would dismiss magical cures would find the occasional miracle quite acceptable, especially when it concerned the well-being of ourselves or of someone close.

Dr C.G. Jung, the Swiss psychologist, recognized our fears when he wrote of his own new ideas: "I had the feeling that I had pushed to the brink of the world; what was of burning interest to me was null and void for others, and even a cause for dread.

"Dread of what? I could find no explanation for this. After all, there was nothing preposterous or world-shaking in the idea that there might be events which over-stepped the limited categories of space, time and causality." (*Memories, Dreams and Reflections*)

The magic of science

Dr Jung would not have been surprised to see how modern science itself has become so complex that it spills into the realm of the magical.

Nuclear physicists speak of mysterious energies, and genetic engineers attempt to recreate the miracle of life. Scientists and mathematicians can now give us logical insights into what were previously considered to be impossibilities. The study of topology has revealed the secrets of some "impossibilities." The topology of the tennis ball is one such example.

The impossible tennis ball

Topology is often called rubber-sheet geometry and is concerned with factors that remain the same when an object is deformed by bending, stretching or twisting. It was a blind mathematician who first analyzed how a tennis ball could, by a series of unbelievably complex mathematical twists and turns, be turned totally inside out, yet remain intact.

Most ordinary, non-mathematical people would dismiss such a suggestion as impossible. It is easy to see how half a ball could be turned inside-out... but to turn a whole ball inside out! That idea is in the realm of the abnormal, a magical idea. The fact that it has happened more than once, and been witnessed, is incredible. All we can do is accept the possibility, or dismiss the whole thing as a trick.

The person who witnessed this extraordinary event was British scientist Dr Lyall Watson, who, in 1979, opened his book *Lifetide: A biology of the unconscious* with the story of the topologically everted tennis ball.

Dr Watson was visiting an Italian family in Venice. Their five-year-old daughter, Claudia, was able to do something very strange.

Her father gave her an ordinary, fluffy, white tennis ball from a new pack. She held it in her hand and stroked it as any child would stroke a small animal. Suddenly there was a popping sound, like a cork being drawn from a bottle, and the ball was rubbery and bald. Claudia seemed unconcerned.

The ball had not just been shorn of its fur. It had been turned inside out, yet the laws of physics said this was impossible. The everted ball bounced and still contained air pressure, as it had before. Dr Watson sliced it in half with a knife to find the outer cover was still intact on the inside. What he called reality was no longer the case.

2 Contagious magic: things that have been in contact continue to influence each other when separated.

The navel cord, for example, was used for contagious magic by the Incas of Peru. They preserved the cord with great care, and it was given to the child to suck whenever he or she fell ill. Since the cord had kept the baby alive in the womb it would cure later illness.

In many primitive communities it was common practice to clean and preserve the object that had caused a wound to ensure that the wound healed.

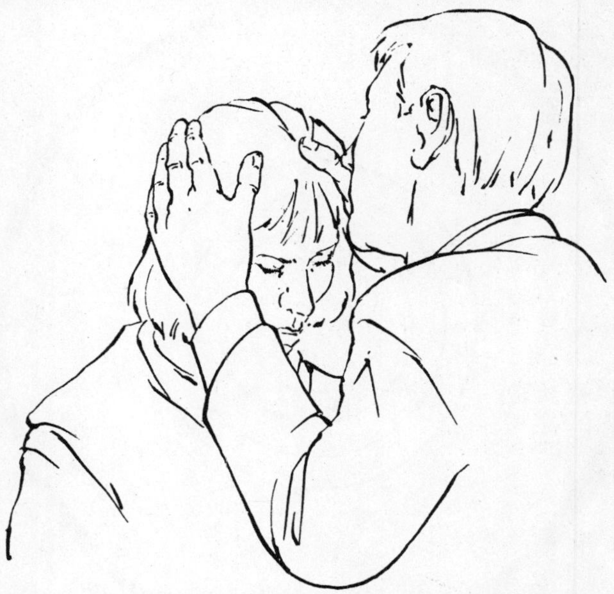

The laying-on of hands was healing by contact with the hands of a healer or a saintly person

The creative cycle

Creativity involves change from one situation to another. A creative change in clothing fashions may mean, for example, a change to a new hem length, or a new fabric.

A cycle is the pattern of repeated occurrences. Some cycles are smooth, even processes like the cycle of the phases of the moon. However, more often the cyclical occurrences are uneven processes that only over a broad period of time can be seen to form a fairly regular cycle, for example, weather cycles and economic cycles.

Diagrams of cycles
Cycles are usually represented as waves rising and falling from a horizontal line, called the base line because it marks the change from positive to negative. The length along the base line usually indicates the length of time taken to complete the cycle.

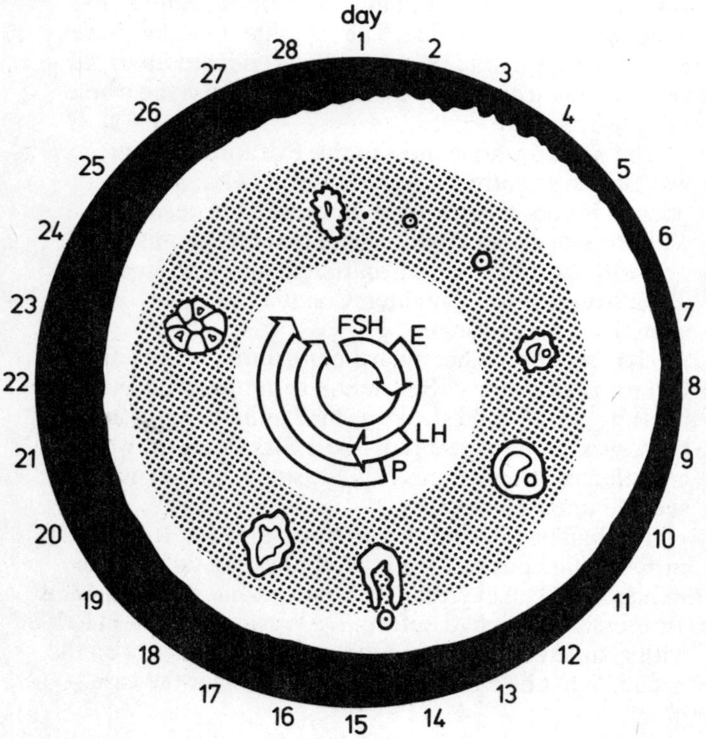

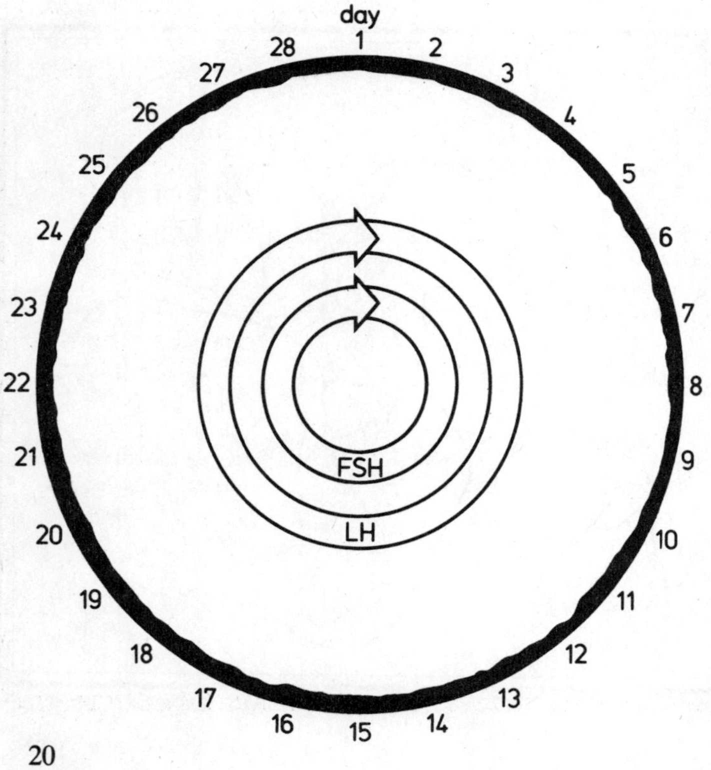

THE MENSTRUAL CYCLE
The natural monthly cycles of the human body are an intrinsic part of female existence and everyone has other cycles, which some people call biorhythms. The intellectual cycle, the emotional cycle and the physical cycle are said to start at birth and continue through life. REFERENCE: For more about biorhythms, see **Section Seven: Diagnostic alternatives 2** (pp.146–147).

The top diagram illustrates the normal 28-day menstrual cycle. FSH and LH hormones (produced by the pituitary gland at the base of the brain) stimulate one of the ovaries to release a ripened egg into the nearest Fallopian tube, so making that egg available for fertilization by male sperm. Meanwhile the follicle inside which the egg has developed is producing hormones too, first estrogen and then also progesterone. These cause the lining of the uterus to thicken in preparation for implantation if the egg is fertilized. If the egg is not fertilized, the thickened lining breaks down, and the woman experiences her menstrual period.

The cycle breaks down
After the female menopause egg production ceases entirely, but small quantities of FSH and LH are still produced by the adrenal glands.

Key
FSH Follicle stimulating hormone
LH Luteinizing hormone
E Estrogen
P Progesterone
■ Uterine lining

The sexual orgasmic cycle

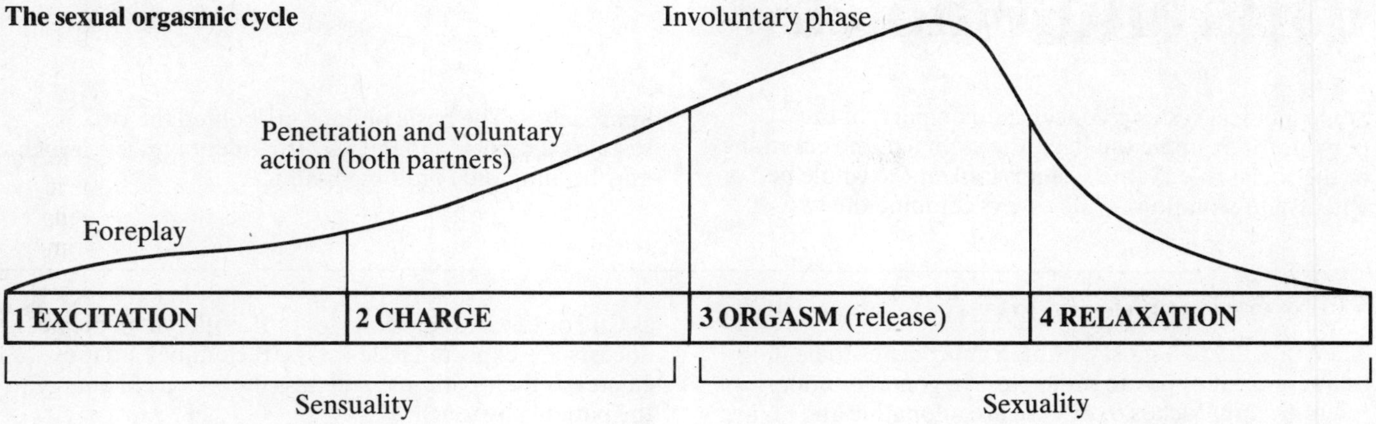

THE CREATIVE CYCLE OF WELL-BEING
The human body is also subject to interdependent cycles which are far too complex to illustrate here. As with all cycles, the human cycles are not always at a peak and nor does good health mean the body is always at its peak. Any serious sportsperson knows the body has its natural ups and downs.

Each day the body has its own cycle. For some people the morning is an up period compared with the evening. Others are evening people who take time to get going in the morning. In general the mornings are better for logical brain activity while in the evenings our senses become sharper when perfume, wine and soft lights come into their own.

The creative orgasm cycle
The most creative cycle of activity in which human beings become involved is the orgasmic cycle, which is generally linked only with sexual intercourse but which occurs as a result of many different kinds of stimulations, such as visual delights, music, exercise such as swimming and dancing, and the many pleasures of family life and hobbies.

There are many levels and types of orgasmic experience but all are part of a natural cycle of activity and relaxation that helps to keep the body healthy. The sexual orgasm is the most focused of all orgasmic experiences but sensual experiences of delight, bliss, pleasure and other ecstasies are just as health-giving and keep the body energy flowing. Hence, a life filled with too much sex can be just as harmful as a life empty of all pleasures.

Typical phases of the orgasm cycle
Phases are not always the same for all people nor for any one person all the time. The orgasm cycle is creative, i.e. there are qualitative differences. Phases one and two can be continued for a long time (hours) for increased pleasure if both partners learn the techniques.

Oriental medicine
Traditional Chinese medicine is based on the cycle of body energy which makes all the organs interpendent.
REFERENCE: For further information, see The pentagram of health (p.10) and **Section Two: The Way of the Orient** (p.32 onwards).

CREATIVE CYCLES
A creative cycle is one in which a change takes place in the quality of the repeated pattern of occurrences, for example, the reproductive and child-rearing cycle which parents undertake. The cyclical pattern remains the same but the children develop different personalities.

The creative cycle of erotic capital
This is a wonderful name given to the extraordinary correlation between changes in fashion and long-term economic cycles, known as Kondratieff cycles.

The brilliant Russian economist, Nikolai D. Kondratieff, died in a Siberian concentration camp in the early 1930s because the Communist regime condemned his work as dangerous. His theory of long-term economic cycles, occurring approximately every 54 years since the late 1780s, was first published in German in 1926. He predicted the peak of the third upwave as 1920 and outlined the decline which became known as the Great Depression.

The erotic level of fashion also moves in a cycle which matches the economic situation. During times of prosperity, rising inflation and peaking commodity prices, women's dresses become more erotic, i.e. they have shorter hems or lower necks. During recessions and depressions the trend is toward longer garments and more cover-up.

Kondratieff creative economic-erotic cycles
Projected to the year 2000 based on the evidence of what has actually happened to commodity prices, the actual year by year picture would show repeated ups and downs, so that the clear downward or upward trend is only seen over the long term, It is similar in fashion. Major conflicts and weather cycles also link with these cycles, indicating how there are many interdependent factors.

Parts and wholes

Some medical systems concentrate on parts of the person, for example the liver, the stomach, the emotions or the social role. Some systems look at the whole person and his life-situation, while others combine the two approaches. The basic philosophy behind the two systems is reflected in the way treatment is given, which may be allopathic or homeopathic.

ALLOPATHY AND HOMEOPATHY

These are the two most common approaches to healing and represent opposite principles. In general, modern scientific approaches to disease are allopathic and many, though not all, alternative approaches are homeopathic.

Allopathy

This is the process of treating a disease by inducing an opposite condition. For example, inflammation would be treated by a drug that reduced the inflammation. Allopathic treatment begins with a diagnosis of the disease via the symptoms and is aimed at removing the symptoms and thus the disease.

Allopathic drugs are disease-oriented, for example, the antibiotics, such as penicillin. They "cure" an infection by killing the bacteria causing it. They also tend to kill many of the body's own protective bacteria, thus leaving it temporarily vulnerable to secondary infections, such as thrush.

Homeopathy

This is the process of treating a disease in such a way that the symptoms of the disease would be induced in a normally healthy person. For example, a fever would be treated by a drug that increased the fever slightly, thus mobilizing the body's own system to fight the sickness.

Correct homeopathic treatment has regard for the whole person and his/her way of life. The assumption is that the body can fight the sickness, so the treatment aims to help stimulate the body to do its natural job. Different treatments are selected for different people, even though they may be suffering from the same disease.

The action of many vaccines could be called homeopathic when they consist of a small dose of the disease which stimulates the body to produce its own antibodies against the disease.

The principle of homeopathy should not be confused with the medical system called Homeopathy, which is only one of many systems based on the homeopathic principle.

Life energy

The life of the body is part of nature. Most civilizations have withdrawn from nature to live and work in man-made environments. Thus there is a need for special activities to mobilize the body and keep its vital energies going.

Sport and exercise serve this purpose in most cultures. The ancient art of Tai Chi, also known as qi gong, is the popular form of exercise in China. Its movements increase the flow of internal energy known as Ch'i or Qi. In some colleges of traditional medicine, doctors are expected to learn the techniques, so they can teach their patients, and pass their own chi energy to the patients by touch.

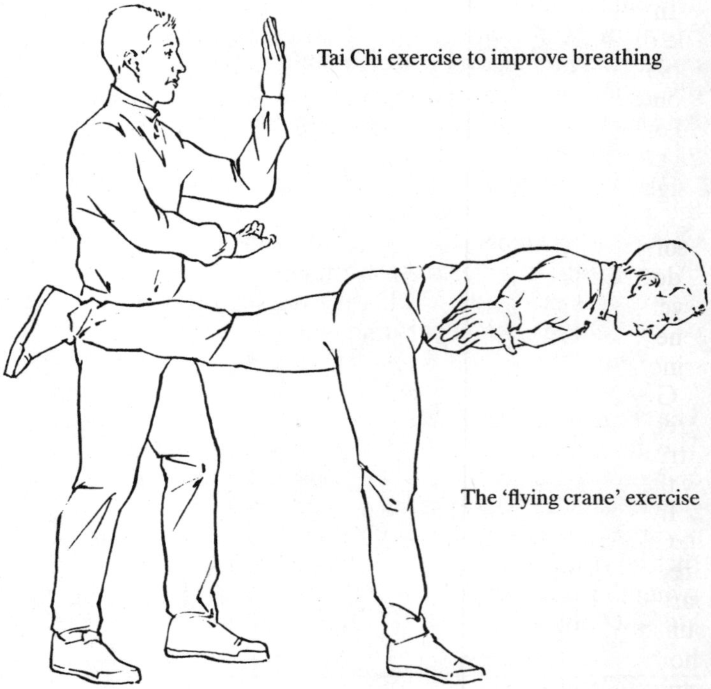

Tai Chi exercise to improve breathing

The 'flying crane' exercise

Living tissues

Proteins are the basic building blocks of the body. The first indication of a new life occurs when protein chains from the male and the female, known as DNA, join together to form the new individual.

It is tempting to speculate that proteins are the life-givers, but DNA, despite its central role in the body, is not the whole, it is only a part.

The modern battle against viruses serves to remind us that the whole is more powerful than the sum of the individual parts, because it takes the whole human body to keep viral intruders at bay.

REFERENCE: Homeopathic remedies are fully described in **Section Six.** The terminologies of alternative, conventional, primitive and Western medicines are defined at the end of this section: **Magical healing methods** (pp.28–29). For more information about viruses, refer to **Section Seven: The best of both worlds** (pp.152–153).

PSYCHOTHERAPY OF THE WHOLE

Gestalt therapy
Gestalt is a German word meaning whole. Gestalt therapies involve the client in the whole situation in which he finds himself in the here and now.

The whole situation may be explored in a group setting, or it can be explored through a medium such as paint or clay. The client is encouraged to use "I" and speak only of current life problems and the actual people involved. He will come across parts of himself which he has not previously acknowledged. It is the aim of gestalt therapy that the client see himself as a whole, and accept these parts into himself without making judgements.

In gestalt dream therapy, a similar approach is made. The dreamer re-tells a dream, taking the part of each person or object in the dream. For example, in a dream about a car, he might choose to speak both as himself: "I am driving to work in an old wreck," and as the car: "I am an old wreck being driven to work." In this way new insights are often gained.

George Groddeck
A doctor and a contemporary of Sigmund Freud, the psychologist George Groddeck (1866–1934) had a general practice in Vienna where he worked on holistic principles. To him mind and body were inseparable.

Groddeck maintained that an unconscious "it" was directing a person's inner life and allowing sicknesses to intrude. He believed that the "it" had to be confronted by the doctor.

In his published case records, called *The Book of the It*, Groddeck describes how, on one occasion, he was tired of trying to persuade a patient to talk about a particularly unpalatable problem and instinctively punched the man full in the stomach. The patient shouted, vomited, coughed, cried, and released many expletives, later declaring how much relief he felt.

Groddeck noted how the man had finally managed to let go of the tension, that had caused so much pain in his stomach, by letting go of the emotions that lay hidden behind the marital problem he had come to discuss.

Groddeck was one of the first Western doctors to recognize that the whole person was affected even if only a small part seemed to be the problem.

Reichian therapy
Dr Wilhelm Reich, who emigrated from Vienna to America and died there in 1957, also linked physical and emotional disturbances. One of his theories proposed that the character defense of a person is reflected in the muscular armoring of the body. In simple terms, chronically tense muscles indicate a chronic attitude of mind, such as anxiety, hostility, prejudice or an exaggerated self-image.

Bioenergetics
One of Reich's New York students, Dr Alexander Lowen, devised a series of stress exercises, known as bioenergetics, to release these chronic tensions. While in a bioenergetic stress position, such as the basic bow position, emotions connected with the tense muscles would be released as screams, sobs or shouts and the patient would also bring to consciousness associated parts of personal history. This holistic release, i.e. physical, emotional and mental, would clear the way for a fuller flow of bioenergy and consequent good health.

Many other doctors and psychologists from traditional Western medicine have done work in this holistic field, which is still developing. Incorrectly applied by amateurs, bioenergetics and other similar techniques can cause more harm than good.

Chronic stress serves its own purpose
It should be remembered that a chronic tension did not appear overnight for no reason at all and removing it can be a major problem to the body that has become used to it. Just like withdrawal from drug addiction, withdrawal from our chronic tensions can require us to face the very problems that tension was designed to protect us from in the first place.

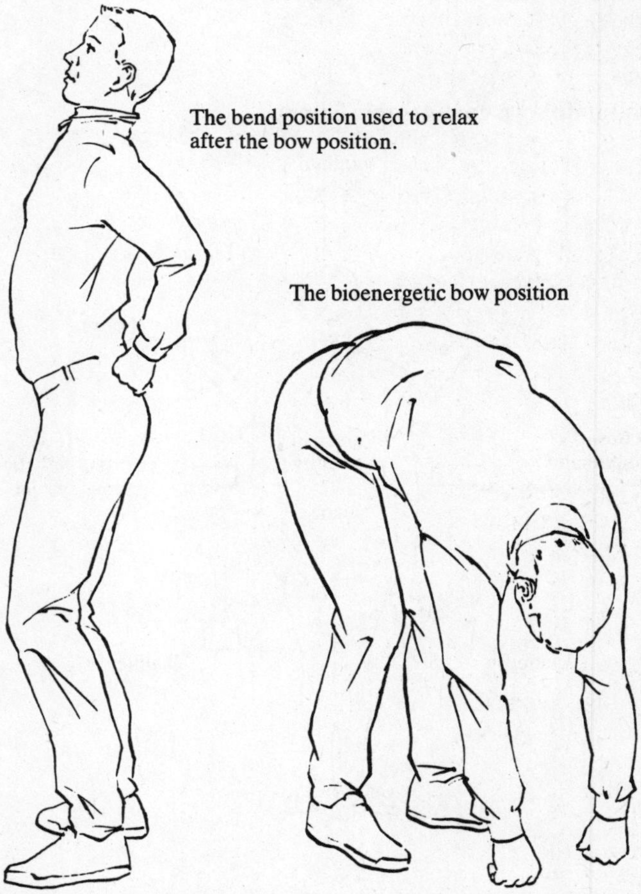

The bend position used to relax after the bow position.

The bioenergetic bow position

Energy states

There are many forms of energy at work in the human body, for example, mechanical, chemical, nervous and metabolic energy. All these dynamic processes produce certain conditions in the body, some of which are shown on the diagram below: Maintaining a comfortable balance, on this page.

Each condition has a natural opposite, for example acid is the opposite of alkaline. As in all things human, a balance is maintained when neither one nor the other dominates all the time. If there is too much alkalinity in the cells for too long, the surrounding tissues will adjust by becoming acidic.

Catabolism breaks down substances to produce energy while its opposite, anabolism, makes substances to build the body and replace old tissues. Too much of one or the other upsets the body leading to illness and discomfort. The loss of balance between any of the opposites has similar effects.

Many medical systems other than the Western allopathic system attempt to stimulate the body to regain its natural balance of energy states. Influencing the senses through the use of sounds, rhythmic movements, visual shapes, colors and perfumes is one of the approaches to good health.

In the past, people did not know about these energy states in today's scientific terms, but they were remarkably accurate in their diagnoses, often done by pendulum dowsing, muscle testing (kinesiology) and a range of other methods as described in **Section Seven.**

Maintaining a comfortable balance

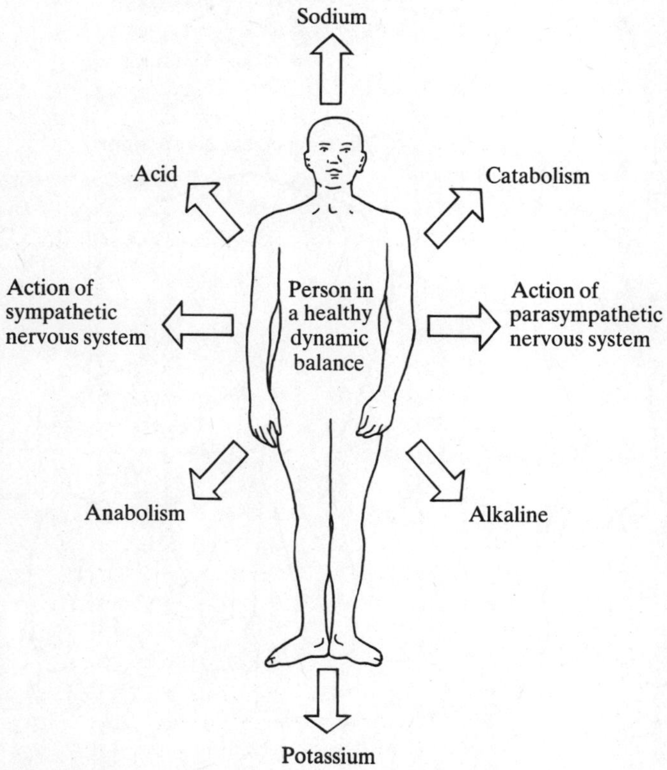

ANTHROPOSOPHY

A holistic approach to health and education was put into practice by Rudolf Steiner (1861–1925) who founded the School of Spiritual Science at Dornach, near Basle in Switzerland.

Steiner came to medicine late in life and saw illness as a disturbance of the hidden inner life of instinct. He believed the unconscious working of the "I" showed itself in individual biographies and important illnesses and accidents. He used movement to music he called eurhythmy as a very effective therapy for healing both physical and mental sickness.

Sounds that heal

Steiner also believed in the healing power of spoken verse that had a regular meter and he was the inspiration for contemporary research into the healing shapes of sounds. When sounds of different wavelengths vibrate through powders and metal filings, each sound produces a different pattern. The healing effect of the various sounds and the images they induce have been researched in London by musician Lawrence Ball and healer Isobel McGilvray. They have produced recordings that have a healing effect, utilizing sounds and their shapes.

Acoustic images	Description	Effect of image
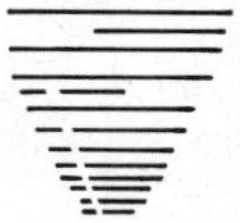	Lines	Clears the mind
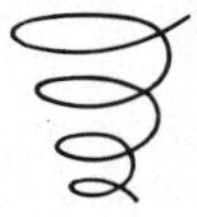	Helix	Stimulates
	Rose	Soothes
	Four-leafed clover	Brings hope
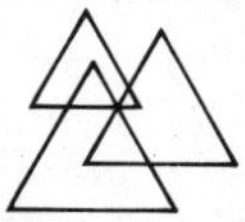	Triangles	Releases emotion
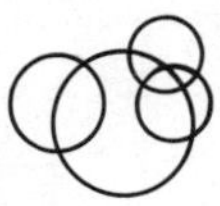	Circles	Nourishes
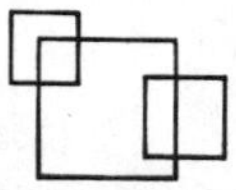	Squares	Reassures

AROMATHERAPY

One of the oldest and more consistently effective herbal medical systems discovered, aromatherapy has also been used cosmetically. The therapy utilizes the aromatic essential oils from flowers, roots, resins and leaves of plants, for example, the essential oils of lavender and rose are from the flower; of rosemary, from the leaves; of sandalwood, from the bark; of calamus from the roots; of lemon from the rind of the fruit and of myrrh from the resin of trees of the genus Commiphora.

Treatment may include taking the oils internally or by inhalation, but it is the absorption of the essential oils through the skin itself that is central to effective treatment. Thus massage is the main activity associated with aromatherapy.

The essential oils

The essences of a plant are the aromatic oils that appear from different parts of the plant at different times of the day. For example, the oil that is extracted from flowers in a morning may have different properties from oils extracted in the late evening. Orange oil from the rind of the fruit is different from the orange oil extracted from the flowers.

The extraction of these oils is a long, painstaking process which makes them quite expensive. It takes, for example, 2000lb of rose petals to produce one pound of essential rose oil by a process known as enflueurage or by a comparable distillation process.

During enfluerage, flower petals, are spread on filters and placed in a bowl of cold-pressed vegetable oil and left for days while the odiferous molecules become absorbed from the petals into the oil. The flower essence is then separated from the oil by a volatile process. Alcohol is never used as it destroys the properties of the essences.

The production of synthetics is attractive, but research has shown that the exact properties of natural oils cannot be reproduced. Essences also differ from the extracts used by herbalists. An English herbalist's catalogue of 1722 recognized the difference and listed 13 separate essential oils.

The ancient Egyptians were devoted to the use of aromatic oils for medical and cosmetic purposes; when Tutankhamun's tomb was opened in 1922 it contained many scent pots, including large amounts of the very expensive frankincence and myrrh.

How does aromatherapy affect the body-balance?

There are many records of the wonderful healing effect of aromatic oils. The term aromatherapy was first used at the beginning of the twentieth century by a French chemist, M. Gattefossé, who poured some lavender oil over his badly burned hand and was surprised how quickly it healed. He published the first book on aromatherapy in 1928.

In 1938 another Frenchman, working in Los Angeles, was treating wounds, skin cancers and gangrene with essential oils and getting good results. A third Frenchman, Dr Valnet, used the essences to heal wounds and reduce scarring during World War II and published his work in 1964.

Until recently, nobody had any idea why the oils worked. Then a study carried out in 1970 showed that lemon oils, well known for their clearing effect on the lungs, worked best when the dose was so dilute as to be undetectable by smell. This lead to a theory that many odiferous particles are ions and their therapeutic effect was similar to that of ion therapy.

Some therapeutic effects of some essential oils

Angelica: a general tonic and aids respiration.
Bergamot: antiseptic, anti-bacterial; aids healing.
Cinnamon: aphrodisiac; stimulates heart and lungs.
Cypress: astringent, diuretic and aids sweating.
Lavender: heals and stimulates the nervous system.
Myrrh: heals, is antiseptic and cures skin diseases.
Neroli: calms anxiety; stimulates anti-viral activity.
Clove: pain relief, e.g. toothache; antiseptic.
Eucalyptus: clears the lungs; aids respiration.

Ion therapy

Ions are particles that carry either a negative or a positive electrical charge due to the loss or gain of an electron.

The air we breathe has a natural, very small ion content, the balance of which can easily be disrupted by pollution such as fumes or by central heating and air conditioning. Some natural phenomena also cause negative ion-depletion: pre-thunderous weather, during solar radiation, humidity and temperature changes, and in certain warm winds such as the Föhn in Germany and the Sharav in the Near East.

All of these are known to cause a general malaise, sometimes called "serotonin hyperfunction syndrome" because the neurotransmitter serotonin moves out of its bound form in the cells into a free form in the body fluids. This results in stress reactions, depression, constricted breathing and other unpleasant effects. Increasing the negative ion proportion in the air will reverse these effects by causing the serotonin to return to its healthy bound form inside the cells of the body.

The atmosphere can regain its own ion balance, given a lack of pollution, and natural weather changes help to achieve a balance. High concentrations of negative ionization exists naturally near waterfalls, on the coast, in some mountain areas and wherever there is fresh air and a fine rain.

Ionizers, using a high electrical voltage to produce a flow of negative ions, can be used in rooms, cars, by the bed or in the office to keep the ion balance healthy. Aromatherapy may be another way of increasing the negative ion balance in the body.

Handling pain

Although the threshold beyond which pain is unbearable varies slightly from person to person, pain is a sensation most humans try to avoid. A few very unfortunate people are in pain all their lives and a few, at the other extreme, are so insensitive to pain signals that they can be seriously hurt and not know it.

Methods to relieve pain include the use of pills, injections, rituals, anesthetics, herbal remedies, alcohol, exercise, music, electrical stimulation, heat, witchcraft, exorcism, massage, beating, bathing and sweating. Surgery is also used to remove the specific part where the pain is located, such as a gangrenous foot, to remove the cause of the pain, such as a bullet, or to cut some of the nerves which carry the pain-message.

All these methods are described in detail elsewhere in the book.

PAIN IN THE BODY

When an injury or disease threatens the well-being of the individual, a sensation of pain is carried along the nerve pathways and through the spinal cord by a neuro-peptide into the brain where it is interpreted as pain and reactions are initiated.

The pain-message can be modified or stopped by the presence of the body's natural painkillers known as encephalins or endorphins, which can travel through the body in the bloodstream. Absence of endorphins allows the pain to continue.

Many of the methods used to control pain stimulate the production of endorphins, and some drugs, such as morphine, have a direct effect similar to that of the endorphins. For example, rubbing, massage and movement are natural responses to the pain that is felt when we receive a hard knock or get backache carrying too many heavy boxes. This is because these activities stimulate the circulation of endorphins, and loosen tight muscles (another cause of pain).

Pain and the emotions

Emotions themselves do not cause physical pain but contemporary research is proving that emotional expression can relieve certain aspects of severe physical pain.

For example, an uncomplaining patient, in agony from pain he could still feel in his amputated leg, was visited by a neuro-specialist. The patient was clearly putting on a very brave face and making jokes to hide his feelings. After a while the doctor quietly and gently asked his patient, "Have you ever cried?" There was a brief silence before tears began to run down the patient's face and soon he was sobbing as though his heart would break.

An hour later, the sobbing had subsided and he was chatting with a new joy on his face; the pain had diminished. The specialist explained that while cracking jokes gave some small relief, the man had to experience the whole grieving process for the loss of his leg.

Grieving would involve expressing his anger, fear and terrible sadness for that part of him that had been taken away. As he grieved, a process that can take two years to reach the stage of readjustment, the pains he felt would be reduced and possibly disappear.

The specialist explained that holding on to emotions is like trying to hold on to a ledge with one's fingertips. Fear of losing control contracts the whole body, causing more pain to add to that caused by a disease. Release of the emotions relieves pain both by relaxing the contracted muscles and by stimulating the production of endorphins.

Some people also use emotion to hide their true feelings, for example, shouting to hide fears or laughing and making jokes to hide grief. Sometimes these pretences are necessary before a person is able to release his extremely painful inner feelings.

Ritual beating

In primitive societies, pain was believed to be an evil spirit that could be frightened away by beating. Some people believed that the sprit would be attracted to the object used to do the beating, which could then be thrown away, destroying the evil spirit with it.

Among the Yoruna Indians of Brazil, the doctor rubs his patient with a green branch all over the body. When he has finished, he carries the branch outside, makes a groaning sound, and throws away the twig and the pain.

The Yoruna Indians beat the ground in front of a sick person with a stick, and other cults beat each other with leaves dipped in spices and herbal mixtures. Since stimulation of the skin produces endorphins, many of these ritual beatings would successfully relieve the pain.

ELECTRICAL STIMULATION

In AD 46 a Roman medical practitioner known as Scribonius Largus is said to have claimed he could cure headaches using the electrical charge from an electric torpedo fish or an electric eel.

The idea of using an electrical charge to cure pain was not new even then; there is some evidence that it was used by the ancient Egyptians. Mesmerism was another attempt to harness natural magnetism to relieve pain. For more information, refer to **Section Five: A healthy charge** (pp.110–111).

Pain and the TENS machine

Transcutaneous Electrical Nerve Stimulation, or TENS, is a modern treatment used to treat pain. A controlled electrical charge is fed through silicon electrodes attached to the skin with a harmless gel. The charge is produced by a small machine known as the TENS machine. It can be bought on the open market.

The TENS machine seems to work best with chronic or stable, persistent pain and has been researched extensively at several pain clinics. There is an 80–90% improvement in the short term and 35% of patients still have relief two years after using the machine. Some people only need to use the machine for a short period, while others need to use it regularly over a long period of time, or even permanently.

Why is electrical stimulation effective?
Research has shown that the electrical message arrives at the central nervous system before the pain message and prevents it from being received. This phenomenon is known as the gate control theory.

Stimulation by a low voltage electrical charge (the TENS method) is even more effective. It was discovered that TENS, like rubbing, also stimulates the body to produce more endorphins, the body's own natural painkillers.

POSTURAL PAIN

Thousands of people suffer from backache. Some back pains are caused by incorrect posture, which in turn can be due to wearing shoes with heels.

The higher the heel, the more the spine has to be arched and leant upon to maintain an upright position. Backache due to high heels can be eliminated by wearing recessed heel footwear.

Recessed heel footwear
Footwear with a heel lower than the sole was invented by a Danish teacher of yoga, who was interested in how the feet behaved when walking. She observed that when standing barefoot on unpaved ground, such as grass, the heel would sink into the ground, which caused the pelvis to tip slightly, straightening the spine and opening the breathing.

Recessed heel footwear is recommended by doctors and sports experts alike. The recessed heel enables people to stand on floors and walk on hard pavements without getting tired or suffering backaches. They have been particularly helpful to pregnant women and overweight people. They should not be worn by people with Achilles tendon problems or with certain foot or back injuries to which their bodies have adapted.

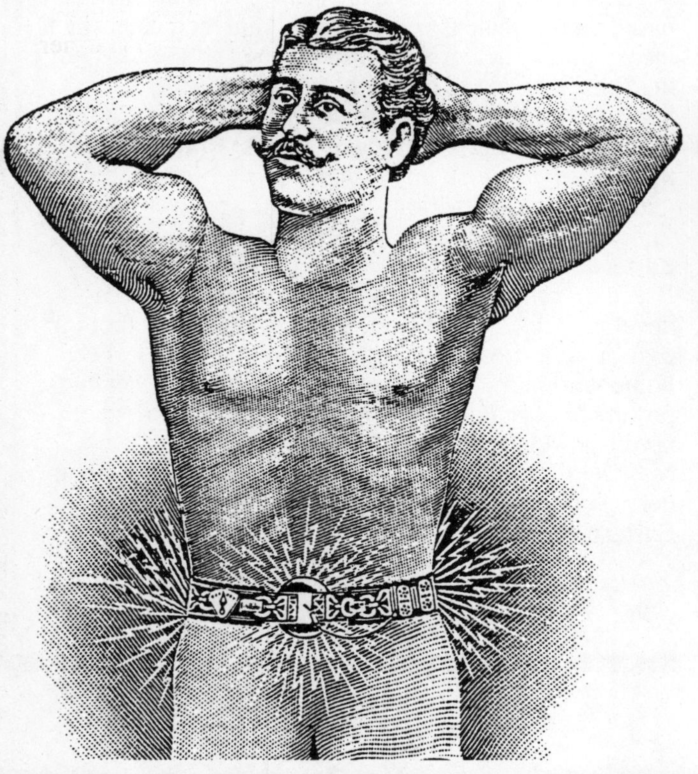

The features of a recessed heel shoe
1 There is a broad area in which the toes can move freely and allow the change of half a shoe size that takes place when the foot bears the body's weight.
2 There is a rocker sole which helps the foot carry the weight forward.
3 There is a contoured, flexible arch support.
4 The level of the heel is below the level of the ball of the foot, on a gentle inclination.
5 There is a well-fitting heel support to prevent the heel slipping off the sole.

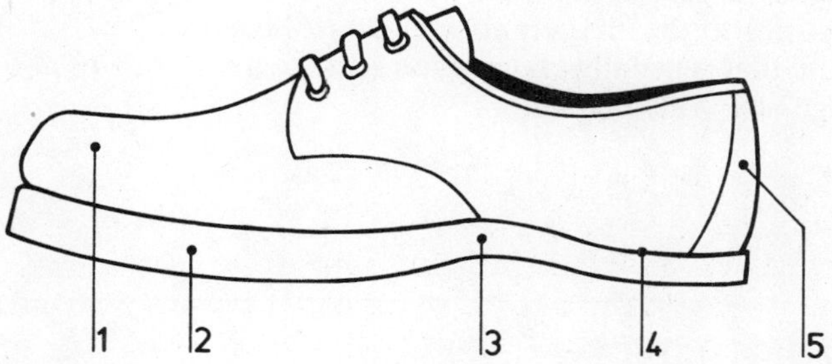

Restraint in the operating theatre
The control of infection, shock and pain were the three most serious problems that hampered the work of the early surgeons. Patients often chose to tolerate the pain of their condition rather than to face the pain of the operating table, so many ran away at the last moment. Once tied down on the table, they were fully committed.

Giant Power Heidelberg Electric Belt for curing all pains, from the 1902 Sears, Roebuck & Co. catalog

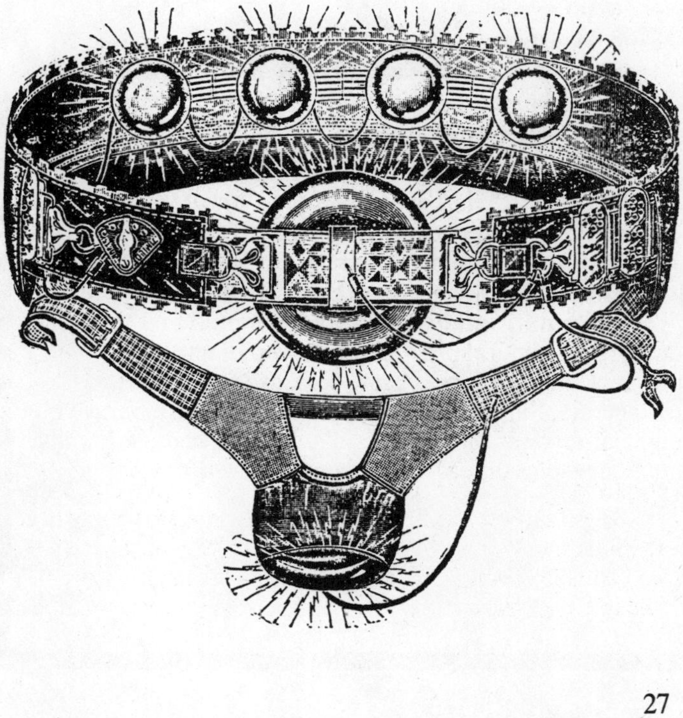

Magical healing methods

Magic is the art of influencing events by inexplicable means. The great majority of medical methods must, therefore, be magical, since knowledge of how each one works is still largely theoretical. Although more is being understood as research reveals how and why the human body operates, most methods are used because they are successful for some people rather than because they are based on scientifically proven facts.

CHOOSING HEALTHCARE

Described, not prescribed, below are a range of healing methods available worldwide. When discomfort, disease and sometimes death threaten, people are apt to try anything to regain their normal state of health. The route that is usually taken when seeking a cure begins at stage one, folk medicine.

1 FOLK MEDICINE

The first resort is to an inherited body of knowledge built up from the experience of generations of lay people and passed down through family groups. If the folk remedy does not work, the patient moves for help outside the family.

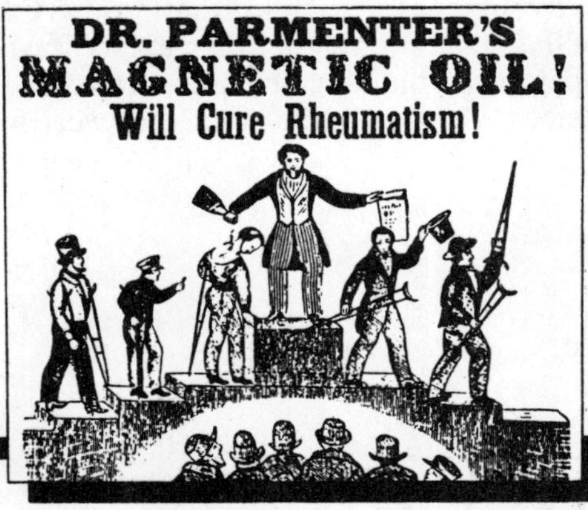

2 PRIMITIVE MEDICINE

This is the traditional collection of therapeutic methods that every culture has acquired over the years. For example, tribal medical traditions have survived to this day in Africa and South America, while shamanism is found in Siberia along with other local traditions.

Each primitive tradition has its accepted first level doctors, or general practitioners, who diagnose, prescribe and, in some cases, dispense traditional treatments. Supporting the medical doctor are para-medical services that usually give the treatments. Family members sometimes fulfill this role as well.

3 FORMAL MEDICINES

There are three formal medical systems, now used in many parts of the world: Western, Eastern and Indian. The distinction between them is still clear, although they have adapted some methods from each other.

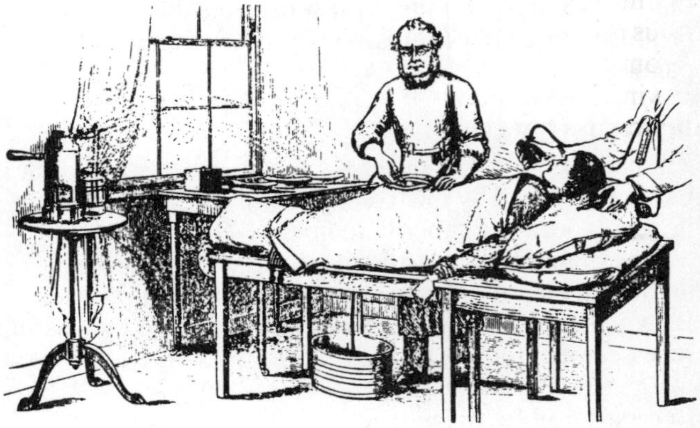

Western medicine

Based on scientific principles, Western medicine is primarily disease-centered and allopathic, i.e. the emphasis is on diagnosis, and the treatment attempts to produce an effect opposite to that caused by the disease. Main methods: chemotherapies, surgery and the use of technical aids. Direct contact with a conscious patient for the purposes of healing is taboo. Some screening and preventive medicine. Division between body and mind, and of the body into parts.

Indian medicine

Based on fatalistic principles, the medical practices developed in the Indian sub-continent are life-centered and include treatments to promote the right way of living which it is believed will bring about good health.

Indian formal medicine includes Ayurvedic medicine based on the ancient vedic texts, Unani medicine which incorporates ancient Arabic medicine and the Siddha medicine developed in Southern India.
Main methods: massage, breathing, meditation, herbal remedies, bathing, and surgery. Direct contact for the purpose of healing is encouraged. Preventive medicine mainly through nutrition. Body/mind seen as a whole.

Eastern medicine

Based on principles of balance, the medical systems developed in China, Japan, Tibet, Korea and other far eastern countries are person-centered and are largely homeopathic, i.e. they engage the body's own healing powers by stimulating a condition that makes the body use its powers to re-balance its systems.
Main methods: acupuncture, massage, diet, movement, herbal remedies, and physical manipulation. The Eastern medical system is preventive in principle.

4 ALTERNATIVE MEDICINE

If the first three stages have failed to produce a cure, the patient may look for an alternative, which will most likely be from one of the other two of the three formal medical systems or be based on the philosophy of that system. Alternatives are also derived from the mainstream of the patient's own formal system. Some are of mixed origins and may derive directly from various primitive methods.

From the point of view of Western medicine, the following are samples of alternatives, all of which and more, can be found in this book.

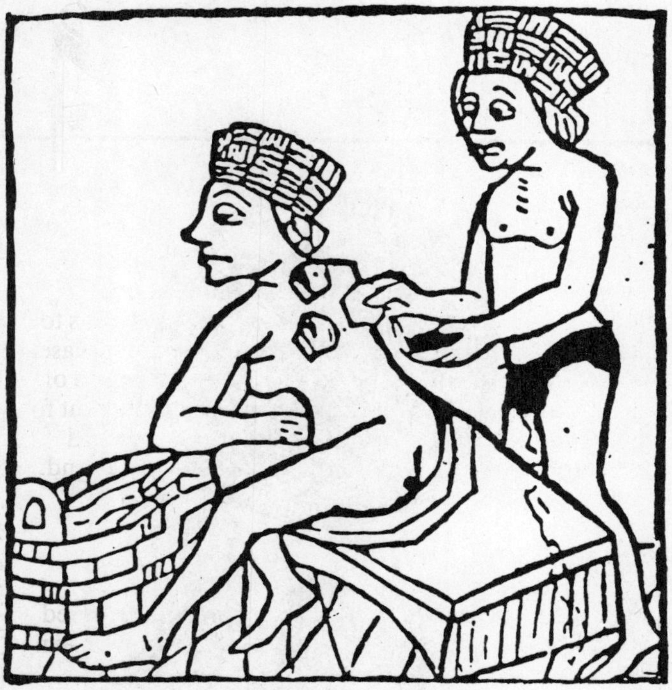

ALTERNATIVES BASED ON EASTERN PHILOSOPHY

i.e. the philosophy of balance

- acupuncture
- acupressure
- electro-acupuncture
- shiatzu
- t'ai chi
- bioenergetics
- Bates eyesight therapy
- psychoperistaltic massage
- chiropractic
- polarity therapy
- reflex healing
- reflexology
- zone therapy
- macrobiotics

ALTERNATIVES BASED ON INDIAN BELIEF

i.e. the belief in life

- Anthroposophical medicine
- Alexander Technique
- Feldenkrais exercises
- laying on of hands
- massage
- bonding
- aromatherapy
- hydrotherapy
- thalassotherapy
- fasting
- osteopathy
- meditation
- breath therapy
- music therapy

ALTERNATIVES BASED ON WESTERN THEORY

i.e. the scientific method

- Ion therapy
- TENS
- magnetic therapy
- bone-setting
- traction
- alchemy
- sauna
- poultices
- cell revitalization therapy
- new psychotherapies
- Bach flower remedies
- biochemics
- mesmerism
- hypnosis

ALTERNATIVES OF MIXED ORIGINS

- blessing
- scapegoating
- balneology
- charms
- amulets
- shamanism
- dance therapy
- thermalism
- mud baths
- leeching
- cupping
- faith healing
- incubation
- urine therapy
- herbalism

5 COMPLEMENTARY MEDICINE

When an alternative medicine is combined with a formal method it may be called complementary medicine, since one fulfills the other's shortcomings. This only comes about when the consultant formal physician, or the alternative practitioner, has an open mind and can step outside the confines of his/her own discipline.

6 HOLISTIC MEDICINE

In an almost perfect world, everyone would get holistic medical care, for this would mean taking account of the whole situation, i.e. the whole person as an undivided body/mind, the person's life-style, family inheritance and environment, and choosing treatment from the whole range of medical systems.

Holism means that the whole is greater than the sum of the parts, and as this is a tendency in nature, it would seem reasonable to expect that if the whole person is treated the whole will have a greater effect in self-healing.

Some alternative practices do attempt to take a holistic view of a patient and complementary medical practice will inevitably move toward holism.

Section two

CREATIVE TOUCH

Touching is a very emotional activity; some people love to touch and be touched while others try to avoid any kind of contact. Many people are particular about the kind of touching they give and receive for it is the quality of touch that stimulates good health and aids healing.

A distinction must be made between caring touching and careless touching. The former is done with concern for the person being touched, and the latter is done inappropriately, without concern. It is also worth remembering that while touching is very often erotic, sexual foreplay and intercourse are only one of many directions touching may take.

Because touching excites the body and produces pleasurable sensations, some unfortunate people learn to mistrust any kind of touch. To some, being touched signals danger; to others it means sex and there are no gradations in between. However, most people are glad to enjoy the pleasure and stimulation of being touched and gain from it.

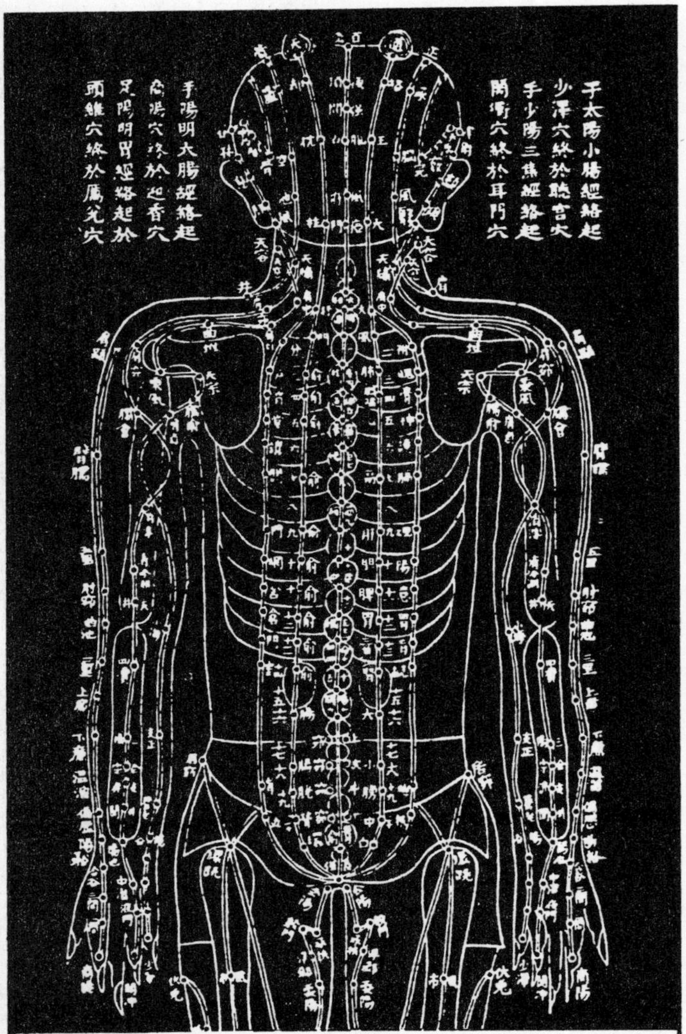

Acupuncture: Chinese diagram of points at which needles are applied. A woodcut of 1935.

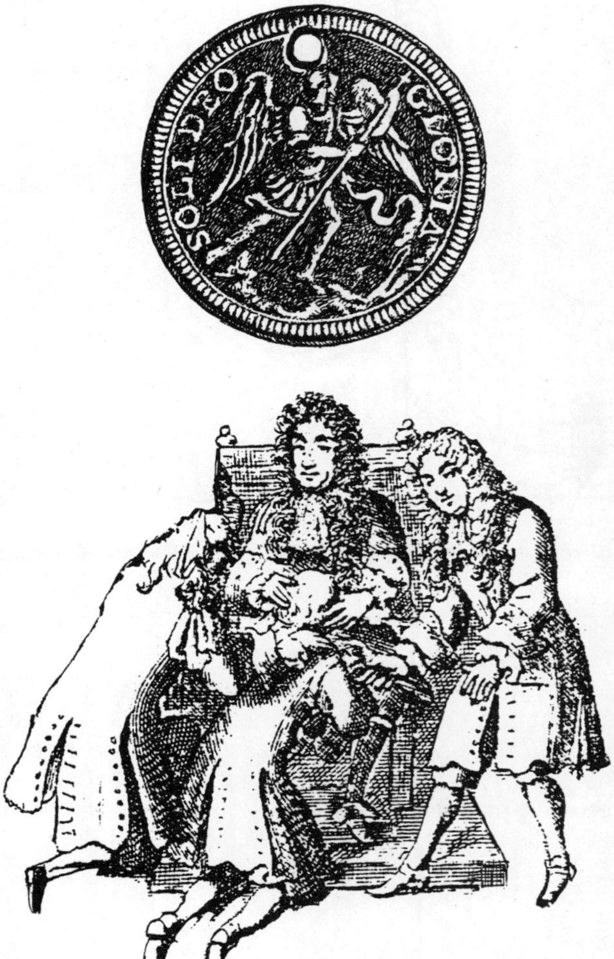

Touch healing: (*Above*) A George III (18th century) touchpiece coin bestowed on a sufferer who had had a royal laying on of hands. (*Below*) Charles II of England touches a sufferer of the King's Evil, or scrofula; a swelling of the lymph glands especially in the neck.

Probably the most popular healing touch has been massage. Known to have been used by the early Egyptians, Greeks and Romans, it still is popular among the survivors of lost civilizations, such as the North American Indians. Patting, stroking and rubbing movements come naturally to most people when they comfort a hurt child or give themselves first aid after bumping or banging themselves.

Other forms of touching for healing are explored in this section. They range from very precise touches, such as pricking acupuncture points, to the all-over stimulation of structured exercises during which the body massages its own internal organs.

Bonding between parent and child or between sexual partners is built through touch. Miracles of healing have taken place through the laying-on of hands. The manipulation of the muscle and bone structures of the body through touch are all explored in this section. Used creatively, touch can be an extremely powerful healer.

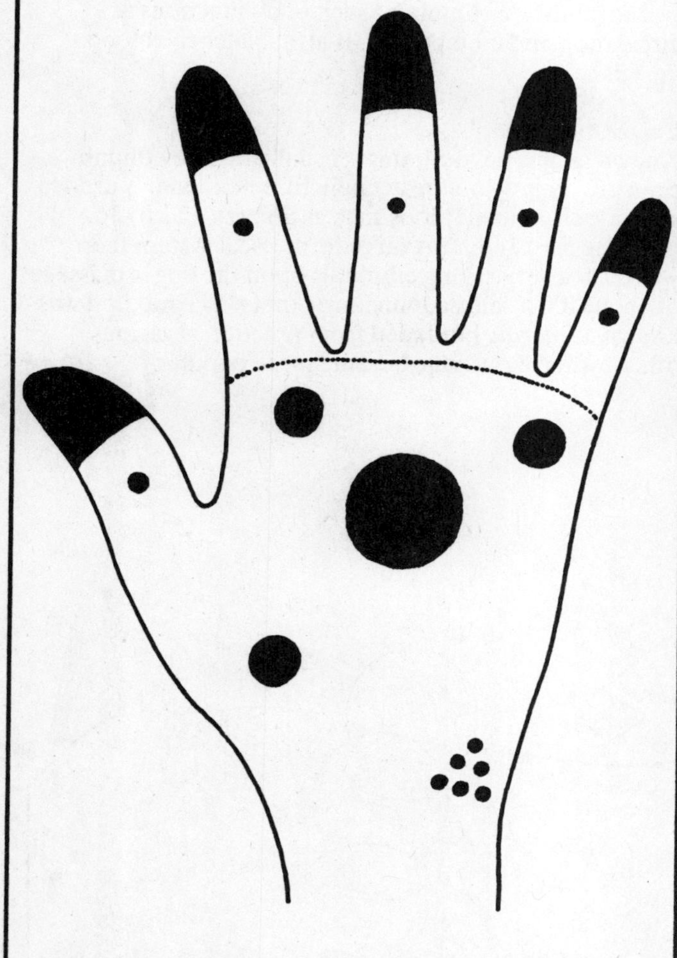

Handwork: Ritual decorations on a woman's hand to stimulate her energies at those points after ceremonial bathing. A 19th century Tantric drawing.

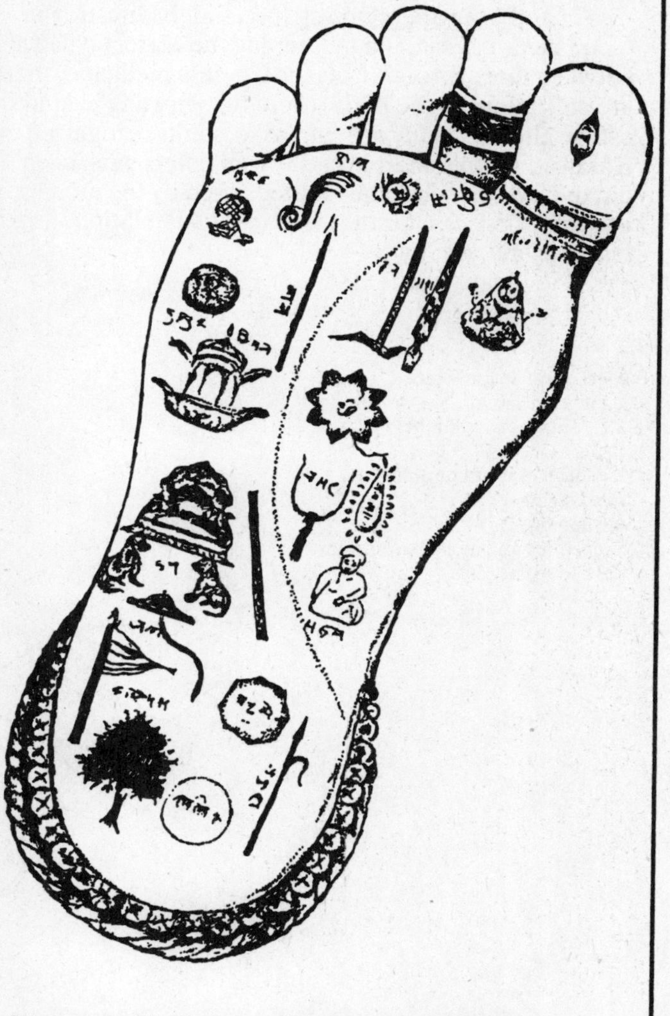

Sole message: The footprints of the Hindu god Vishnu as a cosmic healer, from an 18th century Rajastan gouache painting.

The way of the Orient: Acupuncture 1

In the 17th century, King Louis XIV of France sent some missionaries to Peking to study medical practices. They returned with news of the strange method of needling, which was the focus of Chinese Internal Medicine. It was used for both curing sicknesses and maintaining health. The missionaries called it acupuncture, from the Latin *acus* meaning needle and *punctura* meaning pricking.

Chinese Internal Medicine relies upon touching the surface of the skin to affect the internal condition of the body. Modern acupuncture is the most sophisticated medical system of touching ever devised.

The theory of Chinese acupuncture

It was assumed that the life-force, Ch'i or Qi energy, could be balanced by needling because it flowed around the body in channels, now called meridians. A philosophical model postulated 59 channels, 14 of which are now used clinically. In India a similar idea was popular for a while but was unworkable because the Hindu system had 700 channels.

Yin and yang are opposing forces in the lifestream. Good health is attained by keeping the correct balance between these forces. In classic Chinese medicine, there are 365 points on the body where the yin-yang balance can be altered. Many are similar to points recognized in Karate and other martial arts. More points have been discovered since, but the methods used by the modern acupuncturist remain the same: heat stimulation, finger massage and needling.

Heat stimulation

This is done either by cupping or by moxabustion. Cupping is an old method used to increase the local blood supply. Warm cups, bowls or small drums are placed on the skin; as they cool a parital vacuum is created inside which draws the blood supply.

Moxabustion is heat treatment from the slow burning of the dried leaves of Chinese wormwood, known as moxa, which can be wrapped in small papers and attached to the top of acupuncture needles so the heat travels down the needle. Alternatively, a compact cone of the ground herb is placed over the acupuncture point and set alight so it glows. The cone or moxa burns very slowly and gives out great heat. It is removed long before it could burn the skin.

Moxa can be piled onto a slice of ginger, or leaves of the herb can be rolled into a cigar-shape. The glowing end of the moxa cigar is then held close to the acupuncture point and can be moved along the course of a meridian. Moxa is forbidden at certain points because its effect is too radical.

Moxabustion stimulates such body functions as circulation and metabolism. It also dilates the blood vessels.

Finger massage

Known as acupressure, this is usually done by thumb pressure directly on the acupuncture point and is used in several self-help methods such as Shiatzu and Jo-Jo.

In the East Indian Ayurvedic medical system there was once a very strong emphasis upon the finger massage of about 100 of the acupuncture points. The method was known as *marma* but faded from practice as various other forms of massage became more popular.

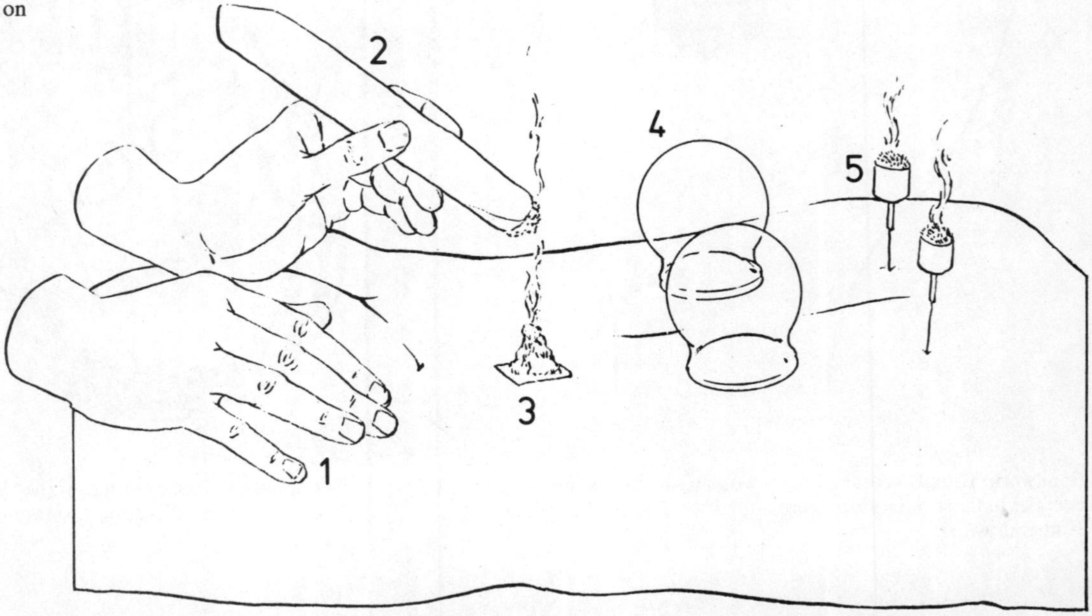

Methods of acupuncture
1 Finger massage
2 A large moxa roll is held close to the skin
3 A heap of moxa burning on a slice of ginger
4 Cupping
5 Needling and moxa burning on the ends of needles

THE BEGINNINGS OF ACUPUNCTURE

Acupuncture is thought to have had its origins in stories about wounded soldiers. It was noticed that many of those who recovered from arrow wounds unaccountably recovered from chronic illnesses.

During the Shang Dynasty (1783–1122 BC), it was realized that massage with sharpened pieces of stone relieved painful areas of the body. Soon, needles were being manipulated at certain points on the body, and, with experience, new points of relief discovered.

The earliest needles were made from bone, horn and bamboo. Later, iron, bronze, gold and silver became popular. The modern fine, flexible needles are made from stainless steel. The first record of successful treatment by needling described how Pien Chuch, who lived from 407–310 BC, cured a very sick prince.

At about 250 BC, *The Yellow Emperor's Classic on Internal Medicine* was written in the form of a dialogue between the Yellow Emperor and his ministers. It was the first Chinese medical book. In it, 132 points suitable for needling are described.

Nine needles described in *The Yellow Emperor's* text

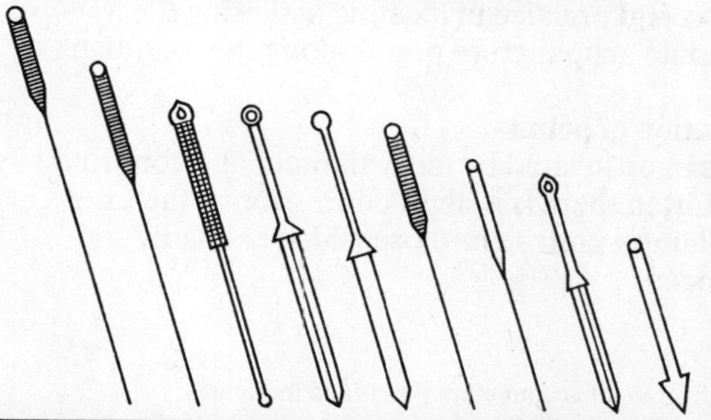

Needling

Modern needles are made of very fine stainless steel and vary in length from ½ inch to 3 inches. Handles are made to suit the preferences of different practitioners. The depth and angle of an inserted needle depend upon the point being used.

The depth of insertion is measured in terms of fens. A fen is one tenth of an ACI or Anatomical Chinese Inch (slightly less than 1/10th of an ordinary inch, see page 36). The insertion may be as little as 1 fen, e.g. in the head, or as much as 30 fen, e.g. in the buttocks.

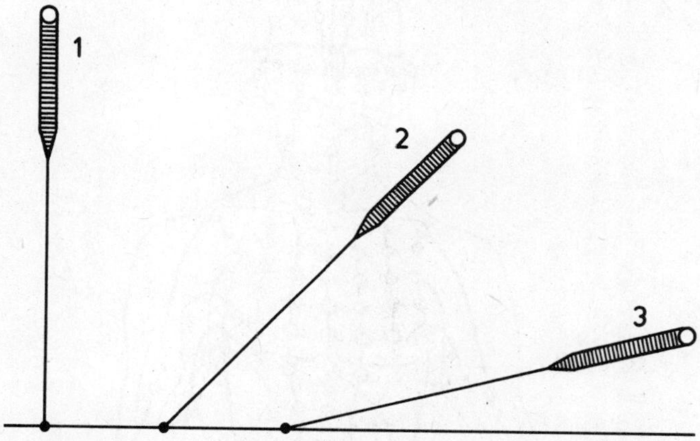

Three angles of insertion using standard slim needles
1 Perpendicular
2 Angle of 45 degrees
3 Sliding along the skin surface

Other acupuncture needles (*bottom right*)

a Prismatic needle
About 2½ inches long, with a sharp head, it is used for acute diseases. It is never inserted for more than 1 fen.

b Seven-star needle
The hammer is 4–6 inches long. The head has a collection of seven, or sometimes five, standard slim needles and is used for gently hammering over the skin surface. It is especially useful for skin diseases and for treating children.

c Inner dermal needles
Very small and delicate, these are used for inserting into points on the head or ears.

d Press needles
These are designed to stay in the skin for several days and can be pressed or manipulated by the patient as required. They are used for chronic conditions. Two points in the ear, for example, are commonly used to help people give up smoking. Press needles are extremely effective when a person needs to resist the temptation to smoke, since the sufferer can apply the extra stimulation required at the exact moment temptation strikes.

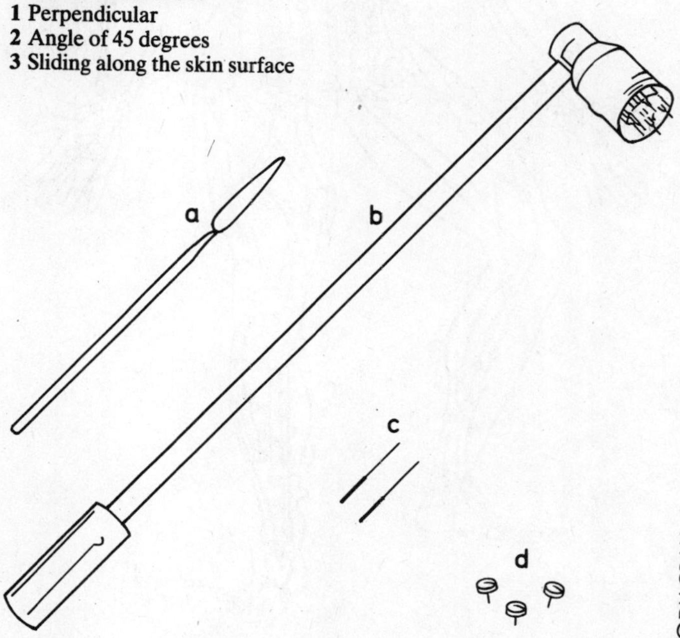

REFERENCE: For more information on acupuncture see pp. 34–35 and **Section Two: The balancing touch** (pp. 38–39). The method of massaging is similar to that used in foot reflexology; see **Section Two: It's all in the sole** (pp. 50–53).

Acupuncture 2

Training as an acupuncturist takes at least six years. The Chinese place great emphasis upon clinical practice and have opened their training hospitals to Westerners with basic medical, paramedical and acupuncture qualifications. Improvement in the health of the practitioner is also given attention. A sick doctor is unlikely to be able to be an effective healer.

A large part of the training is devoted to pulse diagnosis and practice in locating and using the appropriate acupuncture points along the meridians.

The location of points

Points can be located by measurement and confirmed by touch. Often there is a slight depression at the exact point. Painful points are those which are badly unbalanced.

Chinese diagram of acupuncture points and meridians

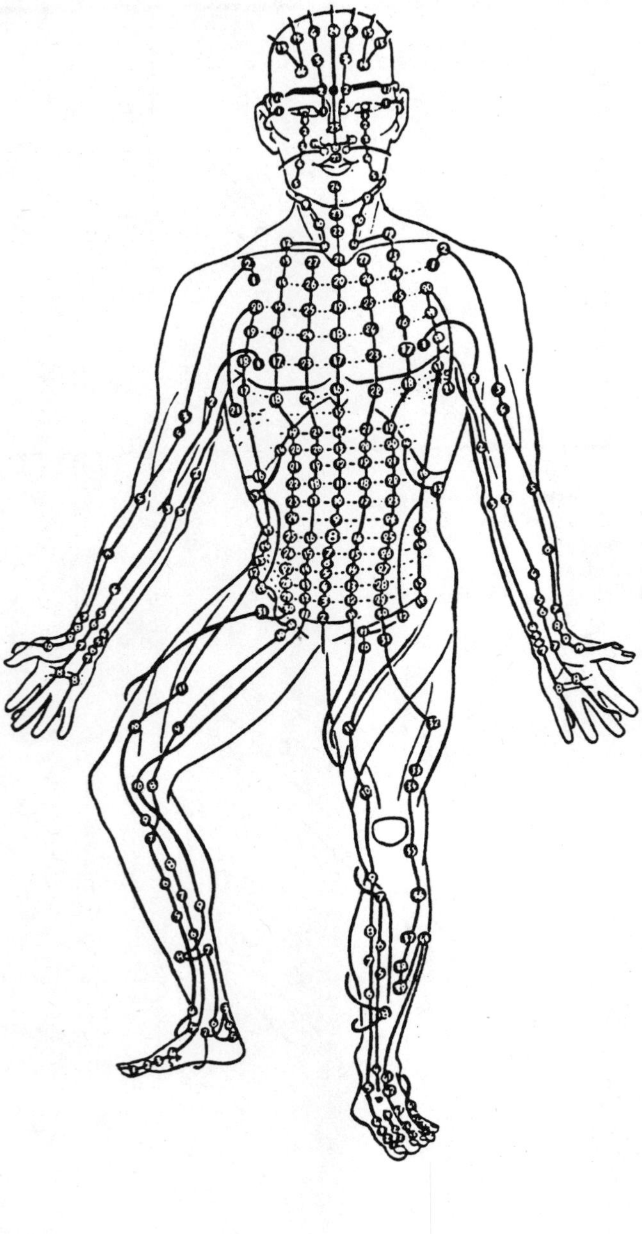

Since acupuncture points have electrical properties, an electronic device, called an acusometer, can be used to locate particularly difficult points. In France it is called a stigmascope and in Russia a tobiscope.

The acusometer measures the impedance near a point. Usually one electrode is held in the patient's hand and the other moved over the skin. The range of impedance in normal skin is from 20,000 ohms to 200,000 ohms and is fairly constant. At acupuncture points the impedance is lower and inconstant, a change that shows clearly on the sensitive scale of the acusometer.

What is the effect of acupuncture?

The skin is the largest and most sensitive organ of the body. Touch can have a powerful effect. The specific massage, heat treatment or needling of acupuncture can excite, inhibit or induce responses, affecting heart beat, blood count, blood flow, hormone secretion and reducing congestion or inflammation.

Needling certain points of the body has been shown to increase the number of white blood cells and intensify phagocytosis. Acupuncture both strengthens the resistance to diseases and stimulates the natural healing processes of the body. The stimulation of certain points inhibits pain and can produce temporary anesthesia.

Responsive disturbances

Some diseases and disturbances are particularly responsive to acupuncture. These include the following:

- Arthritis, in all forms. Very effective for children and at least relieves pain in cases of chronic damage in elderly patients.
- Rheumatism and muscle, tendon and bone diseases.
- Gynecological problems, such as irregular menstruation, pre-menstrual tension, birth control, sterilization, and abortion.
- Neurological diseases, such as epilepsy, sciatica, polio.
- Stomach and intestinal problems, such as acidity, ulcers and digestive disturbances. Very effective as a preventative by catching problems in early stages.
- Infectious diseases, such as malaria, dysentery, influenza and diarrhea.
- Painful conditions such as toothache, headache and migraines can be relieved until further treatment is given.
- Many other conditions, such as angina, bronchitis and kidney disease, are very responsive to acupuncture.

Modern Chinese practitioners tend to adopt some Western methods into their clinical practices, thereby enjoying the best of both worlds.

ACUPUNCTURE AND WESTERN MEDICINE
Chinese and Japanese acupuncturists who combine Western medicine and acupuncture claim high success.

Western medical opinion states:	**Claims of combined medical practices**
Limbs severed for up to 6 hours can be reattached but may not function.	Limbs severed for up to 24 hours have been reattached and became fully functional.
Burns over 80% of the body are normally fatal.	A woman with 98% burns was saved and had new skin grafts.
The paralyzing after-effects of polio are incurable.	People paralyzed by polio for years have been able to walk again after acupuncture treatment.
Deafness and mutism are incurable.	New acupuncture treatments now can cure deafness and mutism, especially in children.

Three types of acupuncture practice:
1 Acupuncture for prevention and cure.
2 Electro-acupuncture: the manipulation of needles by electric impulses rather than by hand. This is used for improving chronic diseases where 30 minutes of continuous stimulation through the needles is necessary at each treatment.
3 Acupuncture anesthesia used for pain relief and in surgical operations during which the patient is totally awake and cooperative but feels no pain.

A report from the Canton City People's Hospital in China in the 1970s said that about 50 visitors from the Trade Fair were invited to watch a Cesarean delivery by acupuncture anesthesia. Two needles were inserted in each leg and manipulated from time to time by a medical worker during the operation, while another worker monitored blood pressure.

The mother, aged 37, stayed totally conscious, calm and smiling, saying she felt no pain at all. The operation took 30 minutes from start to finish and the child was a healthy boy. Of course, there were none of the side effects of a normal anesthetic.

Diagnosis
This is done mainly by reading the 12 meridian pulses. For details refer to **Section Seven: Diagnostic alternatives 2** (pp. 146–147).

There is more information about the meridians on the next page.

1
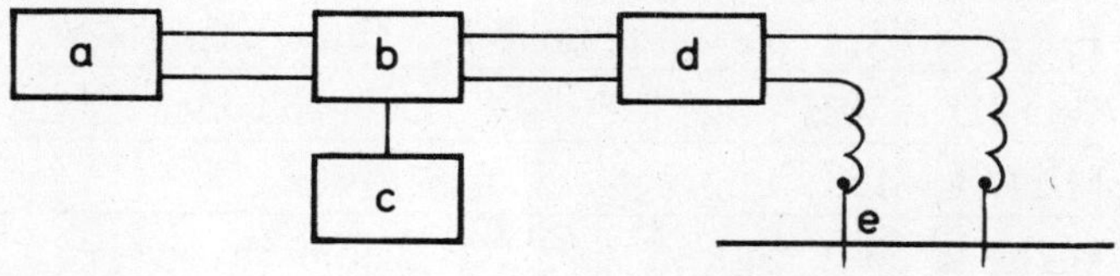

a Power supply
b Pulse generator
c Control of pulse and frequency
d Control of current
e Needles through skin

2
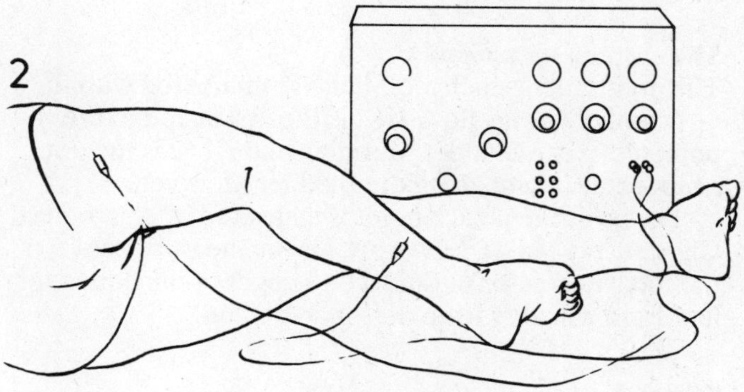

3
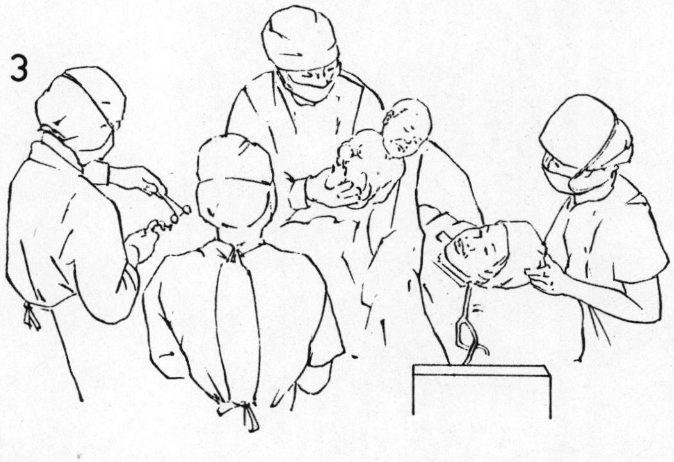

1 The design of an acupuncture stimulator
2 Treating a polio patient with electro-acupuncture
3 Acupuncture anesthesia for a Cesarean delivery

The meridians

According to ancient Chinese medicine, the channels through which Ch'i or life energy flows are 12 paired meridians and two single meridians. The flow of the vital force or life energy can be stimulated by needling at precise points along the meridians known as acupuncture points. The meridians are named according to the areas of the body with which they are primarily associated.

Conventionally, the 12 pairs of meridians are numbered with Roman numerals. According to Oriental philosophy, some meridians are Yin and others are Yang. Each meridian is also metaphorically associated with one of the five elements: fire, wood, water, metal, earth.

The twelve meridians

	YIN (inner)		**YANG** (peripheral)	
FIRE	I	Heart	II	Small intestine
WATER	IV	Kidney	III	Bladder
FIRE	V	Pericardium	VI	Three-heater
WOOD	VIII	Liver	VII	Gall bladder
METAL	IX	Lungs	X	Colon
EARTH	XII	Spleen	XI	Stomach

The two unique meridians
The Conception Vessel (Yin) begins near the anus and flows centrally up the front of the body to the mouth. The Governor Vessel (Yang) begins near the anus and flows centrally up the back, over the head to the mouth.

The acupuncture points
The points along each meridian are numbered with the direction of energy flow. III 1 is the first acupuncture point along the Bladder Meridian and III 67 is the last acupuncture point along the Bladder Meridian.

The position of each point is measured in Anatomical Chinese Inches (ACI). An ACI is the measure between the top two creases of the second finger of the dominant hand and will vary from person to person.

a 2nd finger
b ACI

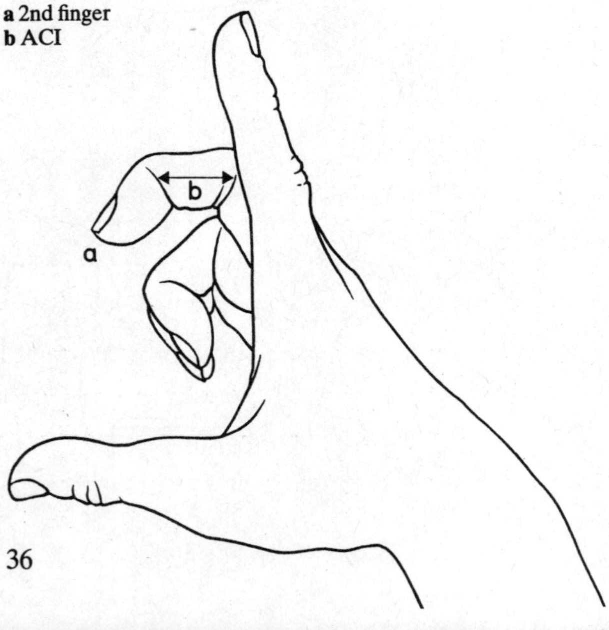

THE MERIDIAN OF THE BLADDER III YANG
This is the longest meridian. In the illustration *below*, the right hand Bladder Meridian is shown on the back. In places it runs close to the central Governor Vessel which follows the median line of the spine.

Diagrammatic location of acupuncture points
a Median line
b Cervical vertebrae
c Thoracic vertebrae
d Lumbar vertebrae
e Sacrum
f Sacral foramen
g Coccyx
h 2 ACI
i 1½ ACI

The meridian begins at the inner edge of the eye and runs over the top of the head

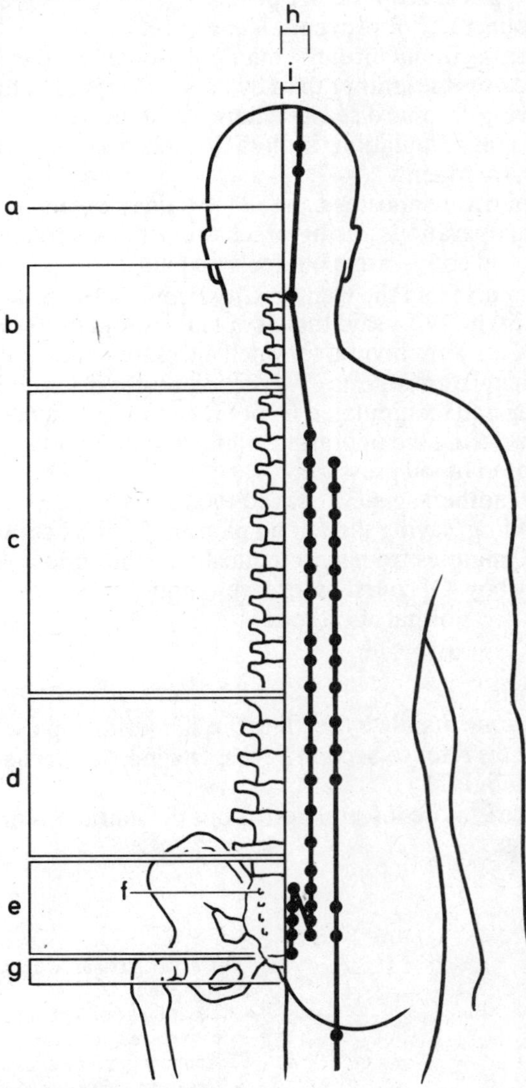

The meridian continues down the back of the leg

THE COMMAND POINTS OF THE BLADDER MERIDIAN III YANG

Most acupuncture treatment is given via points on the arms and legs known as the Command Points. The left or right side will be chosen according to the balance to be achieved.

The Command Points of the Bladder Meridian are shown on the back of the right leg and the outside of the right foot. ACI measurements are shown 0–8 down from the popliteal crease and 0–8 up from the external ankle bone.

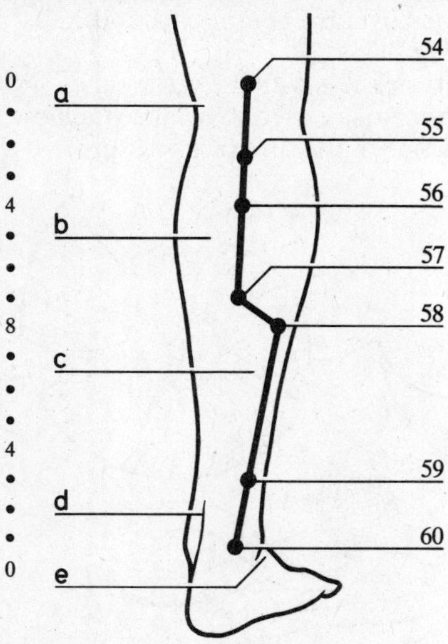

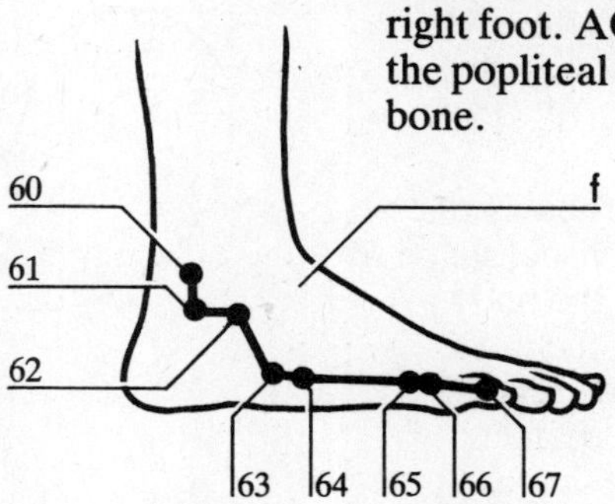

Key to diagrams
a Popliteal crease
b Gastronemius muscle
c Soleus with peroneus longus behind
d Achilles tendon
e Internal malleus of tibia
f External malleus of fibula (ankle bone)

The Command Points	Chinese name
III 54 EARTH. vagabond point. Mx	Wei Ch'ung
III 55	Ho Yang
III 56 Nx	Ch'eng Chin
III 57	Ch'eng Shan
III 58 Junction Point (with IV 4)	Fei Tang
III 59	Fu Yang
III 60 FIRE	Ku Lun

The Command Points	Chinese name
III 61	Pu Ts'an
III 62 Mx	Shen Mei
III 63	Chin Men
III 64 SOURCE POINT	Ching Ku
III 65 WOOD. Sedation	Shu Ku
III 66 WATER. HORARY POINT	T'ung Ku
III 67 METAL. Tonification. Exit	Chin Yin

The Chinese names indicate the value and character of the points, for example, III 63 Chin Men means the Golden Gate of immense power, Chin meaning extreme or great.

Key to table above
ELEMENT: point can boost the named element.
Vagabond point: the point can be hard to find because its position may vary from person to person.
Mx: Moxa forbidden. It is dangerous to use any form of heat treatment on this point.
Nx: Needling is forbidden at this point.
Junction point: links yin and yang meridians (yang Bladder with yin Kidney Meridian IV).
SOURCE POINT: self-limiting in effect.
Sedation: a good point for calming.
HORARY POINT: the meridian's own element point.
Tonification: a good point for stimulation.
Exit: last point on a meridian.

What are meridians?

Meridians cannot be found during a post-mortem, yet their positions can be traced on the living body: the line of a meridian has a lowered electrical impedance. Since this is also a property of nerves, it has been speculated that meridians are nerve pathways. The traditional terminology used in acupuncture is, perhaps, a philosophical metaphor for what we know in scientific terms.

Speculative comparison of terminology

Scientific terms	Traditional acupuncture terms
Nerve system	Meridian system
Nerve pathways	Meridians
Sensory nerve endings	Acupuncture points
Positive and negative ionization	Yin and Yang
Various forms of stimulation and response	The five elements
Wave of electrical depolarization along a nerve	Ch'i energy in the meridians

The balancing touch

The oldest method of healing is by touch. Many ways of touching have been developed over the centuries, but the purpose of touching remains the same: to heal by balancing the disturbed forces inside the body.

At one extreme, balance is achieved by ordering the evil spirit to leave and take its sickness with it. At the other end of the spectrum, sophisticated methods of touching, such as acupuncture and Shiatzu, are used to balance the flow of opposing forces in the body. Shiatzu is the Japanese version of acupuncture, using finger pressure (acupressure) instead of acupuncture needles.

The symbol of the life-force

The symbol, which looks like a curved tadpole or pine-cone, is universal. It combines the on-going flow of rhythmic curves and the mystical spiral, both of which are features of living things.

Called *magatama* by the Japanese, it is probably one of the most potent symbols in the world; its visual shape reflects its meaning. *Magatama* is the shape the body makes when experiencing an orgasm reflex, the most powerful and most pleasurable of all the body reflexes. When male and female bodies combine in a perfect orgasm, they create a whole: two *magatama* shapes make the symbol for yin-yang. When yin-yang are in perfect harmony, they form a whole, a circle.

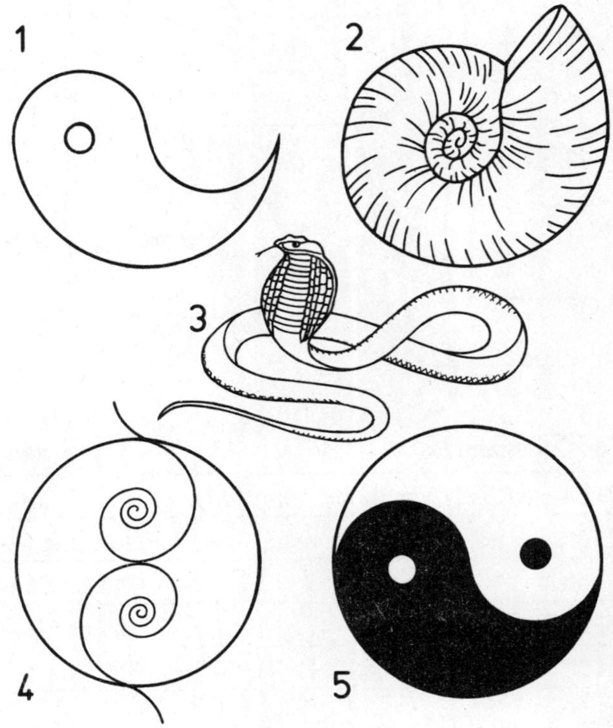

1 *Magatama*
2 The mystical spiral of life in a shell
3 The rhythmic flow of life in snake movement
4 Yin-yang: the combination of rhythmic flow and the spiral of life
5 Yin-yang in perfect balance

The Oriental philosophy of yin-yang

Yin and yang are said to be opposing forces in the flow of life energy. Too much of one or of the other will unbalance the body, and the aim of Oriental medicine is to bring the many yin-yang forces into harmony.

In yin-yang philosophy, the opposing forces must maintain harmony by balancing each other dynamically. Neither must be stronger nor weaker than the other, just as two people leaning on each other maintain dynamic harmony. Some examples of opposing forces are listed here.

YIN	YANG
Female	Male
Noon	Sun
Damp	Dry
Rest	Growth
Cold	Hot
Recession	Expansion
Coma	Convulsion
Acidity	Alkalinity
Inhibition	Stimulation
Forces biologically linked with the sympathetic action of the autonomic or involuntary nervous system.	Forces biologically linked with the parasympathetic action of the autonomic or involuntary nervous system.

The balancing touch

All the methods of healing by touch that are described in this section aim to help the patient's body regain its natural balance. Some methods concentrate on the skeleton and musculature while others tackle the blood flow and hormone balance. In all cases, balance by touch is a kind of magic; nobody is yet certain how touch can do all these things.

It is true that the mechanical manipulation of muscles could be expected to release unbalancing tensions, but little is known of how reflex massage, acupuncture or chiropractic actually work. These and other similar methods are described in the following pages of this section.

EAST INDIAN SERPENT MYTHOLOGY AND THE SYMBOL OF LIFE

In this copied painting of *c.*1760, Vishnu, the Creator, is depicted in his three manifestations *(right)*:
a As himself resting between successive creations inside the golden egg of the universe;
b As Ananta-Sesha, the serpent who breathes life into all things when each of its heads curls in the spiral of inspiration, just like the *magatama*;
c As the cosmic ocean of primordial waters from which the breath of life will create living things.

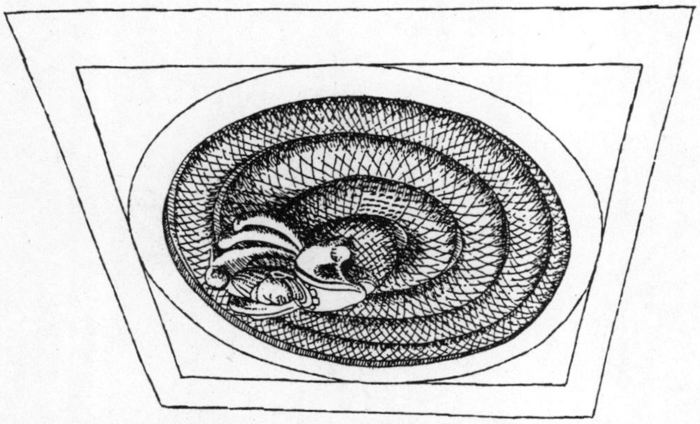

The serpent guardian of the underworld, 6th century carving on a cave ceiling at Badami, India

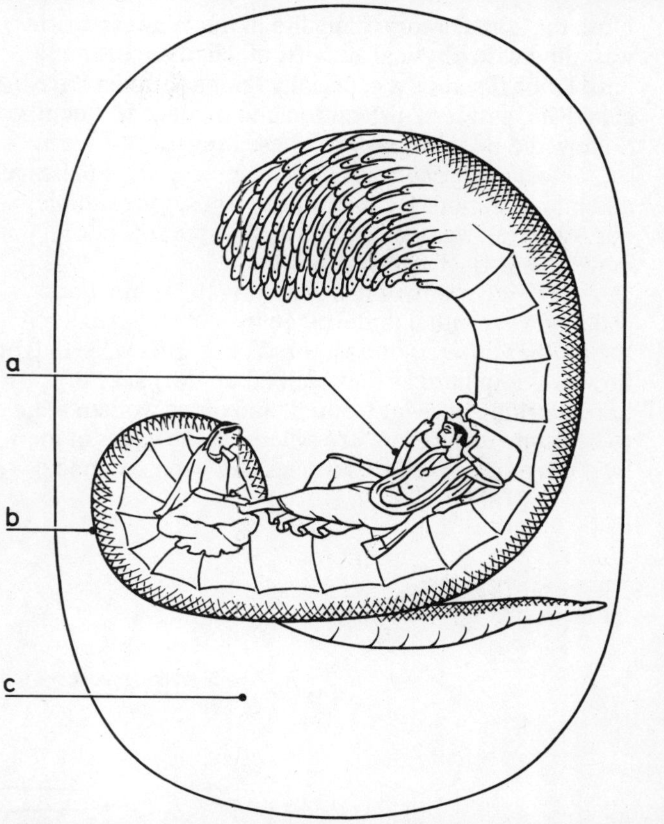

THE PAISLEY SHAWL AND ITS DESIGN

Potent symbols reappear from time to time quite spontaneously. The Paisley pattern is an example.

In the 1770s, officers of the British East India Company would bring back from their travels Kashmir shawls for their ladies. These shawls, twill woven and often patchworked, took two or three years to complete and were extremely expensive. European ladies demanded more shawls, and weavers set up looms, particularly in France and in Scotland, to imitate the Kashmir shawls, copying their designs. These imitations were known as cashmere, in France as *cachemire*.

Some of the most successful weavers were the Scots of Paisley, and their shawls were of high quality. The pine-shaped design they copied from Kashmir became known as the Paisley pattern and has been used in textile design ever since.

The origins of the Paisley pattern

While the *magatama* shape was the symbol of life in the Orient, the Middle East and much of the rest of Asia were developing their own symbols of life.

In Chaldea (Babylon) the date palm was regarded as the tree of life, since it provided food, wine and materials for shelter. The growing shoot of a date palm emerges from a tightly curled bud, similar to the unfurling frond of common bracken.

The shape was used throughout early East Indian and European art. It was called the *boteh* in India, the "tadpole" in France, the "little onion" in Vienna and the pine in Britain, until it was developed as the Paisley pattern.

The *magatama* and the curling shape of the Paisley pattern are both symbols of life.

The Paisley pattern on the border of a shawl

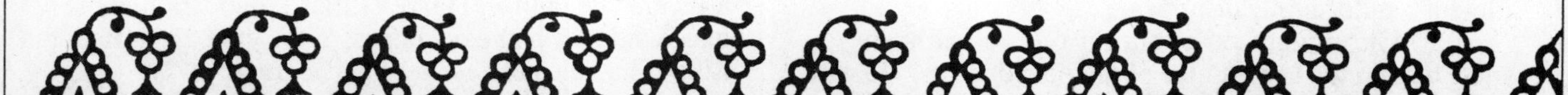

Techniques of manipulation

Until the 20th century, daily life in the Western world was filled with physical activity, much of it extremely hard labor. The body, especially the back, must have ached and suffered dislocation and damage frequently. So how did people deal with these injuries?

Almost everyone was adept at some kind of massage and manipulation. By the Middle Ages, for example, back-walking was well established as part of folk medicine throughout Europe.

An effective way of manipulating the spine, back-walking was a ritual undertaken by women, usually by the mother of twins or a virgin. Young girls were taught how to stamp hard as they walked up the backs of hard-working peasant women, and older women were to be found using their strong legs on the backs of men who were sick or whose muscles had been strained.

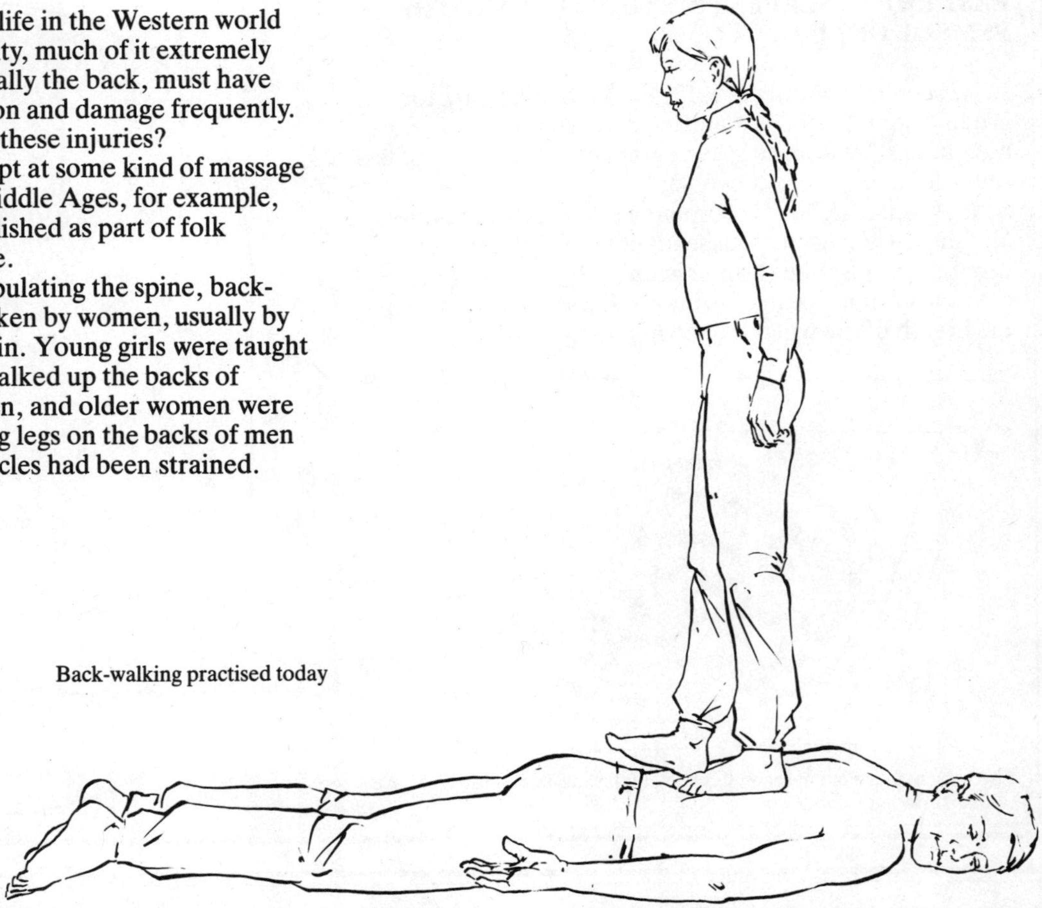

Back-walking practised today

MANIPULATIVE THERAPIES

Osteopathy

In early 19th-century America, Andrew Still was a farming man with a family . . . until tragedy struck. During a meningitis epidemic he lost three of his children. From then on he turned his attention to the problem of disease.

Being devoutly religious, he believed that man must be perfect because he was fashioned in the image of God. How, then, could people fall ill? He concluded that sickness could only occur if parts of the body became maladjusted.

Perhaps it was because he was an excellent mechanic that Andrew Still set about readjusting the body parts methodically by manipulations that often had a miraculous effect. After twisting, pressing and pushing his patient's body around for an hour or so, a chronic ailment would simply disappear.

In 1874 he announced his theory of osteopathy in order to gain the acceptance of medical doctors. He was rejected by them, denounced by his Methodist minister for being in league with the devil and forced to leave the area. He moved to Kirksville in Missouri to open the first school of osteopathy in 1892.

John M. Littlejohn, from Glasgow, Scotland, attended Andrew Still's school. He had already studied physiology for three years at Glasgow University as part of a course in forensic medicine. Later he put osteopathy on a firmly physiological basis and opened the first British School of Osteopathy in 1917.

The modern osteopath is expert in the diagnosis and treatment of malfunctions in the musculo-skeletal system.

Chiropractic

In 1895, Daniel Palmer was living in Davenport, Iowa. Born into a farming family, he became a mesmerist (early hypnotist) but he was disillusioned with the poor results he was getting.

One day, on entering his apartment block, he saw the janitor limping miserably. Enquiring what was wrong, Palmer had to shout his question loudly before he got an answer. The janitor, Harvey Lillard, had strained his back while lifting heavy boxes. That was bad enough but Lillard had also lost most of his hearing.

Palmer took Lillard to his apartment and massaged his back, a new technique he had been trying. Lillard was a large man and his neck was particularly painful. Palmer used quite a lot of force, pressing hard with his thumbs on the most painful spots, as if digging out the pain.

Back stretching
Two people could manipulate each other's backs by linking arms, back to back, and lifting each other in turn. This both stretched the spine and opened the ribs, and it is an exercise that is often used by modern practitioners of bioenergetics to deepen the breathing.

The bone-setters
An advanced form of manipulation was called bone-setting; it was not related to setting broken bones (although bone-setters later became skilled at this too) but involved pulling and pushing the body to reorganize the skeleton.

Usually, bone-setting was a special skill passed down through a farming family. It was believed that pains were due to one small bone, often one of the vertebrae, being out of place. The bone-setter manipulated the bone into place. The click of the neck, wrist or back indicated that the devil causing the pain was being forced out.

Even today the tradition continues. Danny O'Neil, a cattle farmer living near Borris in Eire, treats backaches and dislocations in people and animals alike without any fuss or special equipment.

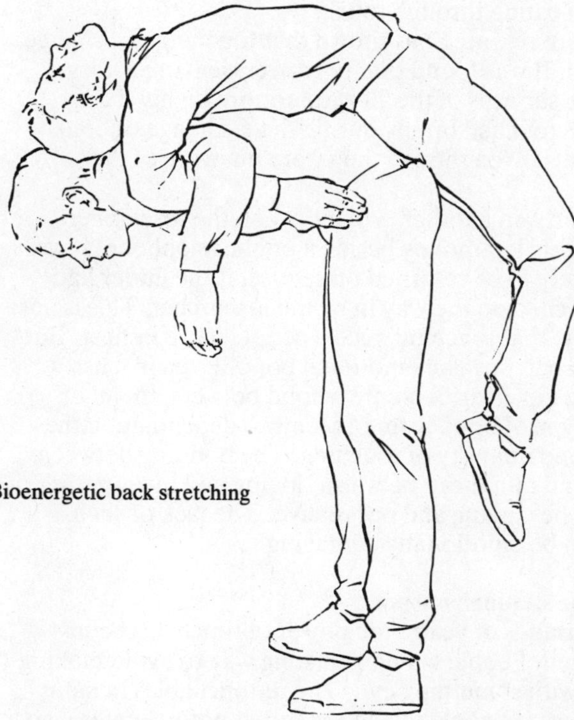

Bioenergetic back stretching

©DIAGRAM

To his surprise and to Lillard's delight, the pain subsided, and over the next few days his hearing improved. After several similar treatments, Lillard could walk without pain and his hearing returned.

From then on, Palmer studied anatomy and physiology and began to formulate a new method of massage which he called chiropractic, from the Greek *cheiro* and *praktikos* meaning "done by hand." He claimed that many diseases were caused by neuro-irritations due to abnormal or strained muscles.

The modern definition of chiropractic is a system of manipulation of the vertebrae to restore normal functioning of the body.

The loss of massage traditions in the West
In 1563 at Trento, in North Italy, the Council of Trent produced a long declaration designed to help the Roman Catholic Church regain its status lost during the Reformation. Many practices were denounced as evil, including surgery, massage and bone manipulation.

What a sad day that was for the Western world! Modern surgeons no longer use their hands for massage, as was common in the 16th century, and while manipulations are tolerated for limited purposes, massage is considered by many people to be either an indulgent pleasure bordering on the immoral or a downright dangerous practice. Yet in Eastern countries, massage and manipulation are taken for granted, and in China they even provide employment for the blind, who are trained in special schools.

Modern massage invitations

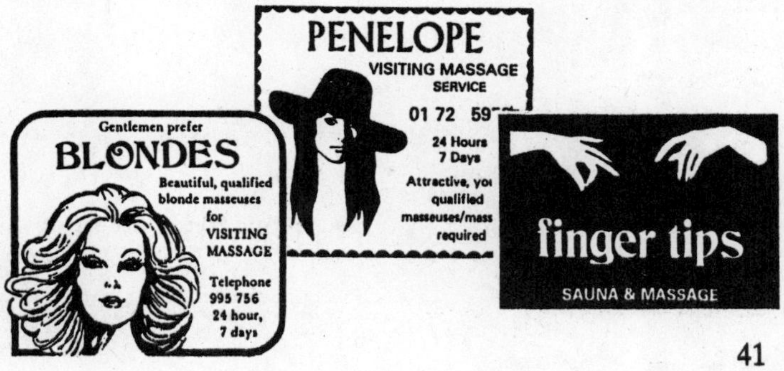

The laying-on of hands

Touching has a profound effect on the whole person. Leaving apart the many taboos about who may touch whom and how, a touch stimulates the nervous system and is a message without words. Most people pick up instant information about the character of a stranger as they shake hands, and lovers do much of their communicating through touch.

Modern research has shown that touching can change attitudes. It was found that borrowers leaving a library rated the services of the librarian more highly if they had been touched briefly during the exchange of books and tickets, even though they were unaware of the contact.

Similarly, in another project, when the researcher deliberately left money beside a public telephone, it was more likely to be returned on request if the finder had been touched on the way in by the researcher. This is not to suggest that touching makes people more honest. But touching can form an emotional bond. Even in a fist fight, the adversaries create a bond between them.

The type of bond formed seems to depend upon the quality and quantity of touching. The bonding between parent and infant can be warm, loving and invigorating, or it can be cloying and oppressive. The lack of such a bond can be emotionally damaging.

Touch me... touch me not

For thousands of years, the power of touch has been recognized. People would go a long way to avoid making contact with something evil. The untouchables in many cultures were people of a lower order, unfortunates who were often sick or severely disabled. To touch them meant risking the sickness-demon leaping into oneself.

Similarly, people would make every effort to be touched by a person they believed to have power or influence. Touching a powerful person meant that some of his good fortune, power or spirit-goodness would leap into oneself.

Giving blessings

Holy men such as buddhas, messiahs, priests, shamans, kings and their chosen disciples often gave blessings by placing hands on the heads of supplicants.

Fathers and schoolmasters also adopted the habit of patting their children and pupils on the head. The meaning of head-touching can vary but in all cases, the toucher is recognized as being more powerful, so that the touched feel blessed.

Touching for healing

When a person is sick, touching the head is a universal method of soothing and healing. Have you ever stroked the forehead of a sick child or friend? If so, you too have used an ancient method of magical healing by the laying-on of hands.

In the Middle Ages, tubercular disorders were commonplace and showed up especially in the glands of the neck (an illness known as scrofula). For centuries, European monarchs undertook the ritual of touching the sick on the head to show their power. People suffering from this sickness believed that being touched by the King would cure them. The disease became known as King's Evil and the ritual was called "touching for King's Evil."

Famous for his healing by the laying-on of hands was Jesus of Nazareth, the messiah of the Christian religion. In the Gospels, which describe his work, there are several occasions when he cured people of paralysis, blindness, leprosy and various crippling diseases. Sometimes he did this by touching; sometimes simply by commanding the sickness to leave.

One famous story tells of Jesus ordering the evil spirits that were making a man insane to jump into a herd of swine that consequently ran off screaming into the river. He also brought some people back to life from recent death. His healing activities were called miracles; to anyone witnessing such acts they must have been sheer magic.

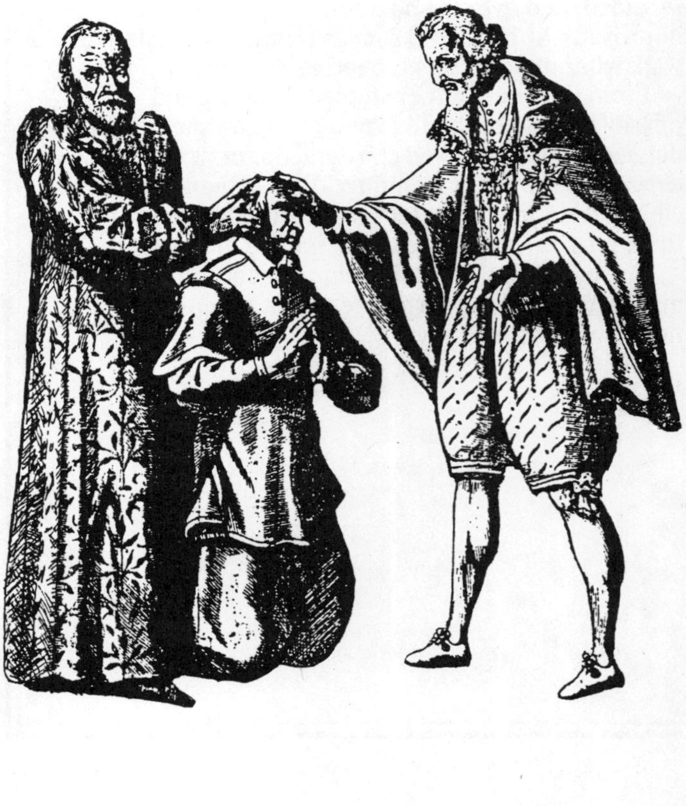

Henry IV of France touching for King's Evil

Healing by drawing out the sickness
In primitive times, an object was often used to draw the evil spirit of sickness out of an ill person. The Eskimo shaman, or medicine man, would go into a trance while holding his medicine stick, a carved piece of wood. Wood was in short supply and came from a living tree, so it was regarded as magical. The magic was activated when the shaman went into a trance, when he would place the magic stick on the forehead of the sick person and draw the demon sickness out.

When sudden, violent sickness strikes in western Borneo, the physician, who is usually an old woman, carves a human doll-image out of wood and touches the patient's head seven times with it, while commanding the sickness to pass over into the image. The wooden image is then staked into the ground at the spot where the sickness is thought to have first entered the person. Using rice, salt and tobacco, the old woman then further invokes the spirit to release the soul of the sick man and plague the image instead "for it is prettier and better than he."

An Eskimo shaman drawing out the sickness from his patient's head

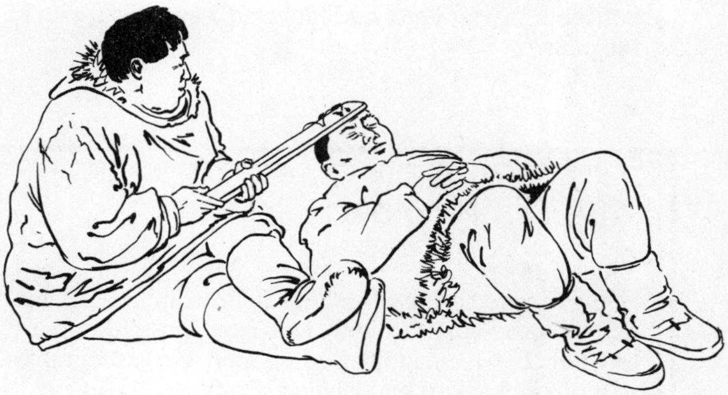

THE HEALING MASSAGE

Many tribes among the North American Indians used a back massage to cure most ills. The sufferer would sit cross-legged with his back upright. If you want to use this massage yourself it is easier on the masseur if you sit on a stool and hold the back of a chair to support yourself.

The massage is given by making wriggling strokes with the thumbs in the direction of the arrows shown on the diagram. The technique is to press with the thumbs upright and then wriggle a little distance with the thumbs flat. If the thumbs find this a strain, the palms of the hands can be used instead. The massage should not hurt the giver or the receiver, so the amount of pressure should be adjusted accordingly. This massage can be given with the person fully dressed, providing clothes are not tight fitting.

Begin at the base of the spine. Massage along the lines as numbered one to four. Proceed slowly; both people should breathe easily and regularly. Never give a massage if you are tense or uptight yourself, as you will do more harm than good to both people involved.

The Indian massage position

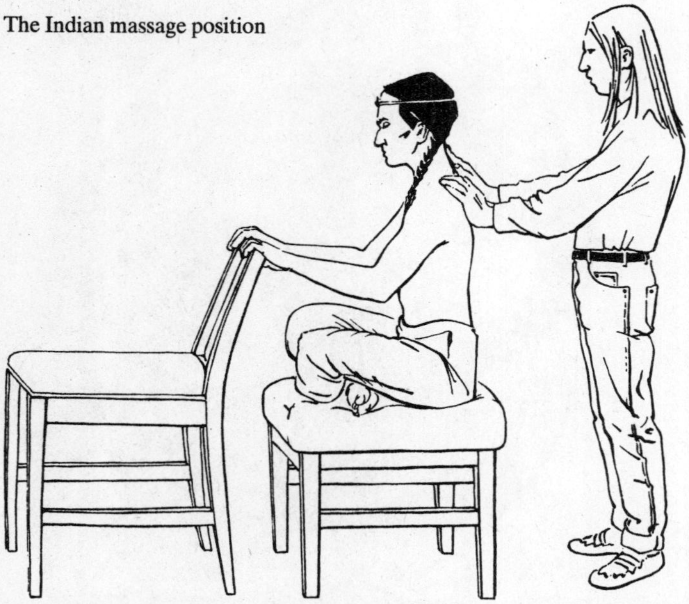

The Indian massage technique

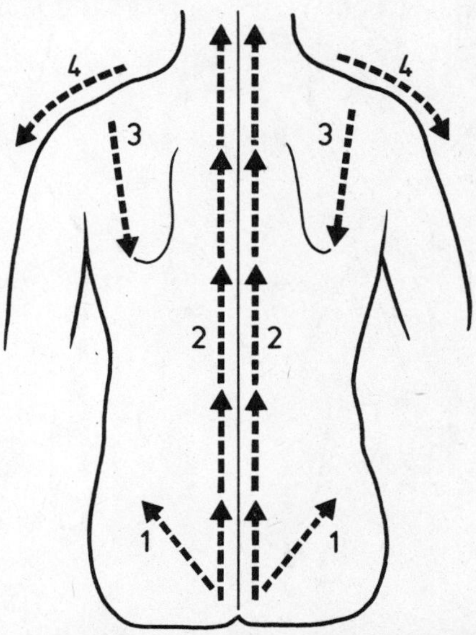

A loving touch

In 1777 Captain Cook, the explorer, landed in the Pacific island of Tahiti. During his stay he complained of severe rheumatic pain down one side of his body, hip to toe. One day, while resting on board his ship, he was visited by a dozen women, some from a family who had befriended him. They said they had come to cure him of the pain.

He wrote that he lay down on the deck and the women crowded round him, each taking a part of him in their big, strong hands and squeezing him from head to toe. After some 15 minutes he was glad to get away from them, although he felt much relief from the pain. The women repeated the squeezing before he retired to bed and twice again the next day, after which the pain had

STIMULATING CONTACT

Touch and sex
Being touched arouses feelings. Unfortunately, many people associate touch only with sex; consequently, touching between adults is often limited to acceptable pats on the back or handshakes. Some people even withdraw when they are touched, fearing to be aroused or "possessed." Others cannot get enough of child-like contact. To enjoy a pleasurable, healthy balance between the two is the aim of mature, platonic contact in some self-development programs.

Getting in touch is a healthy activity; but men have greater difficulty in sharing a non-sexual loving touch than do most women. This is probably due to their historically different sexual and social roles.

Humans enjoying non-sexual contact

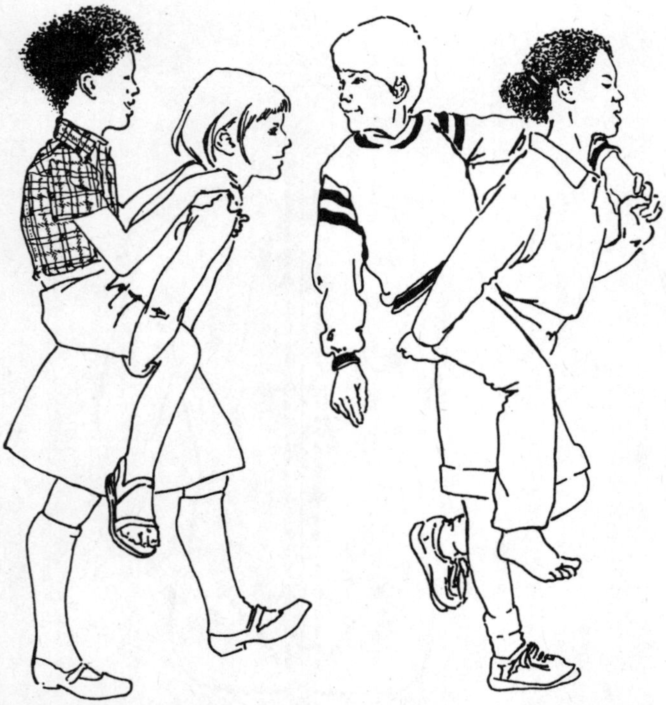

Bonding
The link made between parent and child by good physical contact in the early months of life is called bonding and is essential to healthy development. Separated from the mother at birth and left in isolation, baby monkeys fret, refuse food and display totally neurotic behavior. Given a piece of blanket to hold, these babies perk up considerably but remain nervous. The lengthy absence of contact with a parent monkey would seem to have a devastating effect on development. The same has been found to be true of human babies.

Newborn babies of normal birth weight can survive in isolation without food or water for over a week. After the Mexican earthquake several were dug from the ruins of a maternity ward as much as 10 days later. It remains, to be seen if they show any neurotic tendencies, as they grow up because of their initial separation from human contact. It may be that plenty of healthy contact during childhood will make up for their early loss.

Chimpanzees resting in contact with each other

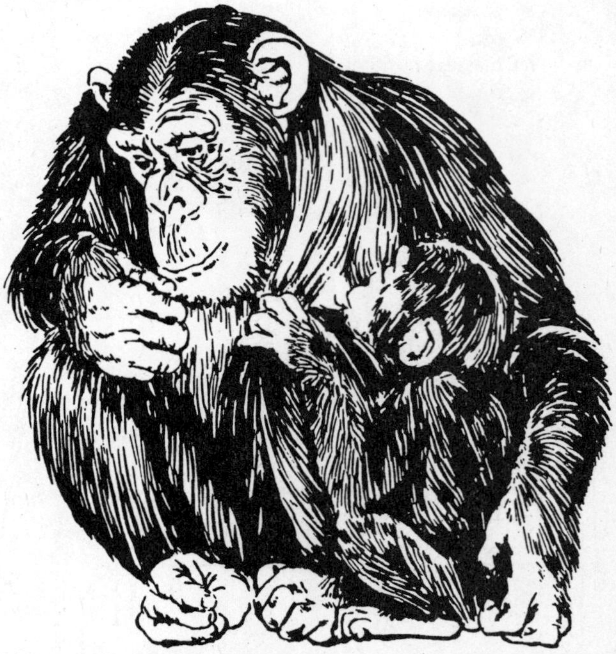

completely disappeared. These women asked for no payment; they simply gave their "loving touch" freely.

Touching with caring has been used for centuries to heal. Modern research has shown that touch need not always be with a human being. Stroking an animal or a soft toy can have a relaxing and healing effect and is recommended to people under stress.

Skin stimulation through touch

Premature babies living in incubators may also be adversely affected by lack of stimulating contact. It has become common practice in many hospitals to place incubator babies on sheepskins. When this was first tried it was observed that babies grew faster and slept more restfully than they had before the sheepskin was introduced.

Similarly, in a maternity hospital in Bogota, Colombia, where incubators were too costly to install, premature babies survived and thrived very well slung between their mother's breasts, which kept them in a constant temperature. It also kept them in physical contact. The practice is spreading to the West, not because incubators are unavailable but because the closeness between parent and baby is satisfying to both parties.

Physical contact is crucial to satisfactory early development of the very young. Known as the tenderness phenomenon, it was taken to greater lengths by Dr Frédéric Leboyer, a French doctor, who advocated birth without the violence of harsh lights, cool temperatures and ungainly handling, such as the old-fashioned practice of holding babies upside down.

He encouraged fathers to hold their newborn children gently in warm water and the mother to hold her baby resting face down on her body. The practice has now been extended to the mother giving birth in a large tub of warm water, with the whole family present. This was a common practice among primitive peoples.

In addition to its health-giving properties, touching has a socializing effect; for example, the social activity of grooming involves much touching.

In some parts of Borneo, babies were carried around until they were two years old, and most primitive people carry their babies in slings in close contact with the mother.

Parents hold their baby close

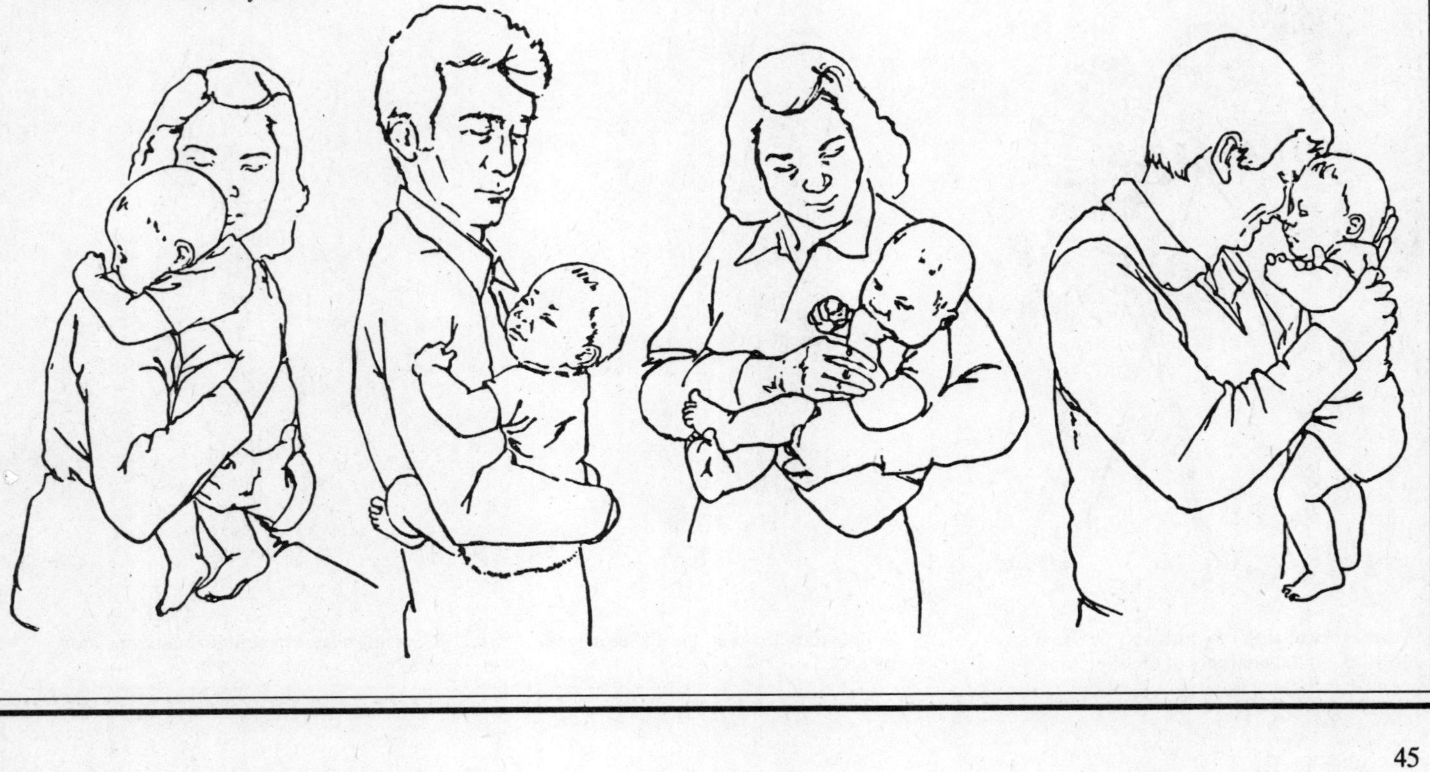

Any old bones

Over the centuries, every culture has developed ways of relieving pain and improving health by realigning the bone structure. Since all the bones of the skeleton are held together by the cartilage and ligaments at the end-points of each muscle, it follows that any chronic misuse of muscles will eventually distort the skeleton, especially the position of the head. This in turn will affect the nervous system, the circulatory system and other organs of the body.

POSTURE

Bad posture (*near right*)
a Tired outlook
b Stiff neck
c Round shoulders
d Restricted breathing
e Lower back pain
f Tight pelvic area
g Easily pushed off balance

Good posture (*far right*)
a Positive outlook
b Supple neck
c Capable shoulders
d Full breathing
e Pain-free back
f Swinging pelvic area
g Can keep a balance

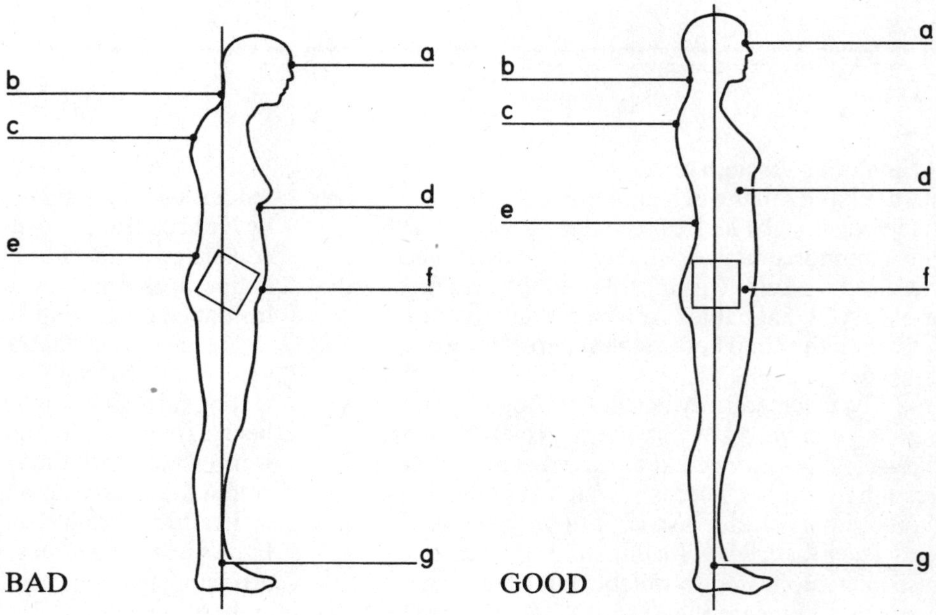

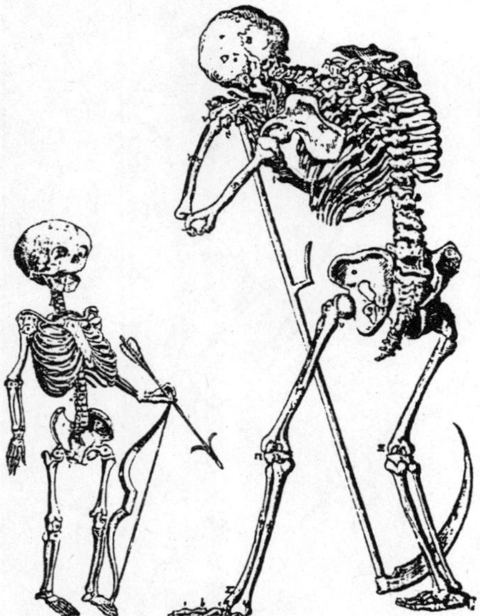

An allegorical view of youth and age from an old work on the anatomy of the skeleton

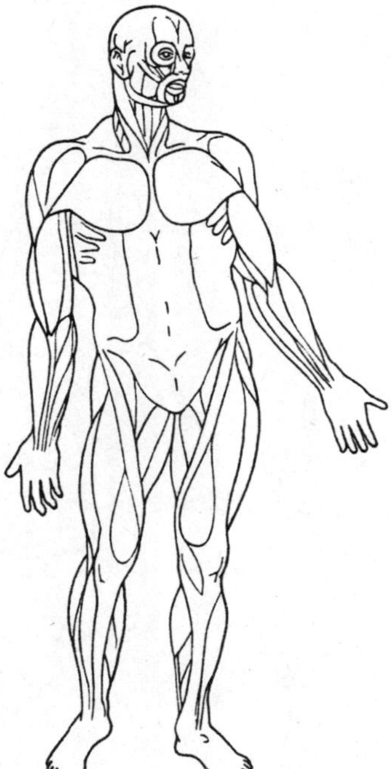

Supple muscles keep the skeleton well-balanced

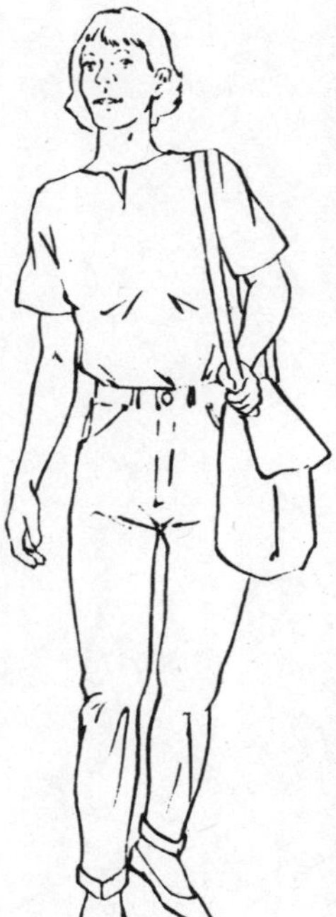

Carrying a heavy shoulder-bag can distort sideways

METHODS TO REALIGN THE BONE STRUCTURE

The Alexander Technique
F. M. Alexander (1869–1955) was an Australian actor with voice problems. He watched himself in the mirror and noticed how he tightened his throat muscles when speaking. Then he taught himself to change the habit and never lost his voice again. His program of re-education demands awareness of the body's position in space and a conscious effort to change the habitual position, thus removing the source of distorting tensions. It is a gentle technique, under personal control.

Feldenkrais exercises
Moshe Feldenkrais was an Israeli Judo teacher who combined Alexander principles of awareness with the movement of Oriental martial arts to produce a series of movement exercises designed to realign the skeleton. He introduced new approaches to simple activities such as walking and crawling.

Structural Integration or Rolfing
Developed by the American Dr Ida Rolf, originally a biochemist, Rolfing is a series of deep tissue massages to free and soften chronically tight connective tissues so that the skeleton rides easily, and the whole body feels lighter. Particular attention is given to the head, which should sit easily on the spine.

Traction and pressure
Traction is used to relieve the pressure of the vertebrae on the spinal cord. The illustration below shows how traction was achieved by the Ancient Greek doctor Hippocrates. The bindings are pulled on sticks used as levers, and a man tramples on the back muscles . . . a common way of giving massage.

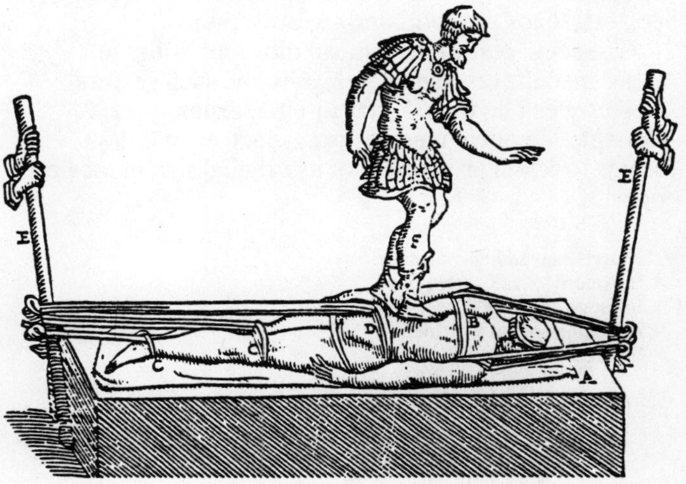

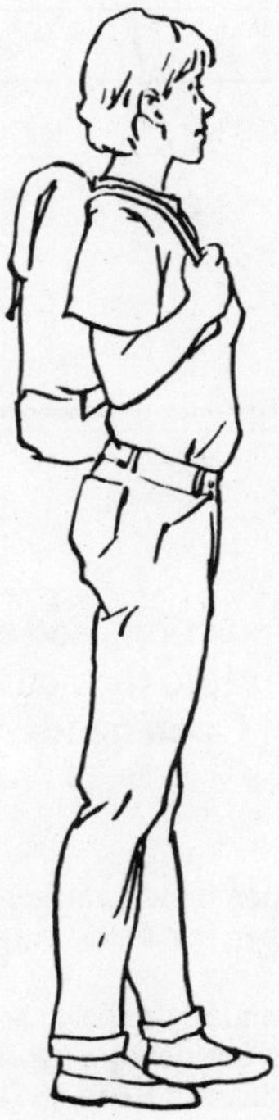

The best way to carry a bag is rucksack style

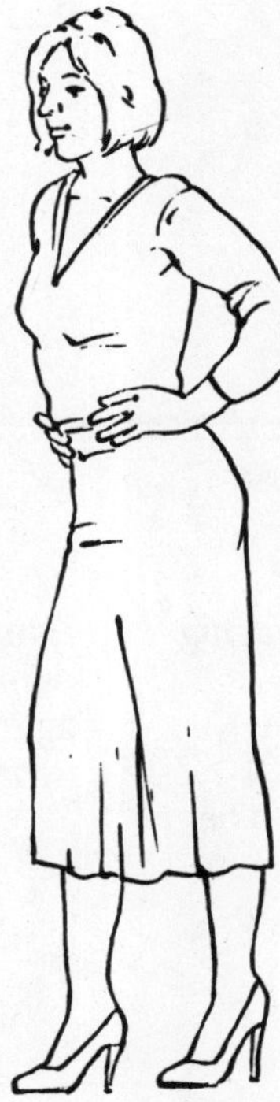

High-heeled shoes throw the pelvis forward and the spine develops a curvature. It may be sexy but it will lead to tense muscles and back pain

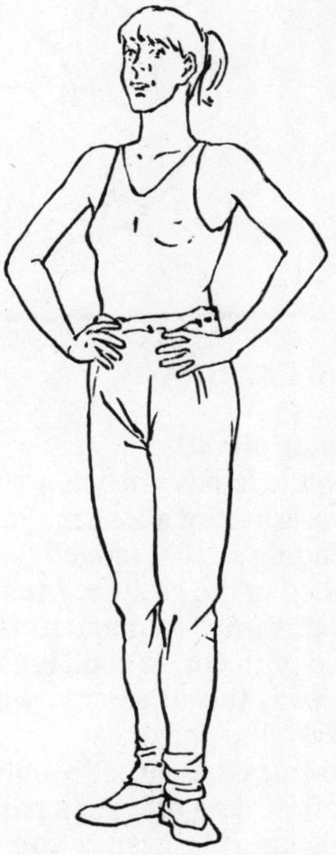

Flat shoes or bare feet help to keep postural balance

Handwork

Ever since man has stood erect, people have used their hands to communicate, for example by writing, carving, making gestures or touching. All communication flows along an energy channel, such as light, sound and heat, so the hands are channels for the passage of different forms of energy, which are interpreted as messages.

Often people are unaware of the original source of a gesture that is in common use; for example, the V-sign so often seen at pop concerts and protest marches was first used by Sir Winston Churchill during World War II to signify victory. Fifty years on, this gesture is understood worldwide and has appeared in sculpture, posters, logos, symbols and advertisements.

The same gesture may mean different things in different cultures, the circle sign is one such gesture. Gestures can be traced back into the distant past, for example the open hand gesture, which even today seems to retain an element of its original sign of magical powers.

The circle sign and its meanings

- In America – OK, great, fine
- In Japan – money
- In France – zero, worthless
- In Greece – an insult

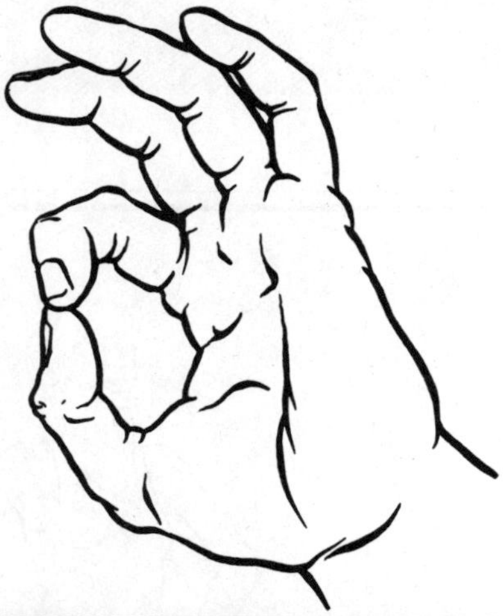

The open hand gesture

To show an open palm to a stranger has always been associated with showing that no weapons are being carried. The open palm is vulnerable to attack and yet is a sign of appeasement . . . rather in the way a domestic dog or cat will roll on its back, exposing its soft belly.

The open palm is also open to self-revelation… the parts of the hand and the lines on the palms are used in palmistry to read the personality and personal destiny.

The main areas of the hand used in palmistry

a Mental
b Practical
c Sensual
d Pleasure
e Will
f Logic
g Sexuality
h Lifeline
i Love
j Hardwork
k Creativity
l Ideas
m Heartline
n Headline
o Art
p Destiny
q Imagination

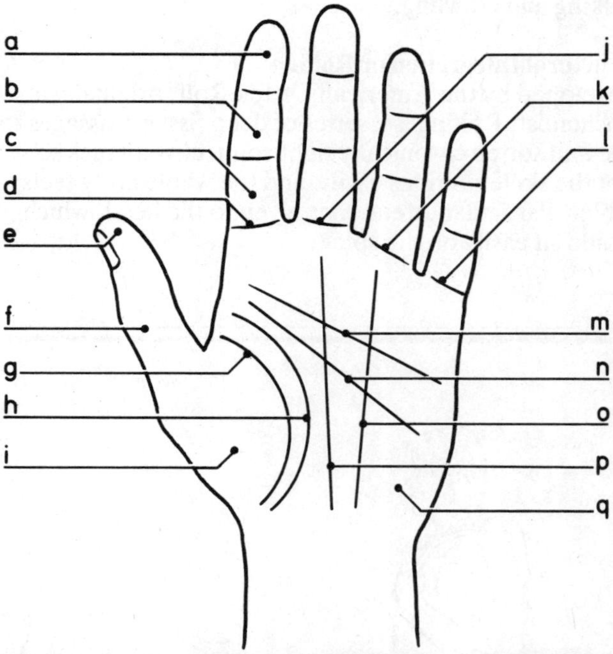

HAND LANGUAGE

Warding off evil

When the hands are held up and wide open, palms facing outwards, there is automatic protection against impending attack; indeed the whole forearm may be included in the gesture. Men, women and children all react this way when under threat or being attacked. The spread of the open hand is usually as wide as possible, to push away the attacker or whatever danger is about to overtake the person.

The message given by outward-facing, open hands is one of warding off evil, a passive indication of aggression. The gesture could very easily be transformed into the downward-facing palm position used to demonstrate magical influence or into the active aggression of overarm throwing. Open hands, facing inwards, are only defensive.

1 Open hands warding off attack
2 Open hands showing magical influence
3 Amulet, or charm against evil, from Sarajevo, Yugoslavia, of the hand of Fatimah (daughter of the Prophet Muhammad)
4 Jewish amulet, a part of religious folklore

The influential hand

The formal use of this wide open hand to ward off any form of evil is common and can be traced back to Egyptian and Byzantine times, and even beyond. The open hand is found in several cave paintings and is thought to have been placed there to ward off the evil eye and protect the tribe from disease and danger.

The same open hand is seen in a Greek car-sticker called the *moutza* which takes the warding off of evil a step further into the realm of abuse. In Greece, the open hand is a gestural relic used to insult others. In the car it means "keep your distance," with the equivalent strength of an obscene word.

Pushing the flat palm directly into the face of another person is a modern form of insult in many cultures, though in Greece it is the most offensive gesture possible... hence its use at a relatively safe distance in a car.

The origins of the open hand as insult are in the custom of throwing dirt in the faces of criminals as they were dragged through the streets to execution. Probably those in the stocks would have had many hands pushed into their faces.

The modern open hand

In everyday life, the open, outward palm is a universal symbol of power with still a small touch of magic about it. Traffic controllers stop vehicles, and religious or political leaders demonstrate their power by raising outstretched hands, as do many people to indicate their agreement in large gatherings such as pop concerts, union meetings and evangelical communions.

Hands and the messages they send are not just practical things; they have a communicative power and magic of their own which is recognized universally. The raised, open, waving hand is a sign of greeting, farewell and goodwill throughout the world. Hands are not just flesh and bone but the source of a power that can perform the magic of communication, healing and protection.

1

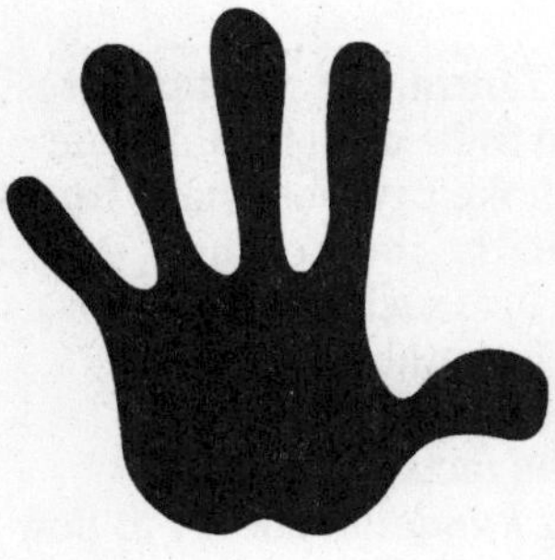

1 Greek *moutza* insulting car-sticker.
2 Paleolithic painting from the Pech-Merle cave. The hands warding off evil can be seen just above the dappled painting of an animal

2

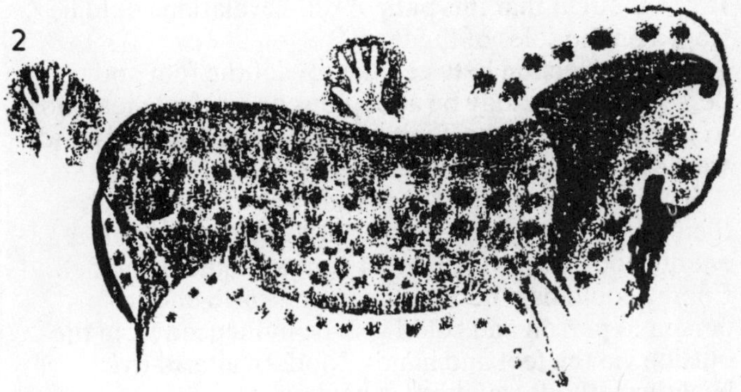

3

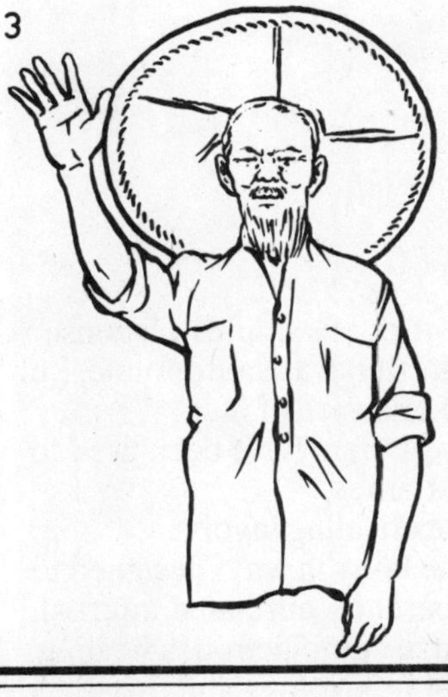

3 The open, waving hand of greeting.

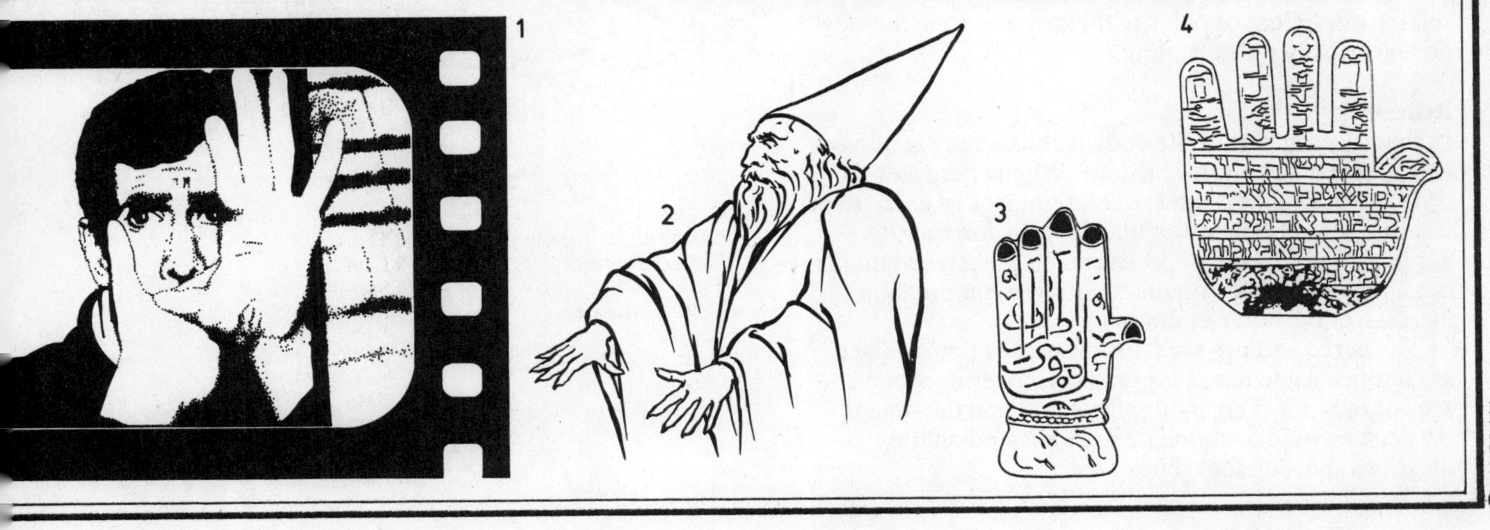

It's all in the sole 1

In the Indian religious cult of Tantra, the great pictures, known as *tankas*, are intended to be used to stimulate particular mental states and evoke psychosomatic forces. Tantra throws people deep into the roots of their identities and obliges them to face such human truths as birth, death, sex, social roles and other personal realities.

By making believers face the facts of life, tantric practice enables the life-giving *kundalini* energy to flow unobstructed through the body, bringing enlightenment. It was thought that this path of self-revelation could be traced on the soles of the feet.

The connection between the sole of the foot and personal destiny may be a religious or magical metaphor; to many ancients, the Tantrikas included, feet and hands were very significant.

They were not merely flesh and blood, as we see them; rather, they were those parts of the subtle or energy body with which direct contact could be made. Energy could pass between man and earth and from person to person and could also be influenced from the outside via the feet and hands. Modern alternative healing methods call it reflex healing.

SOME REFLEX POSITIONS ON THE FEET
These positions are approximate

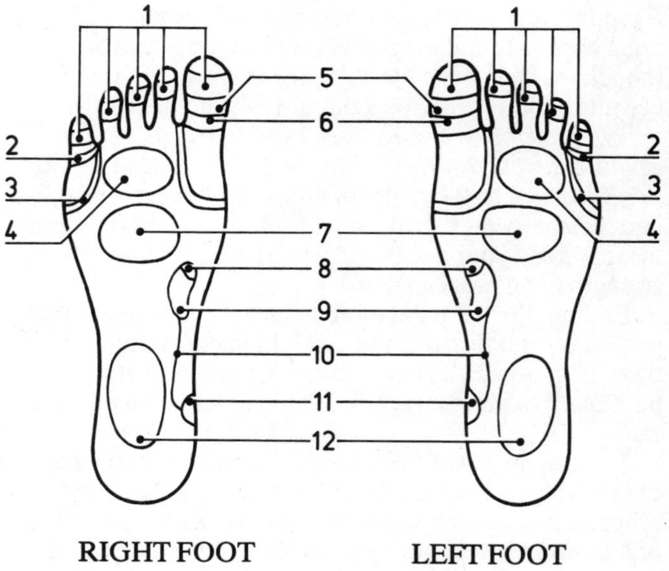

1 Sinuses
2 Armpit
3 Shoulder
4 Lung
5 Pituitary gland
6 Thyroid and neck
7 Solar plexus
8 Adrenal glands
9 Kidneys
10 Ureters
11 Bladder
12 Small intestines

Reflex healing
The body has an intricate network of stimulus-response reflexes, such as the knee-jerk, which are autonomic, i.e. they bypass the brain. We are unaware of most autonomic reflexes, but many of them have been used to stimulate healing since earliest times.

The various systems of reflex healing involve massaging a surface area of the body in ways designed to stimulate a response in an apparently unrelated internal organ. Acupuncture and Shiatzu combine reflex healing with other methods, while foot reflexology and the related disciplines of polarity therapy and zone therapy are exclusively reflex healing.

Reflexology
In theory, each part of the body is connected via nerves to several end-points on the foot. When energy levels drop, through illness, bad circulation, lack of exercise or wearing shoes, then crystalline deposits form at the nerve endings. These deposits can be broken up and the health-giving reflex stimulated by deep compression massage at the nerve endings.

The nerve endings are known as reflex points. Each main reflex route has many endings, covering a small area of the foot. The main reflex areas and the organs they can be used to stimulate are indicated on the diagrams showing foot reflex areas.

INSIDE RIGHT FOOT
The same points are on the inside of the left foot

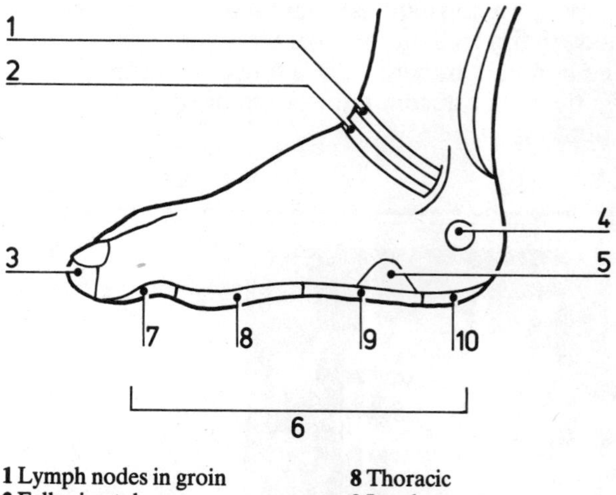

1 Lymph nodes in groin
2 Fallopian tube
3 Top of head
4 Uterus, prostate
5 Bladder
6 Spine
7 Cervical
8 Thoracic
9 Lumbar
10 Sacrum, Coccyx

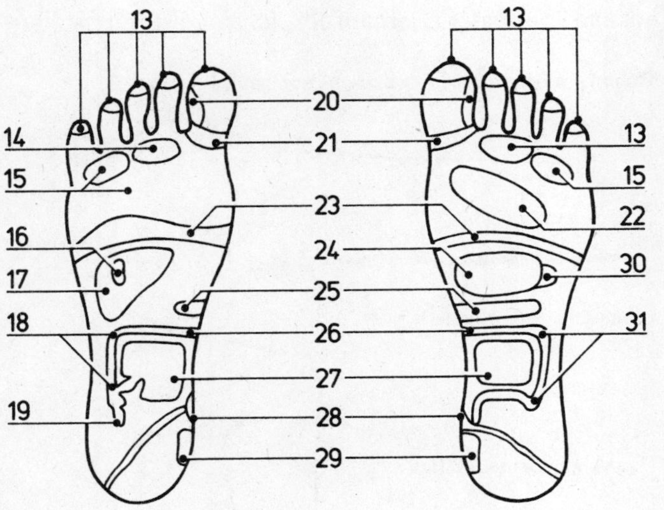

RIGHT FOOT　　　LEFT FOOT

13 Head
14 Eyes
15 Ears
16 Gall bladder
17 Liver
18 Ascending colon
19 Appendix
20 Voice
21 Neck, throat
22 Heart
23 Diaphram
24 Stomach
25 Pancreas
26 Transverse colon
27 Small intestine
28 Sciatic nerve
29 Coccyx
30 Spleen
31 Descending colon

OUTSIDE LEFT FOOT
The same points are on the outside of the right foot

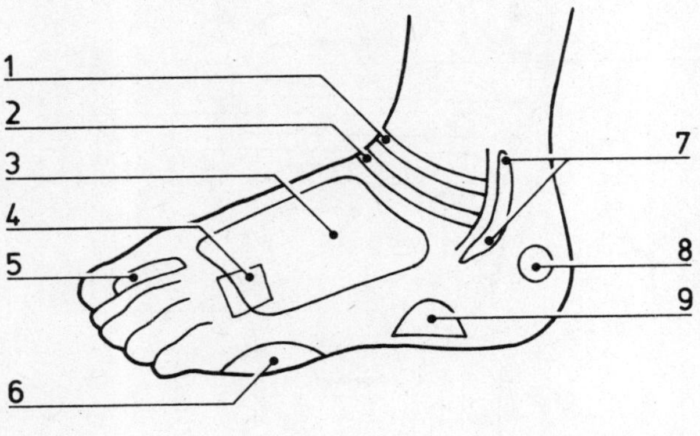

1 Lymph nodes in groin
2 Fallopian tube
3 Lymph glands on front of body
4 Breast
5 Lymphatic system drainage
6 Shoulder
7 Hip, sciatic nerve
8 Ovary, testicle
9 Hip, knee, leg

RELATED THERAPIES

- **Polarity therapy** uses the same reflex points as foot reflexology.

In theory, when any reflex point is stimulated there is a polar reflex response in both sides of the body, bringing the two sides or the back and front of the body into balance.

- **Zone therapy** divides the feet and body into horizontal and vertical zones. Massaging a particular zone on the feet is said to affect all the organs in the same zone in the rest of the body.

The horizontal body zones

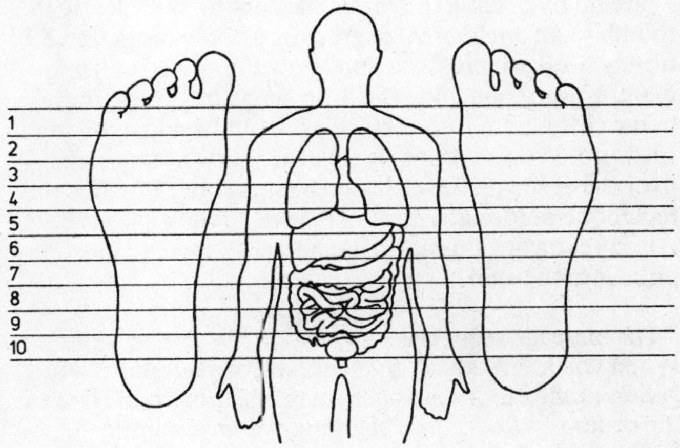

The vertical body zones

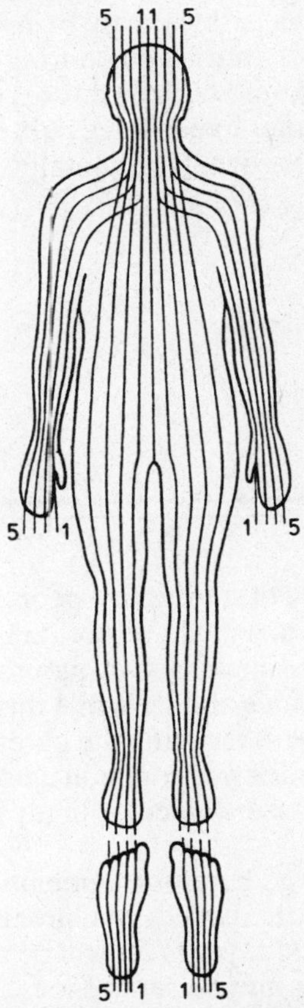

It's all in the sole 2

While the use of foot reflexology for the therapy of severe disorders should be left to trained and qualified practitioners, everyone can perk up their system by giving their feet a regular reflex massage to invigorate the whole body. Couples and friends may like to massage each other's feet.

If you don't want to massage your feet, then a good soak in hot and cold water alternatively can be most refreshing.

How to give a general reflex massage

1 The technique

The method of touching involves finger pressure combined with a gliding massage movement from one pressure-position to the next within the prescribed area. You should not put pressure on any areas that are painful; it would be better to consult a doctor or a qualified reflexologist.

Begin by placing the thumb flat on the skin. Raise the thumb to an angle of 90 degrees and apply pressure very briefly. Release pressure and allow thumb to return to flat position; then glide it a little way along the skin before lifting it to the vertical again and again applying pressure. Proceed to press, release, glide in tiny steps over the area you have chosen to stimulate. Practice this technique before attempting to give a reflex massage. Also, keep your thumb-nails short . . . the nail must not poke into the skin.

2 The massage sequence

When you are ready to give yourself or your partner a general reflex foot massage, cover the areas indicated in the order shown (*right*), beginning at area number 1.

Proceed with sensitivity; the aim is to break up any crystalline deposits beneath the skin surface and to stimulate the energy pathways, using the natural reflex. People whose reflex pathways are being properly stimulated may feel "turned on" during or after the massage, so you should both be aware of this before starting. On the other hand, some pain may be felt as a blockage begins to move. (Incidentally, tickling is NOT reflex massage!)

Thumb positions for the reflex massage technique

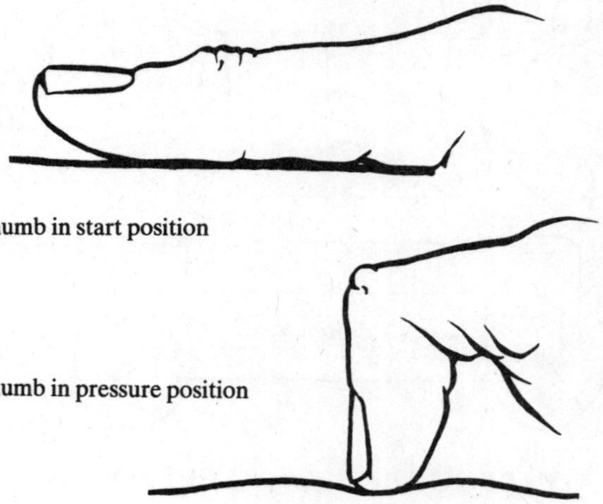

Thumb in start position

Thumb in pressure position

Sequence for general reflex massage

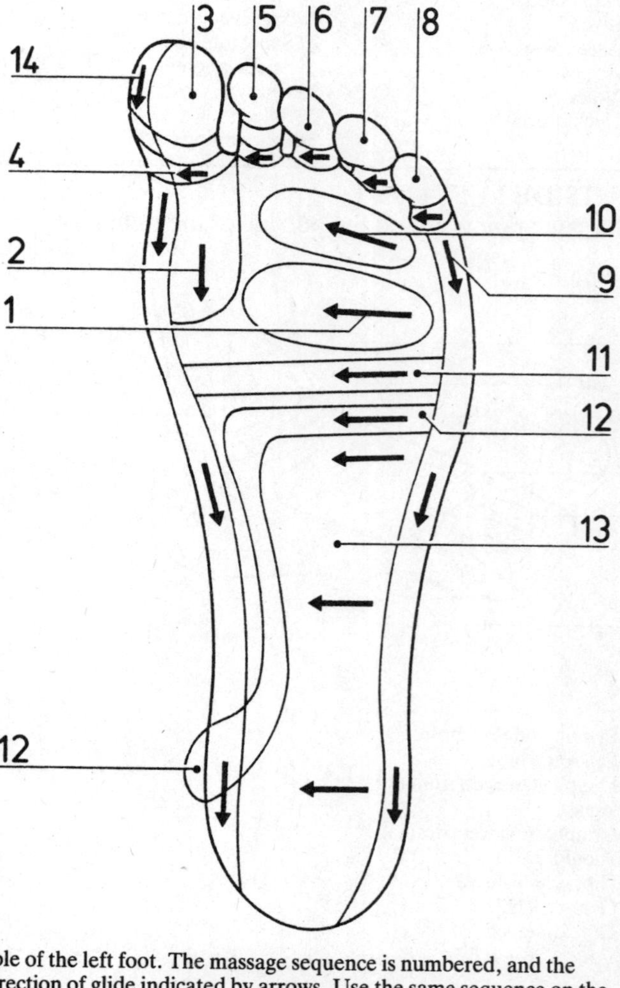

Sole of the left foot. The massage sequence is numbered, and the direction of glide indicated by arrows. Use the same sequence on the right foot

GOING NATIVE

It has been claimed that primitive people remain healthy because they walk around barefoot, thus keeping their feet supple and well-massaged by natural contact with the earth as they move about. While this may be true, there are also hazards awaiting the barefooted. Infection through cuts and bites was common among primitive peoples. Modern hazards include many man-made poisons.

If you decide to go barefoot, remember to acclimatize yourself little by little. Unless you have been without shoes since childhood, your feet will be soft and will also have adjusted their muscle-set to shoes.

SOLAR BREATHING

The solar plexus is a nerve mass just behind the stomach which services most of the involuntary organs and is affected physiologically by deep breathing.

When the general reflex massage (or the alternative soak) has been completed, take your partner's feet onto your knees and apply pressure to the lower part of the solar plexus areas on both feet. As you press, your partner should breathe in deeply through the nose. The breath should be held for a second or two and then released, through the nose, as you release the pressure at the reflex points.

This can be repeated three or four times as you apply the press-and-glide action of compression massage to the whole of the solar plexus areas on both feet. Then your partner might end with a couple of deep, relaxing yawns.

This solar breathing helps to balance all the flow of energy along the nerves which has been released during the general reflex compression massage.

Using both thumbs to press the solar plexus reflex on both feet during solar plexus breathing

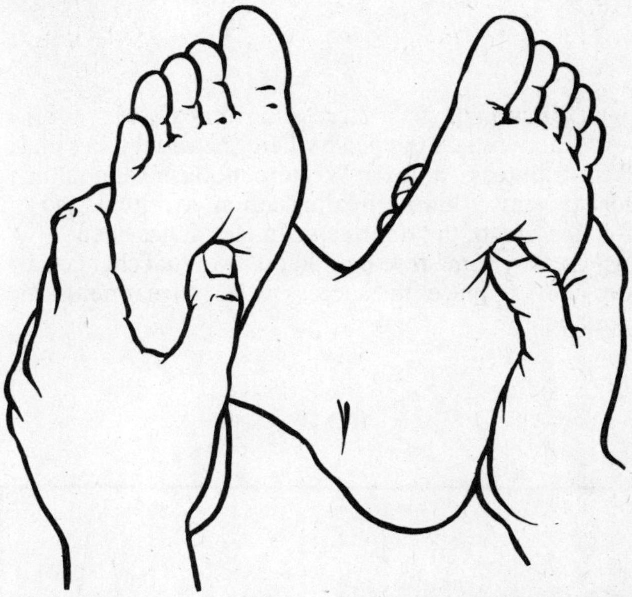

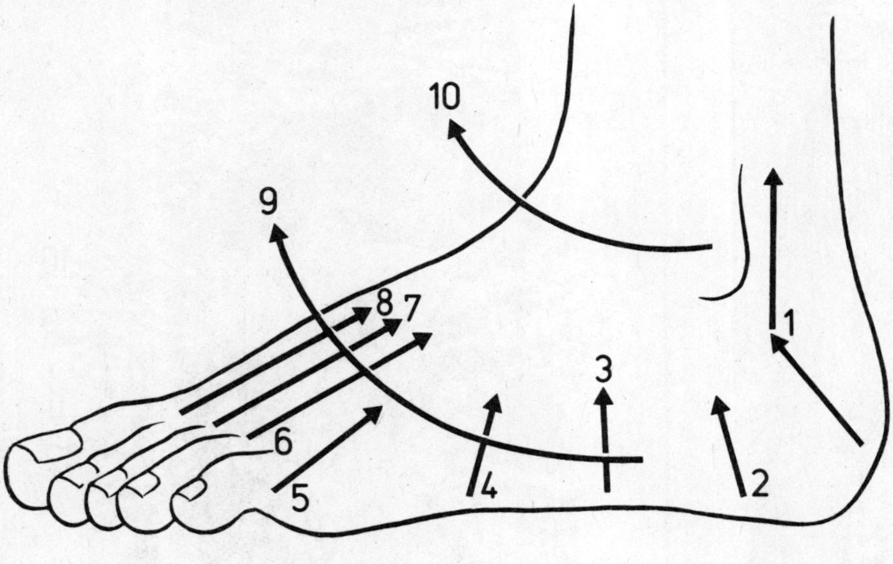

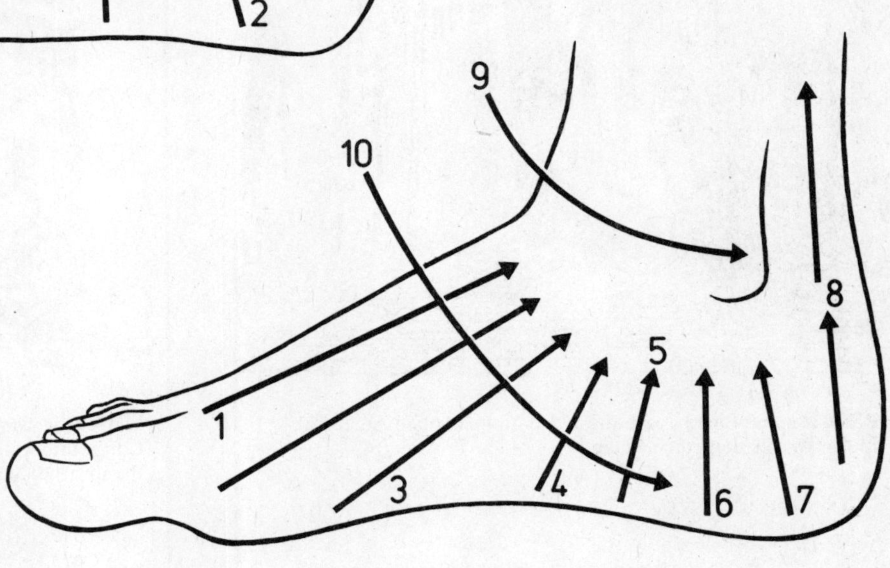

Direction of massage on top and sides of both feet

Section three

RITUAL TRANSFORMATION

Many things make up a successful ritual: clothes, tools, words, actions and the place where the ritual takes place all contribute. In modern Western medicine and in the most ancient, primitive healing ceremony, ritual is an effective part of the treatment. In fact, it has been suggested by some research that if the ritual changes, or does not take place, the success rate of a treatment drops dramatically.

In this section rituals from many times and places are explored and presented for comparison with some of our modern medical rituals. Human beings are creatures of habit, so these rituals seem to play an important role in the treatment process. This is as true for the doctor who draws his knowledge from a scientific background as it is for those whose tradition is that of magic, such as witchdoctors or shamans.

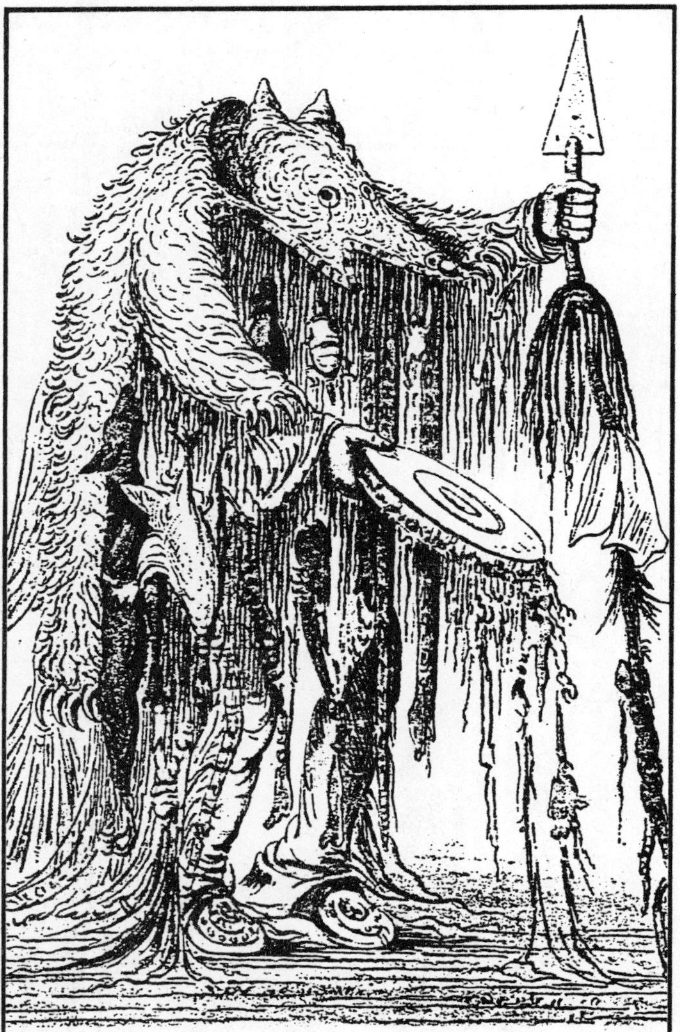

Ritual healing: Bizarre costume and equipment of an American Indian Blackfeet medicine man.

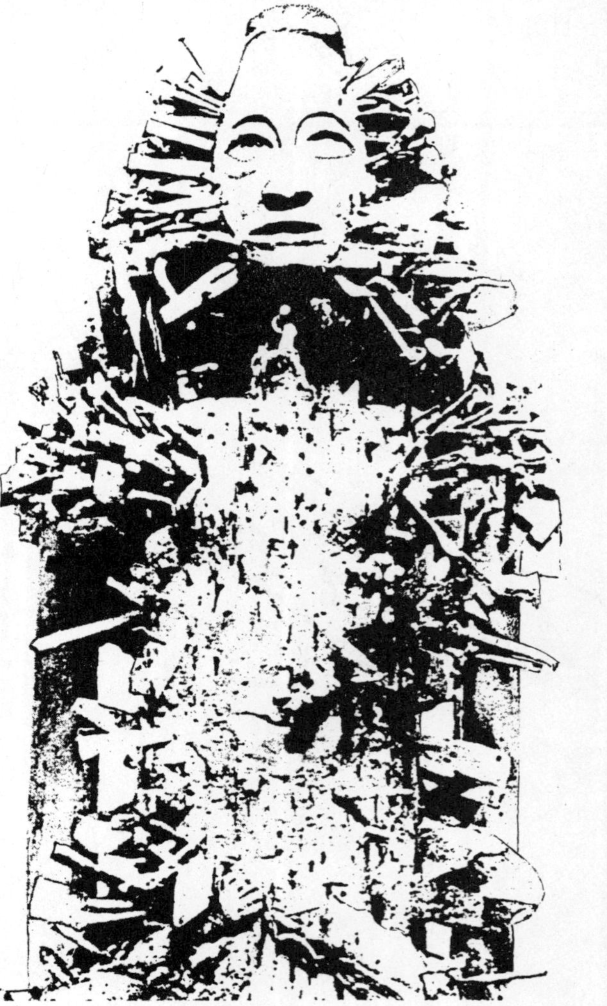

Magic objects: An 1870s Bakongo fetish figure from the African Congo into which knives and nails have been driven as petitions to the spirits to heal sick people.

Many rituals are based on a superstitious belief rather than a scientific fact, and some are performed because they have always been done that way. The use of charms and amulets for healing is part of the traditional rituals of most cultures. Even the preparation of medicines and potions was often carried out by a precise ritual, as in the case of the work of the alchemists.

Enlisting the help of magical beings, such as spirits and fairies, was also a part of the rituals used over thousands of years. By exploring the many aspects of ritual as used for healing purposes, it can be seen that even many modern medical practices have an element of magic about them.

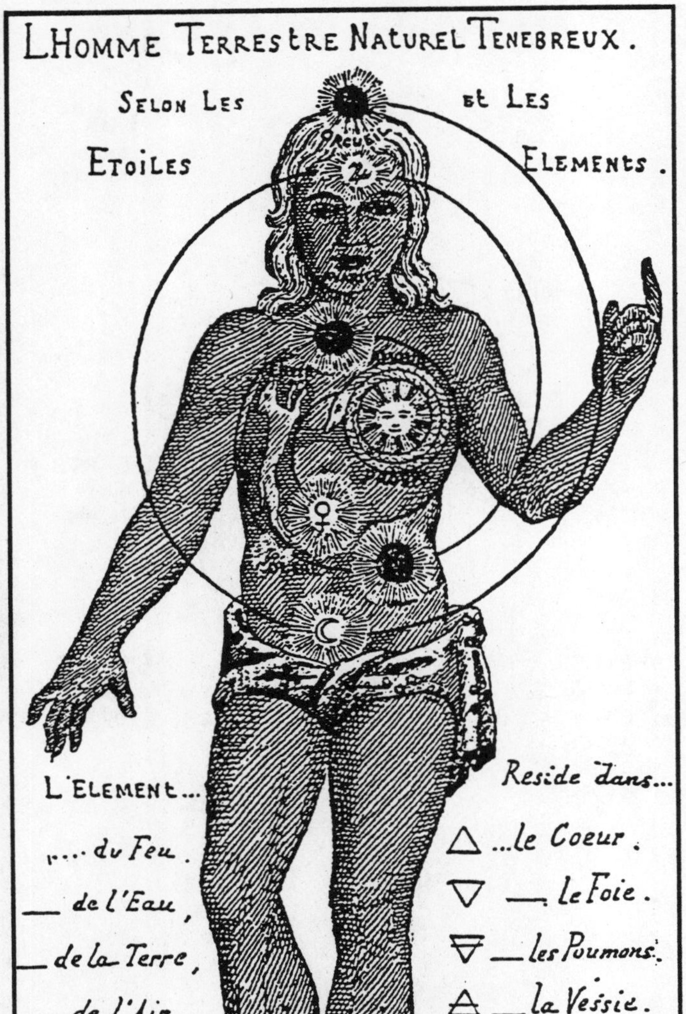

Healing circles: The cosmic spiral related to bodily conditions, 17th century engraving.

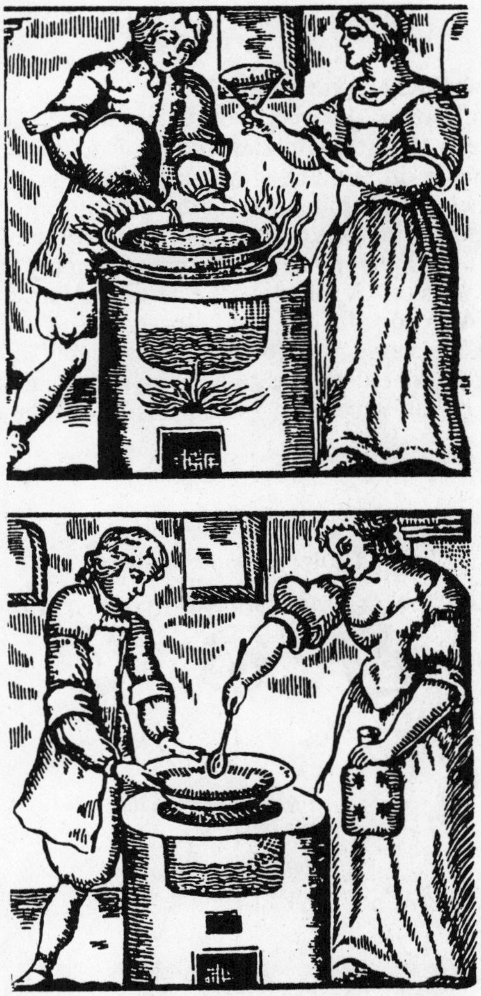

Alchemistical potions: To pour, mix, boil and filter. Alchemists sought cures for common ailments and were predecessors of today's chemists and druggists. Engraving from J J Manget's *Bibliotheca Chemica Curiosa* (1702).

The way of the Vedas

The Vedas are a collection of ancient Hindu scriptures originating between 800 and 600 BC, one of which is the Ayurveda, the science of life. Ayu means life and veda means to attain through knowledge.

Ayurveda is the body of knowledge used in traditional Indian medicine, based on the philosophy that health is a natural state and ill-health only occurs when the balanced flow of intelligence from mind to body is interrupted.

There are many branches of the Ayurveda but one universally attractive characteristic is the gentle, meditative ritual of many of the treatments.

The origins of Ayurveda

According to one of several legends, 50 sages met one day on the slopes of the Himalayas to discuss how diseases could be removed because they were so prevalent and often exacerbated by primitive folk medicine. The sages agreed that the best person to approach was Indra because he had access to the Ayurveda of Brahma, the creator of the universe.

The doctrines of Ayurveda

The philosophical concepts of the physical medicine of Ayurveda are intertwined with religion and ritual and may vary in different geographical areas. The basic doctrines included ideas about the constitution of the universe. Food, for example, was said to be composed of five bhutas or elements. Since food eventually builds the body and makes it function, the correct balance of food is crucial to good health.

The five elements in food are transformed into the seven components of the body, known as the dhatus, which operate according to the principles of the three humors.

The five bhutas of the universe

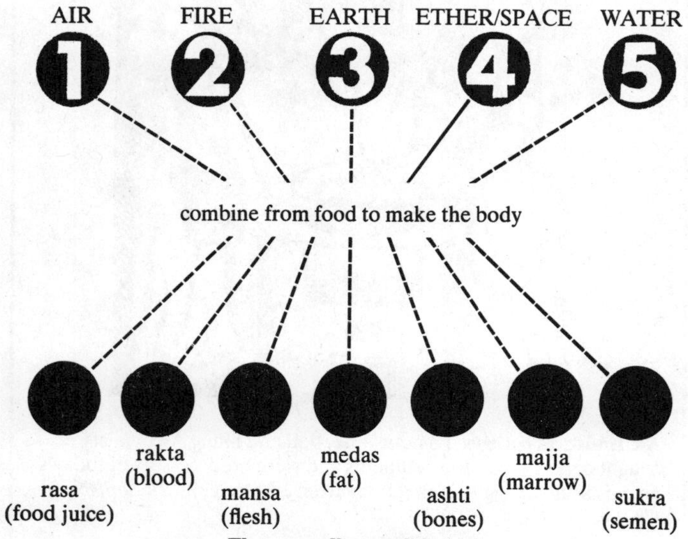

The seven dhatus of the body

THE FIVE BHUTAS OF AYURVEDA

The universe consists of five elements. Each one corresponds to a direction, a planet and one of the five senses. They are similar to the five elements of oriental medicine, except ether/space replaces the wood element of oriental systems. In some traditional Acupuncture systems, metal replaces air.

In some areas, such as among several of the ancient sects who lived on Sri Lanka, Ayurvedic ideas were combined with sorcery to destroy enemies. Using an image of an enemy scratched on the fruit of the ash melon, incantation rituals of 108 mantras were used to upset the balance of the elements, activating the ash melon and thus, by sympathetic magic, throwing the enemy off-balance. It was perfectly obvious to these people that Ayurveda, the life-giving knowledge, could be used in reverse to cause troubles.

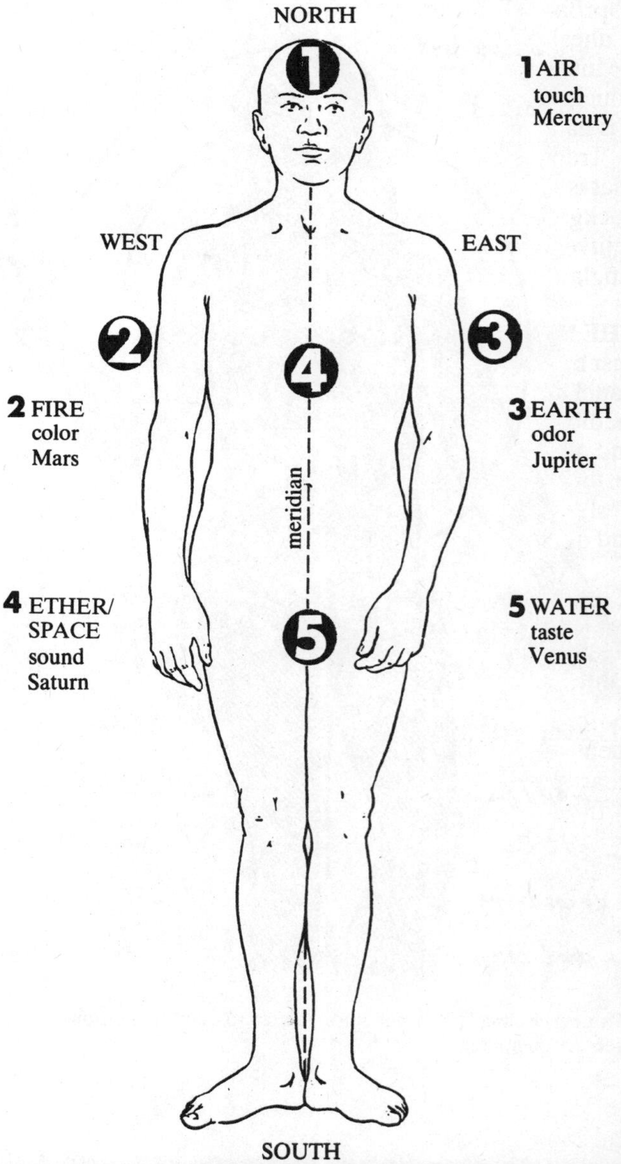

The causes of Ayurvedic troubles
All ill-health was thought to be due to imbalances, the causes of which, in primitive times, were thought to be one of the following:
- an ancestral spirit, for mischief or revenge;
- a demon of the supernatural world;
- the evil eye or evil mouth (of a person);
- the gods, to punish wrong-doings;
- sorcery practiced by your enemy;
- inauspicious planetary influences;
- personal bad karma (debt from a previous life).

Certain other causes were also recognized, such as poison from snakes, insects, plants, etc., or natural disasters such as floods and accidents. However, even natural events were believed to be caused by one of the seven agents listed above.

The Maharishi Ayurveda
Over the centuries, Ayurveda has been changed and modernized, yet the essential philosophy and basic approach to treatment survives. When the Maharishi Mahesh Yogi came to Europe and America in the 1960s, he introduced a modernized version of the ancient art which is now available throughout the western world and has had a profound influence on many people.

Transcendental Meditation is one of the processes that is now used by thousands of people from all kinds of backgrounds. Maharishi Ayurveda healing and rejuvenation programs are available at clinics in England, Ireland and the US.

THE PANCHAKARMA THERAPY
Just one of the many Maharishi Ayurvedic programs, the Panchakarma is widely used for both prevention and medical cure. It consists of a series of relaxing cleansing and purifying procedures which are both eliminative and restorative. A thorough medical check-up includes western diagnostic methods and Ayurvedic pulse-taking and questioning.

A typical Panchakarma program
First there is a week's cleansing, at home, known as the Virechana treatment. This involves taking increasing amounts of ghee (clarified butter) for four days, to loosen impurities lodged in the digestive tract. A day is spent resting before taking a dose of castor oil which clears out the dislodged impurities.

In five days spent at the clinic, gentle and very delicate treatments are given by people of the same sex (to avoid natural distractions) who follow the program worked out by the consulting doctor according to personal need. Even people who are medically fit by western standards will find they are invigorated by the whole process. The individual treatments will probably include the following:

Abhyanga
This is a complete body massage done with great care and compassion by two trained people who work in silence. The massage is done using warm herbal oils prepared to match the patient's constitution and rubbed in deeply to loosen impurities from the cell structure.

Netra Tarpana
A very delicate treatment of the eyes using cool liquid ghee. The relaxed yet concentrated attention given to the patient is total during all the treatments and is a feature of Ayurvedic methods. Much of the healing takes place due to personal attention and active (rather than passive) relaxation.

Swedana
A very gentle herbalized steam bath to stimulate the circulation and clean the pores. The temperature and humidity are controlled to suit personal needs.

Shirodhara
This is a two-hour treatment to calm, settle and balance the activity of the nervous system and bring about a wonderful feeling of happiness. A warm, soothing flow of fine aromatic oil is poured onto the forehead.

Pizzichilli
Known as the royal treatment, because in the past it was only available to kings and queens, this is a lengthy massage on a specially constructed table, during which warm, herbalized oils are applied to all parts of the body.

Basti
This is a painless enema treatment to clean out all impurities dislodged by the other treatments.

A note about semen
Among the ancients of several cultures, semen was the vital life-fluid of both men and women; vaginal secretions were thought to be the same as semen from the penis. It was understood that when the semen of a man mixed with the 'semen' of a woman, new life was created. However, due to this misconception, it was also thought that if the 'semen' of a woman was, somehow, to get into another woman, then two women could also create new life.

Cultural beliefs
The three humors and five elements appear in many cultures around the world and their correspondences vary, usually because of geographical and cultural differences.

To each culture, their body of medical knowledge was sacred and infallible. Their historical manuscripts were accepted because they came from great authorities, none less than the gods themselves. Even today, many people believe the printed word of authority.

REFERENCE: For details of the five elements of other cultures, refer to **Section One: Five life-forces** (pp.10–11); **Section Two: The meridians** (pp.36–37). For more about the three humors, refer to **Section One: The human body** (pp.16–17).

Ritual is magic

Traditional rituals make people feel well satisfied and secure. Consider any ritual in which you participate. It may be religious, such as the Christian Christmas or the Jewish Hanukkah; it may be social, such as a formal dinner or a birthday party; or it may be a ritual in connection with work, such as a board meeting or an apprenticeship. If any aspect of these routines is disturbed, they lose much of their value.

Superstitions, political processes, celebrations and social institutions all depend on rituals to reinforce their meanings. Rituals are so powerful we have learnt how to use them for many purposes, such as advertising, upholding the law and maintaining national identity. Medicine, education, theater, sport and many other human activities each has its own ritual designed to have a specific effect.

In 1967 the Canadian social commentator Marshall McLuhan suggested in his book *The Medium is the Message* that a society is shaped more by the media through which people communicate than by the content of the communications. A ritual with a message implicit in its activity is truly magical. Even a uniform gives a message.

Primitive medicine-men, shamans and witchdoctors use the suggestive power of rituals. In modern medicine, it is the content of the process on which emphasis is placed, yet the ritual itself remains and has been shown to be vital. Without the ritual, the meaning is at risk.

A primitive healing ritual

Ritual magic has some clear features, as shown by Yoruba healers in western Nigeria, who still practiced in remote areas up to the early 1960s.

When a person fell ill, he or she would first try home remedies. If these did not bring about a cure, the patient called in the Yoruba priest, known as the babalawos, who would use his contact with the spirit world (and intuitive psychology) to find the cause of the illness and

COMPARING MEDICAL RITUALS

Yoruba healing ritual	Modern medical treatment
The healer (babalawos) is a special person whom it is expected can influence the spirit world.	The doctor is an expert expected to cure ills.
He uses mysterious language and paraphernalia.	He uses mysterious language (Latin) and paraphernalia (stethoscope, white coat, etc).
He gives an impressive performance revealing the patient's condition and pronouncing the treatment.	He gives an impressive performance diagnosing the disease and prescribing the treatment.
He displays confidence and optimism while increasing the patient's initial anxiety.	He displays confidence and optimism while increasing the patient's initial anxiety ("if you don't do as I tell you, you only have yourself to blame").
Once the treatment is in progress, the patient receives much physical care and attention. The patient participates in throwing off his or her misfortune during abreaction and sacrifice.	The patient receives some physical care but little by actual contact, unless the disease is debilitating. The patient also tends to be passive in the healing process and more active during rehabilitation.
The patient's ego is strengthened by becoming a member of a special group of people who have also been initiated into a cult. Positive images are used during group incantations, such as "the river always flows forward not back, so your illness will never return."	The patient's ego is sometimes strengthened by becoming a member of a support group.
The reputation of the babalawos increases with every cure, especially dramatic ones. If he has several failures, he will lose his status.	The reputation of the doctor increases with every success, especially if it is dramatic like a heart replacement. If he has several failures, he may lose his license or his reputation.

suggest medicines and other remedies. These might inlcude moving house to avoid demons and making sacrifices to appease offended ancestors, spirits or the patient's double.

The Yoruba believe that everyone is born with a physical body and a double, the spirit body, who remains in heaven. A person makes a contract with his double about how he will live his life. To become ill is to break the contract and is a very serious matter requiring great sacrifices.

The babalawos may also recommend his patient be initiated into one of many cults, depending upon the nature of the disease. For example, the Sopono are spirits responsible for smallpox, delirium, abcesses, rashes and many of the psychoses. If a patient has one of these diseases, the babalawos will carry out the initiation into the Sopono cult, which is designed to protect the patient from the Sopono spirits.

Sopono intiation

The Sopono shrine is prepared. In the evening, a sick young woman having boils, delirium and bad dreams is wrapped in a sheet and enters backwards. Family and friends are present throughout the initiation and sing songs and beat drums to call the spirits. The woman is warned of the dangers of being possessed. All female illnesses are thought to be caused by spirits possessing the woman's body while male diseases are caused by spirits masquerading as the man. The anxiety level rises and all those present work themselves into a frenzy, thrashing and shouting.

When the abreaction is over, the babalawos ties a bundle to the woman's head, and she goes out to be washed while the bundle (of bad luck) is buried. Re-entering the shrine, her hair is shaved and she is painted red all over with camwood. She then sleeps.

She remains in the shrine for three weeks and is not allowed to speak for the first week. Every morning she is washed by other initiates, repainted with camwood, and the babalawos sings special incantations to dismiss the spirits and call upon her ancestors and guardian "double" to protect her.

He also orders sacrifices, which are made on the third, seventh, fourteenth and twenty-first days. Usually an animal or bird is used to carry away the sickness after contact with the patient.

At the end of the third week, the patient is dressed in new clothes and black beads and taken to the market by the village elders. People throw her money to mark her acceptance as a healed person.

REFERENCE: for further information about suggestion in healing, refer to **Section Five: Suggestive healing** (pp. 112–113).

Navaho Indian initiation: a young girl is kneaded into the shape of a woman

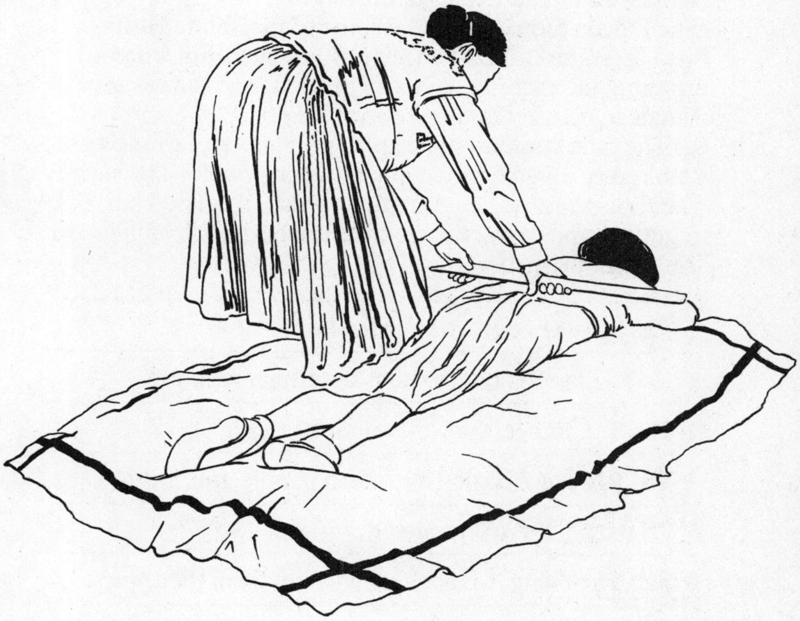

THE WHITE COAT EXPERIMENTS

Research carried out in a hospital during the 1970s showed that volunteers being treated for minor conditions responded well when they were treated by a person who looked and behaved like a doctor, regardless of whether they received real medication or placebos.

On the other hand, people receiving real treatment, but from doctors who did not look the part nor behave like doctors, failed to respond and often felt worse.

It would appear that the medical ritual is a vitally important part of the treatment. The hospital doctor's white coat and stethoscope would seem to be sending a message which says: "when you see us, you will get better."

Suggestion is a strong element in all rituals. An indication of how prone we are to suggestive ritual is that in the final analysis many people place all responsibility for curing illness upon the practitioner.

Magical rituals

The healing rituals of the North American Indian tribes are based on a belief in the power of the Great Spirit and the many spirits which reside in people, animals, plants and all objects. The ceremonies often last several days and rejuvenate everyone who takes part, although the rituals are directed toward one sick and often elderly person.

The seven sacred rituals of the Sioux
The Oglala Sioux tell of the spirit of the White Buffalo who appeared to their ancestors as a beautiful woman, bringing the sacred pipe and knowledge of the seven rituals to be used in times of need.

The pipe contained the spirit of peace and was to be smoked as a sign of goodwill between people. The seven rituals were sacred ceremonies, which, if carried out regularly and correctly, would ensure a healthy and good life for all the tribe.

1 **The Sweat Lodge**, for purification

2 **Calling the Vision**, for boys entering manhood

3 **The Sun Dance**, for renewal of strength

4 **The Rites of Relationship**, with people and spirits

5 **Preparing for Womanhood**, for girls

6 **Ball Throwing**, for seeking wisdom from the spirits

7 **Soul Keeping**, for purifying the souls of the dead

Navaho medicine
In the American southwest, the Navaho is the biggest tribe and has the most colorful and complex rituals. Healing rituals are the most important of the Rites of Relationship, brought about by invoking healing spirits to cast out the evil spirits causing sickness. This meant developing a close relationship with healing spirits through the rituals.

Some Navaho medicine men are first-grade doctors, called hand-tremblers, while others have risen to consultant level. In cases of serious illness, a family may have to call in both kinds of medicine-men, and pay them both.

The hand-trembler is first invited in to diagnose the sickness. He brings with him a medicine bundle of skins, colored stones, seeds, feathers and painted sticks. Holding these objects one by one and chanting in a continuous drone, he contacts the spirit world, searching for possible causes of the disease and chanting them aloud as they occur to him.

The disease may be retribution from an offended god or punishment for wicked sexual activities. It may be the patient sat where a bear had trampled ants, stood where a coyote had urinated or chopped down a tree containing bats (forbidden because bats are the messengers of the spirits). When the doctor's hand begins to tremble he knows he has hit upon the cause of the illness. Finally, he decides which of the 30 Navaho medicine chants is the best prescription.

The family of the patient then have to call in the Navaho consultant doctor. He will undertake the chanting ceremony to cure the disease. A popular ritual is the Hail Chant.

Smoking the Sioux White Buffalo pipe (*below*)

Navaho hand-trembler diagnosing sicknesses (*right*)

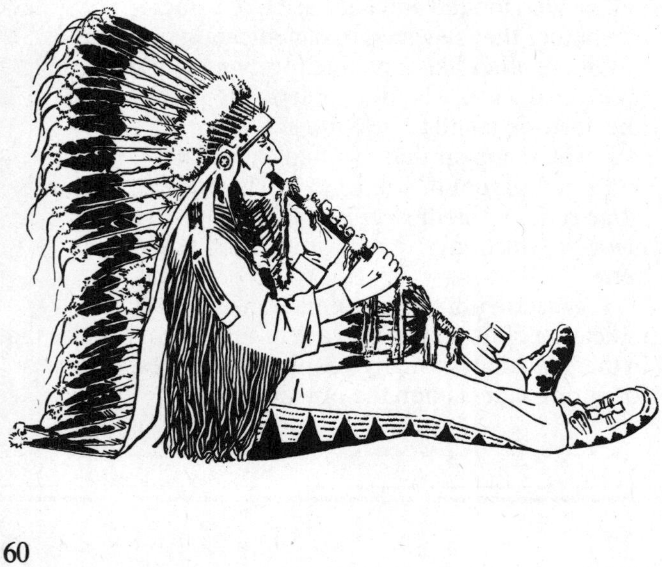

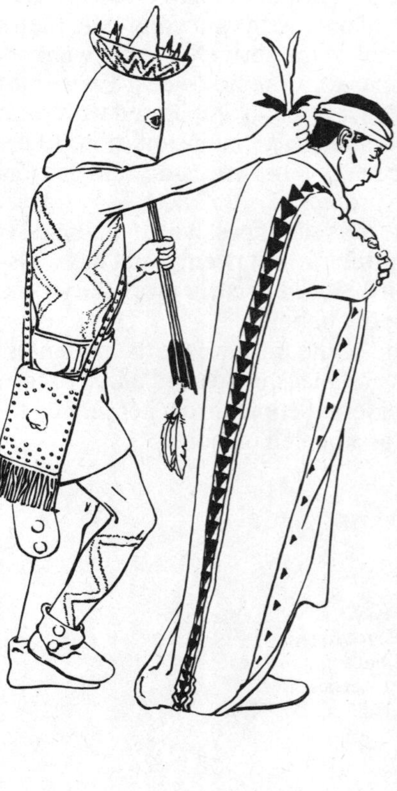

The Navaho Hail Chant ritual

The preparations may take as long as two weeks. A tepee is cleared, and sprigs of oak and corn pollen are placed around the walls. Sacred water is sprayed over the walls and ground, and a herbal fumigation is the final cleansing process. Little cakes made of corn and resembling hailstones are made for relatives and friends who will take part in the ceremony, for no one will be allowed to eat anything else. Many other things are forbidden during the ritual, such as urinating while facing north.

The ceremony begins at sundown, as the world enters the time of dreams. For the next two days, all the participants purify themselves in the sweat lodge. Then the patient is made to vomit and clean out his bowels by taking herbs. The soapy yucca cactus is used to wash him, and he is then anointed with fragrant oils and herbs.

The ritual drumming, rattling and whistling then begins, each sound being made with a special object, to help the patient and make his spirit leap. The patient is eventually emotionally moved to make a spontaneous confession of his misdeeds and the taboos he has violated, i.e. he has an abreaction.

During the third day, songs are chanted while the air is filled with smoke from tobacco, burning herbs and feathers. The chanter tells the ancient Navaho story of Black Rainboy and his sister Blue Raingirl, recounting their many adventures at great length as they are destroyed and then restored to wholeness.

On the fifth day, the patient is kept out of the tepee while a picture of the story is made with colored sands. At sunrise, the patient re-enters and sprinkles cornmeal on the picture and recites prayers. As the chanting and drumming reach fever pitch, the medicine-man puts his wet hand on the sand picture and touches the patient, who instantly becomes one of the holy people. He repeats the words of the chanter, and happiness and feelings of pleasure and beauty flow into everyone present.

On the seventh day, the chanting and drumming reach a final climax and everyone withdraws, leaving the restored patient to rest and return to his whole self. Often many other sick people feel restored to health by contact with him.

REFERENCE: For other rituals see **Section Three: The magic circle** (Sweat lodge ritual, p. 68) and **Section Five: The sounding board** (Calling the vision, pp. 116–117).

Sand picture of the Hail Chant ritual of the Thunder people, who are holding hailstones and lightning.

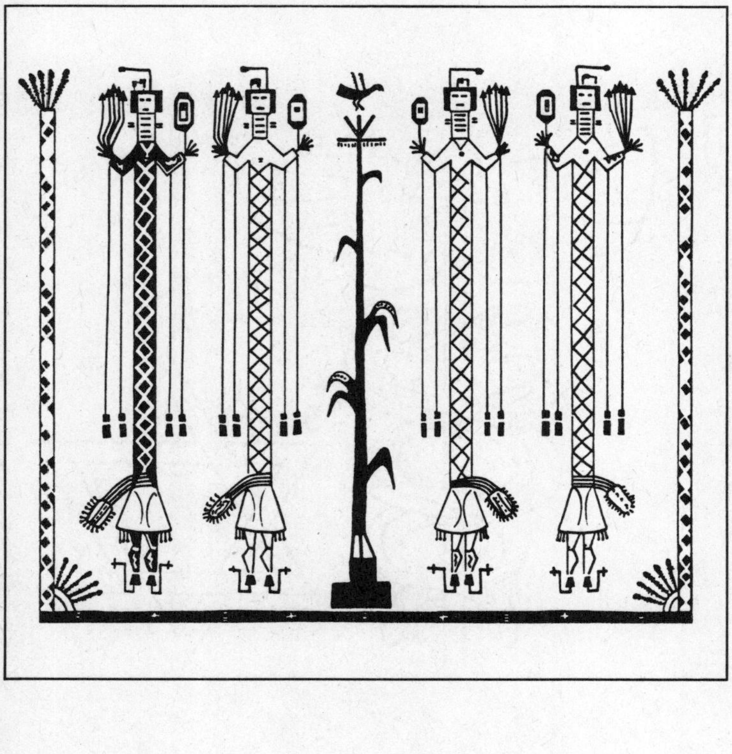

Sand painting of Rainboy and Raingirl; he walks on lightning and she walks on rainbows around a lake at the four corners of which are the sacred plants of corn, beans, squash and tobacco.

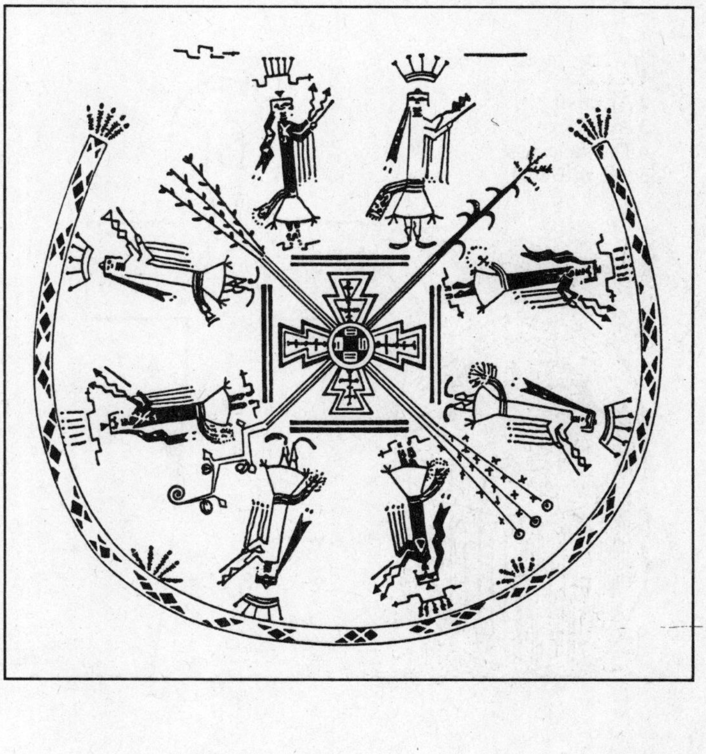

Magic charms

Magical protection from the spirits of disease was big business among communities in the past. Folk medicine would be used only if an illness became a physical reality, but prevention was better than any cure. Charms, amulets and talismans abounded and were not so different from the mascots and charms we use today; they also were intended to stir the spirits of good fortune and bring the wearer luck in the casino of life.

Many charms had a religious origin. The Ancient Egyptians had a pantheon of gods that controlled every detail of daily life. The talismans and amulets associated with their gods were therefore thought to have great powers.

What is a charm?

A charm is anything that will protect against evil. Some modern charms are a sprig of heather, a four-leaved clover, a rabbit's foot or a pendant of St Christopher, the patron saint of travelers.

Charm bracelets are popular with some people, and many objects of personal significance found or received as gifts in special circumstances become charms against personal disaster.

An amulet is an object made of wood, stone, metal or other substance which protects against evil and may be inscribed with magical characters or figures. It is expected to invoke the help of great spirits associated with a culture or religion.

A talisman is an amulet that has been engraved with characters that attract occult influences. Hence the zodiac signs made into rings or brooches could be regarded as talismans.

A mascot is a person or animal, or a thing in the form of an animal or person, that will bring good luck. Regiments have adopted animals such as dogs, cats and goats as their mascots, while individuals who do dangerous work, such as racing drivers, have been known to carry old, fluffy toys as mascots.

Some Ancient Egyptian amulets for health

Amulets were known in Ancient Egypt by the name *udjau*, meaning "that which keeps you safe." Most Egyptian amulets were not only worn by living individuals but were placed in tombs to ensure the souls of the dead would have protection, good health and long life when the time came for resurrection.

One of the oldest and most significant of the Ancient Egyptian amulets is the scarab, which was dedicated to Ra, the Sun God, the giver of life and protector of the heart. The scarab is a representation of the dung beetle, which lays its eggs in animal dung, rolls it up into a ball and pushes it to a place where the eggs will hatch in the sun. The scarab symbolizes how the power of the sun can be harnessed by even the most lowly of creatures.

Another ancient amulet is the *ankh*, which represents life itself. It is thought to be a representation of a scroll of papyrus doubled over and tied with a strip of papyrus. On the scroll was written the spell which restored to life the Egyptian god Osiris.

Two other amulets that were carried to guard against ill-health are the "two fingers" amulet, which would be carried by a person in danger of falling, such as a stonemason, and the *ba* amulet, which was a small, red model of the heart and was carried by people with heart problems. In a tomb it would bring to life the mummified heart.

The color red has had magic properties since prehistoric times. The Romans believed coral to have healing powers because of its pink color. In the Middle Ages in Europe, a cure for sickness was to wrap a clipping of hair or nails from the sick person in a red cloth and bury it in the ground.

1 A scarab
2 An *ankh*
3 An ouser
4 The caduceus
5 Star of David

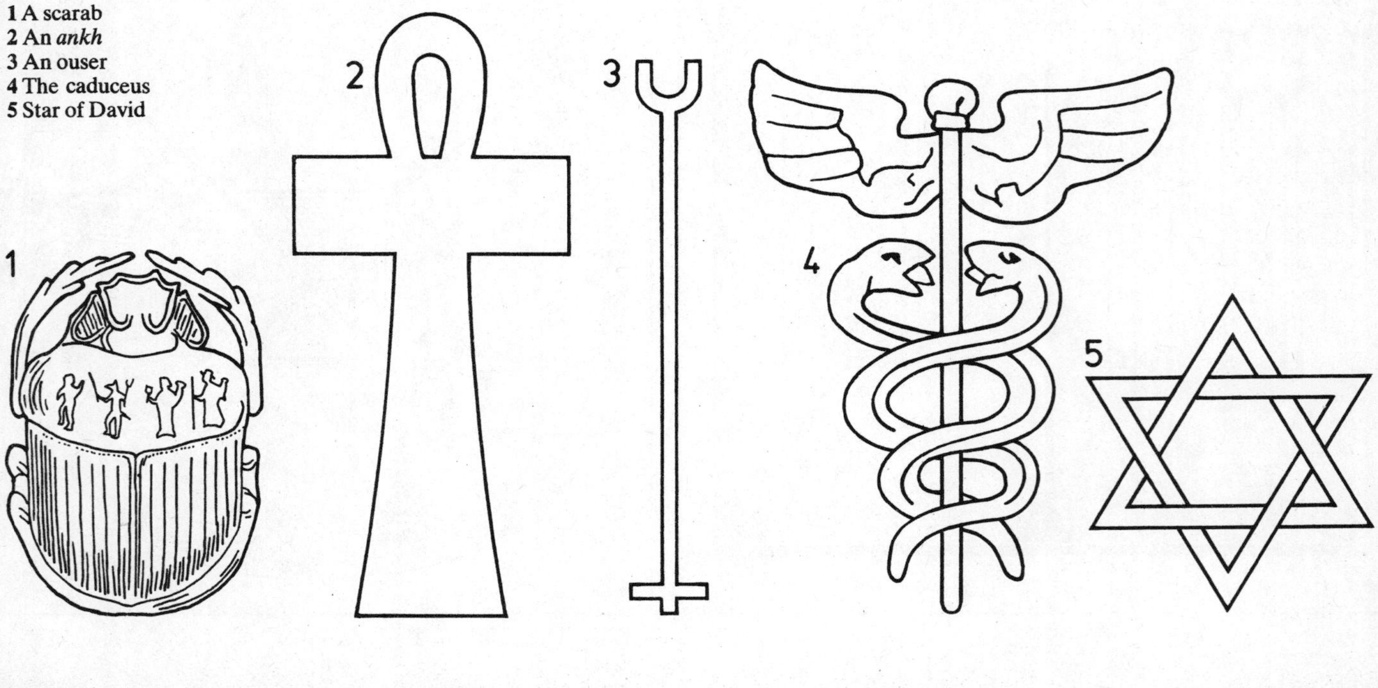

The ouser was a magic wand with enormous powers. In many healing rituals, sick people would hope to be touched by the ouser and its healing spirit.

It was a straight stick about four feet long with two prongs at one end forming a U-shape. At the other end was a T-cross. The magic rod given to Moses to lead the Israelites out of Egypt was probably an ouser. According to the Old Testament stories, he used his rod to turn water into blood, dust into lice and to produce hail, fire and spring water. The ouser may be the origin of the modern magic wand.

Some Jewish amulets
Typical of many protective Hebraic amulets, the mezuzah is a small piece of parchment on which a quotation from the scriptures is written three times. The parchment is rolled and carefully placed inside a small wooden or metal cylinder and fixed to the door of a Jewish home.

In the past, similar amulets were used against specific conditions. In particular, an amulet was always fixed to the door of an expectant mother's room to ensure safe childbirth.

The Star of David, also known as Solomon's Seal, is probably one of the oldest and best known of all Hebrew amulets. A six-pointed star, it is formed by superimposing two equilateral triangles on each other. The symbol has been used in other cultures but is thought to have originated well before the time of King David, who adopted it as the symbol of his royal house. While at Taberah, on his journey with the Israelites, Moses is said to have used an amulet incorporating a six-pointed star to quench a great fire.

King Solomon himself performed miracles using the star. The amulet he used was a ring seal of gold inscribed with the 12 names of God. In the centre was a diamond known as the Shamir gem, on which was engraved the star with the letter Aleph in the middle. The diamond was said to have a soul which made it possible for Solomon to carry out the large range of healing miracles that are recorded in the Old Testament and other ancient books.

The physicians' amulet
The caduceus is a very ancient amulet used for healing sickness, healing quarrels and bringing peace. It appeared in Sumeria at about 2600 BC and was also used in Egypt, India and Ancient Greece. The two entwined serpents are said to represent the balance between good and evil, while in Buddhist terms they are regarded as symbols of the Kundalini, the life-force that lies coiled at the base of the spine.

In later Greek times the caduceus acquired a pair of wings, attributed to the story of how Mercury, the messenger of the gods, calmed the two fighting snakes with his silvery eloquence. The wings are those from the feet of Mercury.

PRIMITIVE HEALING AMULETS

1 Horseshoes were said to ward off nightmares.
2 An amulet made from the hair and dried skin of a deceased person would protect the mourners from pain.
3 Moles' feet would give protection from rheumatism and were carried in a small bag.
4 The Ancient Egyptians wore a glass necklace as an amulet against the evil eye, the cause of all disease.
5 Amulets to prevent toothache and sore or bleeding gums: (**a**) cowrie shells (Russia); (**b**) orris root (Poland); (**c**) a fossil shark's tooth (Holland); (**d**) bag of alum (Russia).
6 Teething amulets served a double purpose as children could also chew on them: (**e**) ivy wood necklace; (**f**) seed necklace; (**g**) shell necklace used in Jersey, Channel Is.

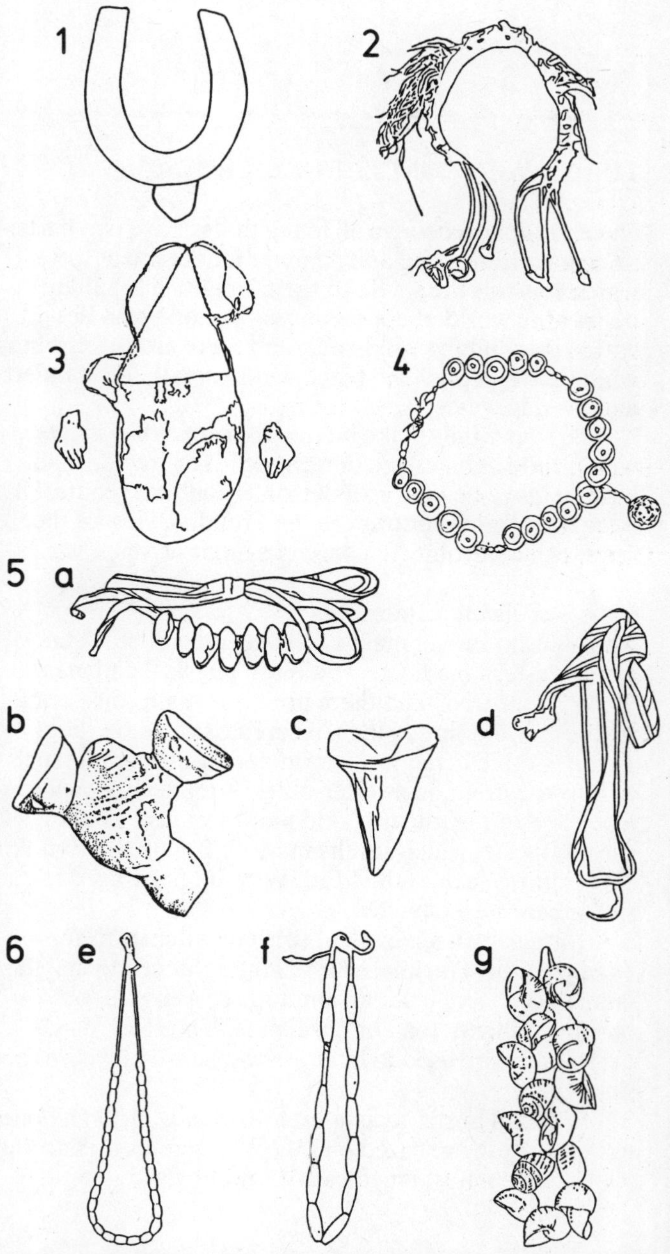

What's in a name?

The modern names for illnesses, such as epilepsy, tuberculosis, carcinoma and depression, serve to identify them and may describe one symptom, but rarely do they explain causes or cures. However, this has not always been the case; among the Navaho American Indians, for example, names for sicknesses are very graphic and unmistakably linked with the Navaho conception of life. Similarly, the name given to the prime medication of the Ndembu of East Africa reveals a different attitude to healing.

A NDEMBU MEDICATION

The Ndembu used to live in circular villages of about 30 people in East Africa, the women normally residing in their husbands' villages. They did not acknowledge any natural cause of disease and believed chronic sickness was due either to punitive ancestors or to envious sorcerers and witches. The ancestors were known as shades who were punishing their offspring for often minor misdemeanors.

Treatment of Ndembu sicknesses involved ceremonies to heal social arguments, quarrels and relationship problems. During the ceremonies, grudges had to be confessed and various herbal remedies taken because they had magical properties. The most commonly used remedy was *musoli*.

THE NAVAHO CONCEPT OF SICKNESS

Navaho Indians believe all living things have two parts: an outer, visible shell and an inner independent form which controls the shell. To them, reality lies hidden behind the world of appearances. The one who lies within is called the wind-soul, and there are seven winds: white, blue, yellow and black winds, small, left-handed and shining winds.

The soul-winds make all the decisions; they arrive with a child at birth and determine his character. The Navaho have no ego, so a person is unable to control his behavior. This is contrary to the Freudian view of the outer ego controling unconscious inner drives.

Causes of Navaho illnesses

The Navaho Indian makes little distinction between what Western medicine would call physical and mental illness. To the Navaho there are three main causes of all sicknesses and three kinds of ceremony to cure them.

1 Undesirable behavior determined by evil winds, such as how the braid on a water-bottle is made or which way a poker is left by the fire, and more serious behavior, such as incest, which results in Moth Craziness. Evil Way ceremonies, such as the Moth Way Sing, are used to cure sicknesses caused by evil.

2 An attack by a malevolent spirit or witchcraft, for example Ghost Sickness, or being frightened by an animal, such as a bear, an antelope or a coyote, or burning a snake, toad or porcupine. The Holy Way ceremonies are used to fight the witchcraft and cure the sickness.

3 Accidental hurts, such as arrow wounds, broken bones or cuts. These are cured by Life Way ceremonies during which some natural medication may be used.

Navaho Moth Craziness

Intermittent fits, during which the patient froths at the mouth, is incontinent and afterwards does not remember what has happened, indicate that the moths have taken over the body and are thrashing about inside.

Moth Craziness is linked with an old Navaho legend which tells of a time when parents refused to give their children in marriage, so the children married each other, breaking the taboo against incest.

When this happened, moths were sucked in by the soul-wind, flew about inside the head, made a nest in the stomach and became more and more violent, making the patient throw himself into the fire.

The cure is to remove the moths by making the patient vomit them out. Ritual vomiting is induced during a Moth Way ceremony when the patient vomits real moth wings.

Navaho Ghost Sickness

Weakness, anxiety, bad dreams, fainting, depression, loss of appetite, night-time terror, delirium and hopelessness are attributed to Ghost Sickness.

This sickness is caused by the malevolent ghosts (bad winds) that inhabit certain plants. If a person picks any of the ghost plants, then the sickness will travel from him to anyone he touches with his hands. When the sickness becomes severe, the patient dislikes everyone and picks fights, although it is not his fault; it is the fault of the bad winds inside him. All evil things are bad winds.

The cure for an attack of Ghost Sickness is the Blessing Way Sing, a purification ceremony during which there is singing and everyone smokes mountain tobacco. The tobacco wind chases away the bad winds from

Ndembu *musoli*
The botanical name for this tree is *Vangueriopsis lanciflora*, and it is not known to have any medicinal benefit. It is chosen by the Ndembu because its name means "to make visible," and what is visible to the Ndembu is good.

Because it has fruit that is eaten by woodland game during the rains, it is said to draw animals into the open so they are visible to the hunter. It is often given to barren women so that their children may be made visible.

Finally, *musoli* helps to make visible and public any hidden grudges that must be revealed during the ceremony. The name of the medication, *musoli*, explains its effect in the context of the Ndembu belief system.

To the Ndembu, death is caused by disgruntled shades or jealous sorcerers, so after a death everyone used to partake in the ceremony and drink *musoli* medication to bring out all hidden social problems lest they cause sickness.

inside. For example, a boy who could not sleep because he pined for his mother who had died some years before, took part in the healing ceremony and smoked the mountain tobacco, which got inside his head and cleared away the bad winds of the Ghost Sickness, and he was happy again.

Navaho healing ceremonies
The patient has the support of the whole community during a healing ceremony; he is not held responsible for his illnesses, except for one, known as Crazy Violence, the sickness let loose by drinking large quantities of alcohol.

The Navaho do not humble themselves, nor do they analyze their own behavior; they believe that a named ceremony, correctly performed, will put the power of the gods at their disposal. The sick person has only to participate in the ceremony to be healed.

The Navaho have a holistic view, and their healing ceremonies work. The cures seem to be due to the power of suggestion and in large part to the concentrated concern of every member of the community. Perhaps our modern self-help support groups are the nearest thing we have to the Navaho communal healing ceremonies.

Navaho Crazy Violence
While alcohol is seen as firewater, drinking it is seen as deliberately self-determined and not the will of the wind-soul. The reason for this is that when drunken Navaho men go on the rampage, they inflict violence on others and often end by committing suicide. Wanton destruction and violence against others of one's community and against oneself is alien to the Navaho belief in the inner reality of the wind-soul, which is a life-positive force. Restraint and isolation are the treatment for Crazy Violence.

The names of the three sicknesses described are more than mere labels. They are related to the belief system of the Navaho people. The names given to herbal medications are often similarly significant.

A Navaho sand-painting used in healing ceremonies

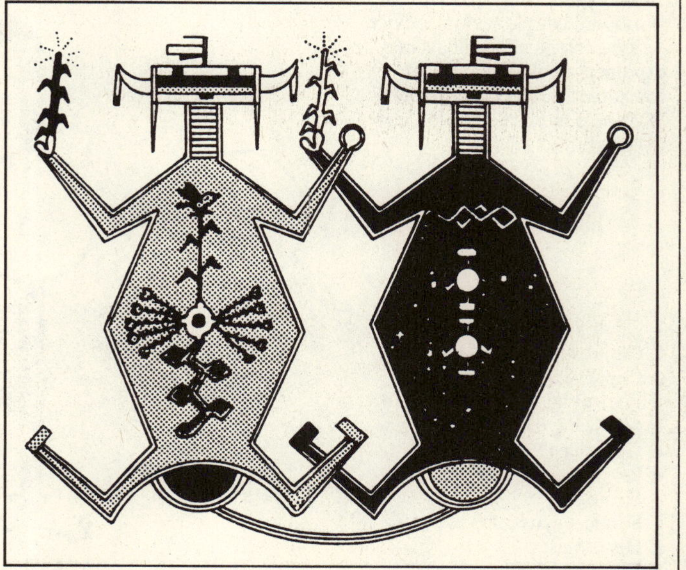

Portents and familiars

When a medical problem arises, a home remedy is tried. If there is no improvement, a doctor may be called on to make a diagnosis and suggest treatment. Should this fail to satisfy, a second opinion may be sought from a specialist. There is nothing modern about this search for a cure. Throughout history, most communities have had a similar hierarchy of consultants, for example, the Balahis of central India.

Balahi medicine

An untouchable caste of servants and weavers, the Balahis live in remote rural villages and have a very strong social identity. They follow a cult of the Hindu religion with their own shrines to gods and other superhuman deities.

When Balahi people fall ill, they first look for a natural remedy among traditional household medicines, which are often effective since they are based on generations of trial and error. Sometimes a village quack doctor will suggest other lotions and potions.

Should the illness persist, then the Balahi have the choice of two kinds of medicine man known as the janka and the barwa. The janka, like a doctor, diagnoses and prescribes. The barwa, like the specialist, uses his own specific skills. Their methods, however, are very different.

A janka reads the portents

The janka is a person of the same caste who diagnoses and prescribes by divining the portents. He or she takes the patient's pulse with the left hand while pulling the patient's fingers in turn with the right hand. With each pull the janka says the name of a spirit or god to discover which caused the disease.

As the finger joints crack, they are counted as portents, and other methods may also be used to discover which spirit is to be appeased. Grass stalks, the flickering of oil lamps, the patterns made by thrown grains as they are fanned and other methods, such as dowsing, may be used to read the portents that reveal both the diagnosis and the treatment to be applied.

Janka treatment

The janka takes the patient and the family to the shrine of the deity who has caused the suffering. The god has to be appeased by gifts made during a ritual.

The janka begins by reciting some mantra (incantations) designed to awaken the deity and impress on him or her the urgency of the case. The mantra begins with the deity's name and may continue: ". . . with folded hands I pray: save and cure this patient. But if you don't cure the patient, I shall dishonor your mother."

To emphasize the message, the janka takes some red string and makes six or seven knots, repeating the mantra with each knot and ending with some hefty curses.

During this ritual, it is the janka's job to discover any way in which the patient has sinned against the deity. This is usually easy to assess, since everyone knows almost everyone else's business in a small Balahi village. If there is nothing specific, there are so many religious laws that can inadvertently be broken that it is simple for the expert janka to use the patient's guilt to reveal a trangression that accounts for the deity's anger.

When the wrong-doing has been discovered and acknowledged, the knotted string is tied round the patient's wrist or neck while the deity is worshipped and given offerings of eggs, chickens, a goat or coconuts.

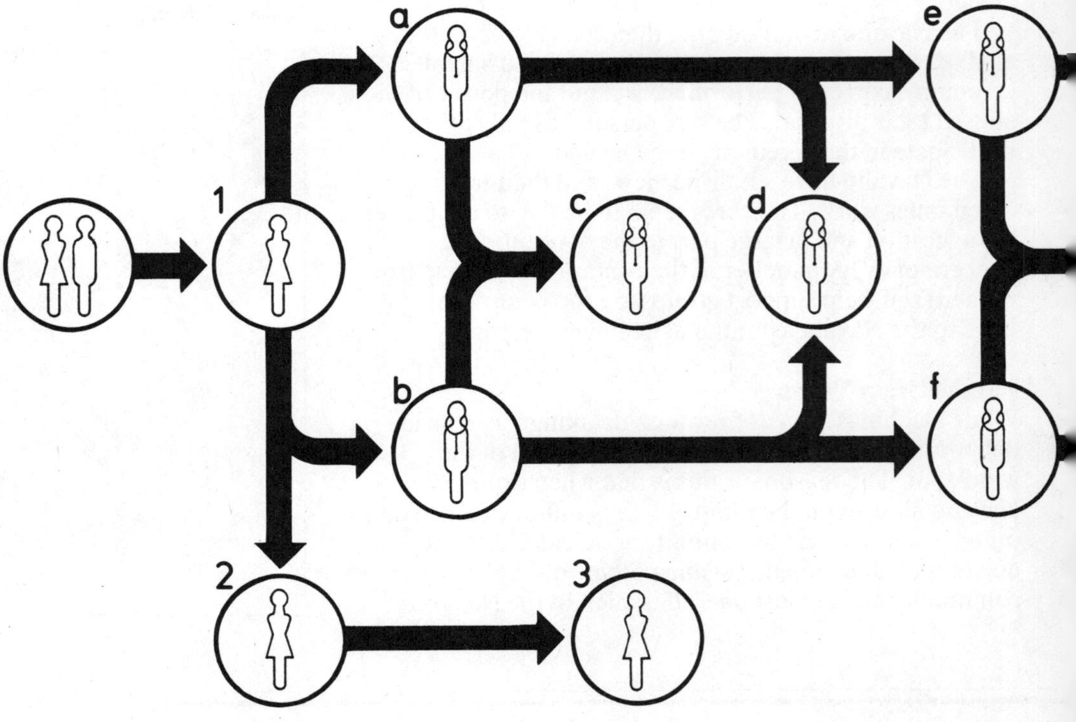

A modern couple seeking advice on gynecological problems may explore a whole hierarchy of consultants via a clinic secretary (1) from a medical gynecologist (d) to a biochemist (j).

1 Clinic secretary
2 Clinic nurse
3 Clinic social worker
a Andrologist
b Medical gynecologist
c Geneticist
d Psychiatrist
e Urologist
f Surgical gynecologist
g Histologist
h Radiologist
i Endocrinologist
j Biochemist

Then everyone enjoys a feast, except the patient, young women and children. The janka demands a fee which is placed on the same dish as the offerings and leaves. If the patient gets worse, or dies, the janka is rarely blamed, as disease is in the hands of powerful deities. The transgression may have been committed by another member of the patient's family or by the patient in his previous life. Whatever happens is fated by a person's karma.

Experienced jankas wisely interpret the rituals as portents of death if the patient is quite evidently suffering from a terminal illness. If the patient lives but fails to improve, the ritual is repeated several times, or he or she may opt to take the case to a barwa.

A barwa enlists the help of his familiar

Barwas are born into the role of mystical medicine man, unlike the Siberian shamans, although the two groups have many similarities.

The barwa is a person who genuinely believes he has magical healing powers that are available through contacting his familiar, i.e. the personality of his chosen deity. He learns how to do this by dissociating himself from his normal personality and entering into his familiar while in a trance.

Trances are deliberately induced. The barwa takes a warm bath, wraps himself in a loin cloth and squats on a sheet in front of an image of his deity. Liquors are often drunk, and hemp or camphor is burnt and inhaled. To the accompaniment of a monotonous drum beat, the barwa chants endless mantras and stares at his favorite deity. Suddenly he begins to tremble, roll his head and glassy eyes at great speed and shout unnaturally. The barwa is now possessed by his familiar, and the deity speaks and acts through him. The process may continue in one of two ways.

1 The familiar gives the diagnosis

While the barwa is in a trance, his assistants ask him questions about the patient's condition. Among his incoherent replies they catch odd words and phrases that tell them which of the *deos* and *matas* (male and female gods) are causing the disease and how they can be appeased.

2 The familiar fights the evil spirit

When a patient is thought to be possessed by an evil spirit, known as a *churel*, the barwa's familiar carries out an exorcism.

A small fire of smoking camphor is lit, and the patient is placed next to it and may be deliberately burnt and whipped (to make it unpleasant for the *churel* to remain in his body). Both the fire and the patient are then covered with a sheet while the barwa recites mantras to induce the *churel* to leave. A violent argument ensues, the patient is uncovered, and has a shoe pushed in his mouth (this is an insult to the possessing *churel*). Finally, the patient is nailed to a tree by the hair which is then cut, symbolizing the final release from the *churel*. After this violent treatment the patient has good reason to get well.

The barwa, too, has an interest in a cure, since his failure as an exorcist will lead to an uncomfortable ritual death. The fee for an exorcism is consequently very high and paid in advance.

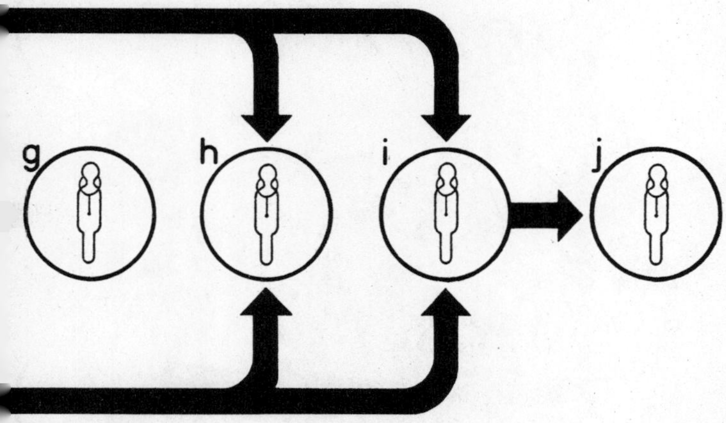

Hindu gods are often depicted symbolizing a struggle between good and evil. Kali, Goddess of Destruction, overpowers her husband Shiva, God of Time among many attributes, in this 18th century Punjabi artist's conception.

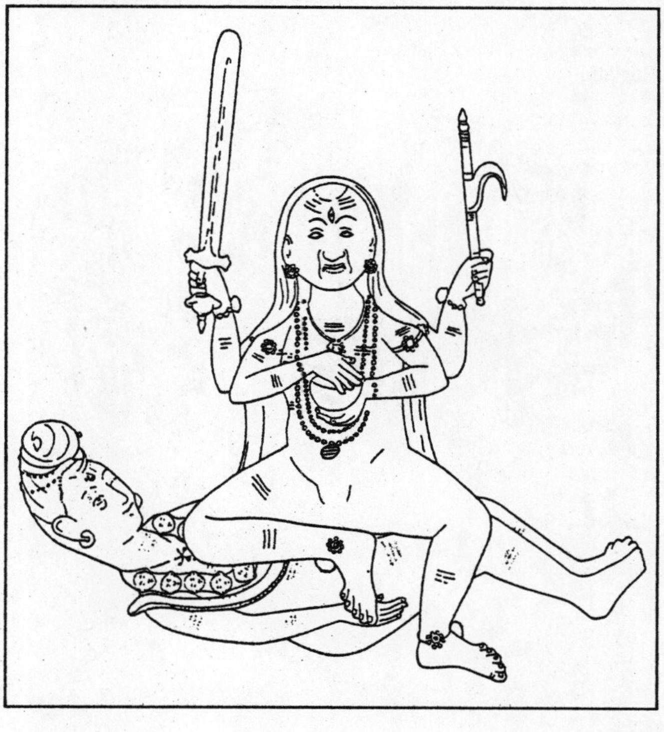

The magic circle

A very old, international folk tale tells how the little people, such as fairies, elves, goblins and other magical beings, will grant a wish. A clearing in the woods must be found, where the grass holds the early morning dew. If you are lucky and find a circle of brighter green in the grass, stand in the middle of the circle, close your eyes and make your wish, for you have found the magic circle of the fairies.

It is rumored in many folk tales that fairies interpret wishes very literally and will play tricks on those who are insincere, impractical or vague, so if you find a fairy circle while out walking in the country, take care how you make your wish.

CIRCULAR MAGIC

The circle, and its variant the spiral, were used in rituals, buildings and symbolism because it they were thought to have powerful magical qualities.

People holding hands in a circle can sometimes detect a charge of something akin to electrical power passing round from person to person through their arms, especially when they are involved in something active like deep breathing or chanting.

The circle can build tension or share group energy, depending upon the collective circumstances. Circular arrangements involve the participants and do not easily allow individuals to withdraw. The circle with a central focus such as a totem pole or a fire is far more engaging than the theater-style arrangement of many modern gatherings, which encourages detached voyeurism.

The circle has appeared throughout history: at Stonehenge, in the Round Table of Arthurian Legend, in tribal dancing rituals, at Hogmanay during the singing of Auld Lang Syne, in circuses, bull rings, football games, Greek theaters, rodeos, parliaments, race tracks, meal tables, cattle auctions and the Olympic games.

The circle appears in the yin-yang symbol unifying opposites and in the medical symbol of the serpent consuming its own tail.

North American Indian tribes, such as the Navaho and the Sioux, use the circular sweat lodge for self-purification at the start of their healing rituals. The lodge is similar to a sauna held inside a tepee, where the participants sit in a circle and offer fire, water, herbs and prayers to the Great Spirits.

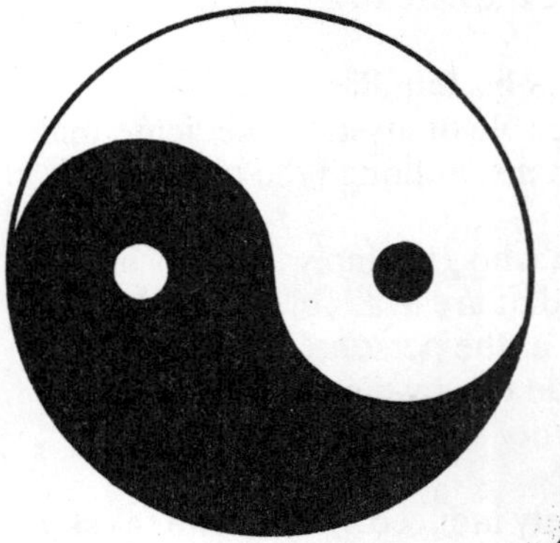

Unifying circle in yin-yang symbol

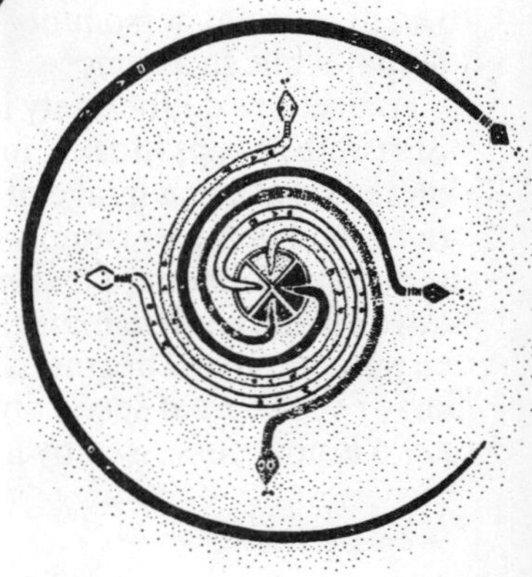

Navaho Indian healing mandala, US Southwest

Stonehenge, Salisbury Plain, England

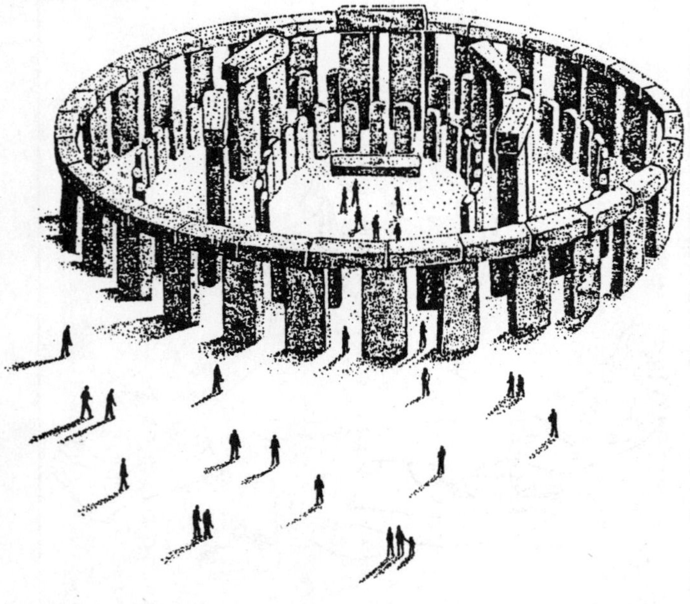

Oneota Indian harvest dance, US Midwest

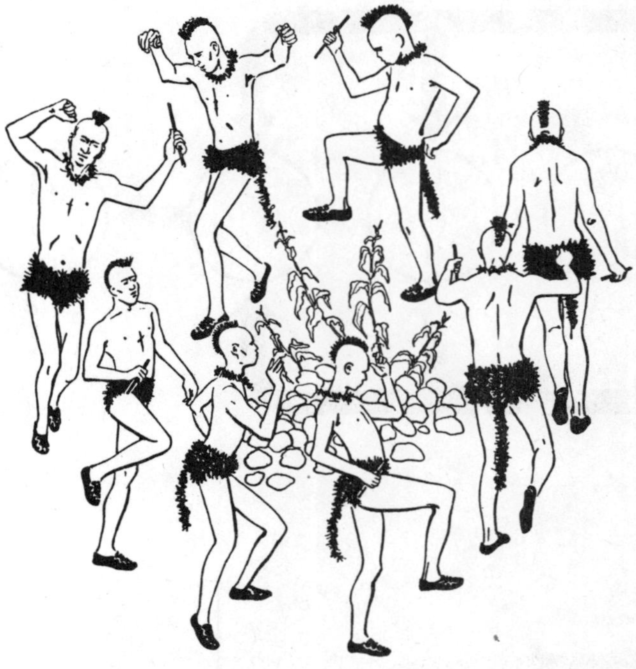

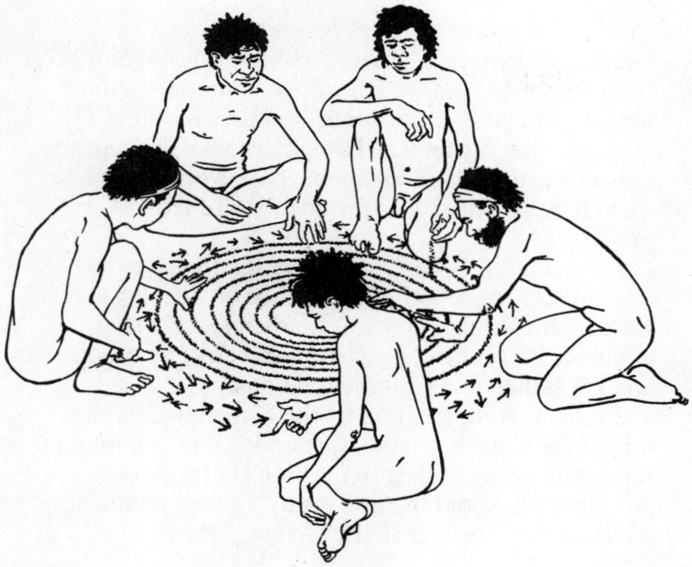

Among the Northern Aranda aborigines of Australia, the sacred gateway leading from this world into the next, is a small waterhole around which concentric circles are drawn in charcoal and ash. The hole represents the place from which the sun and the great ancestor, Karora, were born, and through which Karora returned after his sojourn on earth. The arrows represent the tracks of the mythical emu that accompanied Karora on all his wanderings.

REFERENCE
For more information about suggestion, refer to **Section Five: Suggestive healing** (pp.112–113).

ENCIRCLING AS A HEALING RITUAL

Outlining the diseased part of the body was a very common folklore practice among early communities in South America, parts of North America and Southern Europe.

In some parts of Spain, lung diseases were treated by outlining the whole body. A boy suffering from "air disease" in Pontevedra was taken to the top of a hill overlooking the sea and laid on the ground while a line was drawn round him. The earth within the edge of the line was dug up, carried home with the child and thrown to the back of the fire. When it was burnt, the child was supposed to be cured.

People suffering from tuberculosis had similar treatment. In one case reported from Galicia, a healer scattered sand on the ground and asked the sick man to lie on it. The healer drew the man's outline in the sand. The man was then moved and the line of the drawing was cut away with a knife, to cut away the disease.

In Chilean folklore, the foot is used to represent all parts of the body, its outline being drawn on the bark on the trunk of a tree. This may be done for foot injuries or body problems, such as a hernia. The piece of bark is then cut away from the tree, leaving a bare patch. Healing is said to take place to the extent that the bark grows to fill the space. When the bark is completely regrown, the healing is complete.

Encircling the ailing part is also found in American folklore. In Pennsylvania bunions and other foot problems were said to heal if a piece of turf was cut out round the foot and turned upside down to dry. In Louisiana, childhood croup was cured by taking the child to the south side of a tree where a print of the foot was cut in the bark. In this case the bark was left intact because the child would recover from his attacks of croup when he outgrew the footprint.

All of these methods of outlining the sickness seem to be a form of contagious magic; the person is divested of the sickness by contact with the earth or a tree round which an enclosing circle had been drawn. People relied on these methods for curing certain kinds of disease, so perhaps the real healing came about by the power of suggestion and through a lapse of time.

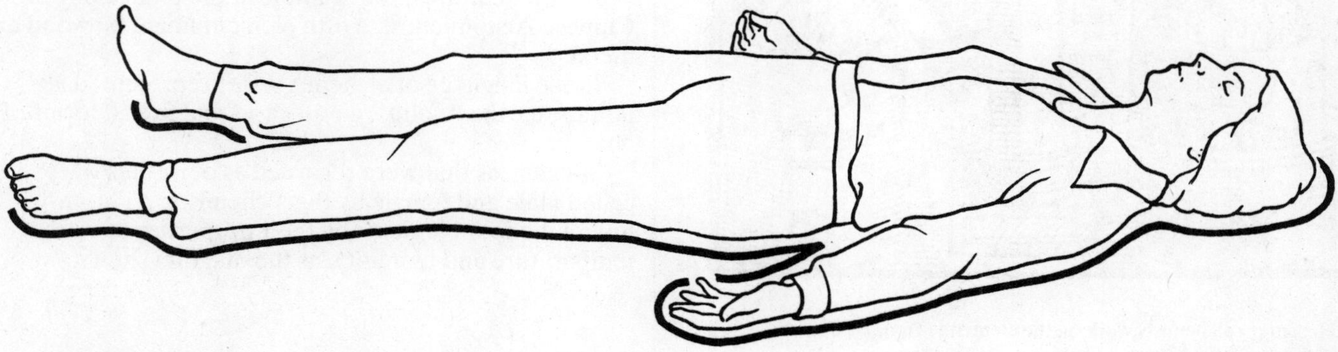

Alchemy

Modern chemistry, pharmacology and metallurgy can trace their origins to the ancient art of alchemy, which had three aims: to find the Philosopher's Stone, to discover the Elixir of Life and to transmute base metals into gold. To achieve all three would be to gain knowledge, eternal youth and wealth. These are not unlike some of the aims of the three modern disciplines already mentioned.

The origins of alchemy

According to one legend, alchemy was founded by the Egyptian god Hermes, who was known as Hermes Trismegistus in his human form. Alchemists called their work the hermetic art and closed their vessels with the seal of Hermes, hence the modern term hermetically sealed, meaning tightly closed.

Several records written on papyrus in the 2nd and 3rd centuries indicated that the Greeks of Alexandria were familiar with methods to make imitation gold and silver from colored alloys, which were commonly used for jewelry and table decorations, as they are today. Over the centuries, alchemical knowledge was also passed between artists and craftsmen whose work had made them familiar with raw substances and chemical processes.

Over a period of a thousand years, the activities of alchemists broadened. The practice of alchemy spread west via the Arab countries. Many researchers also point to similarities between alchemy and esoteric practices in ancient Indian and Chinese religions.

In the west, opposition by the Christian churches forced the alchemists underground and they kept their records in secret codes. In the 16th century some alchemists devoted themselves to creating medicines, while continuing to seek the elixir of life.

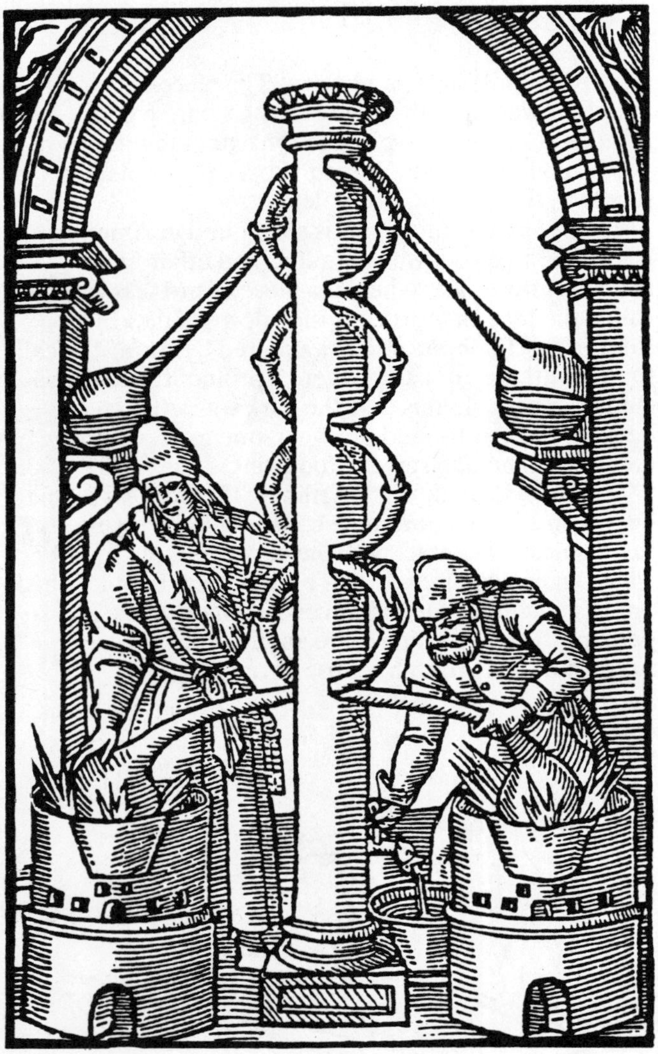

16th century alchemists work on the elements, from *De Secretis Naturae* by Philip Ellstradt (1544)

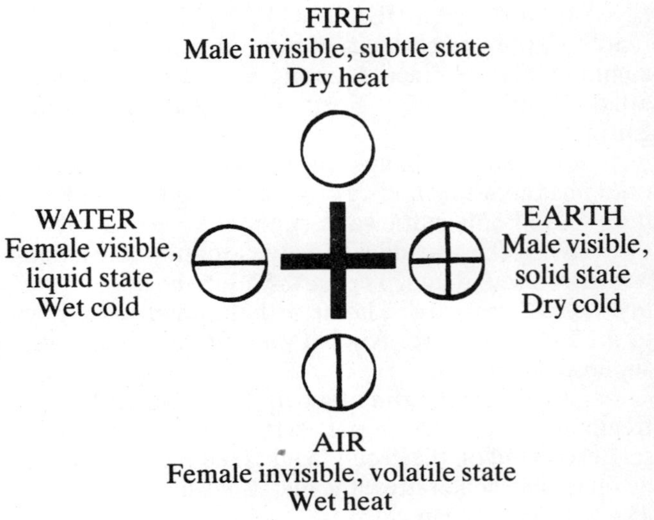

The four elements

According to the alchemists, these are qualities found in all substances and alchemy is the art of converting one element into another. The four elements of the alchemists are earth, fire, air and water.

In other cultures, for example in the philosophy of Chinese Acupuncture, a fifth element might be wood or metal.

In the language of alchemy, water represented all liquids, earth all solids, air all gases and fire all forms of heat.

Substances that were regarded as opposites were called male and female by the alchemists. Aristotle linked the four elements by their properties of temperature and humidity, as the diagram shows.

THE PHILOSOPHY OF THE EARLY ALCHEMISTS

In a treatise called the Emerald Table, written by Hermes Trismegistus, it is stated that everything comes from the One and returns to the One, which the alchemists called the Materia Prima.

It was the task of alchemy to find the Materia Prima and transform it into the Elixir and the Philosopher's Stone. It is thought by some modern researchers that the early alchemists believed this would act as a catalyst when transforming any base metal into gold.

Ourobus, the dragon or serpent who feeds on its own tail, is symbolic of the concept of One to One. Often the length of Ourobus was colored half red and half green. Green symbolized the beginning of the Great Work and red the goal of the Great Work of alchemy.

The Great Work of alchemy

The task of alchemists was to make known, visible and touchable that which is occult, invisible and subtle, and vice versa, using the four elements of the universe and the three principles of alchemy.

The three principles of alchemy

Alchemists work to realize the three potentialities or three degrees of perfection attainable by the Great Work. The terminology indicates complex and lengthy processes which are not the same today.

1 Purification of the Materia Prima: to extract pure mercury, the volatile principle.

2 Digestion of the Materia Prima: to extract pure sulfur, the fixed principle.

3 Fermentation of the Materia Prima: to extract pure salt, the formative principle. Salt was a salt of a substance, not common cooking salt.

The Great Work then proceeded, using the three prepared principles, mercury, salt and sulfur.

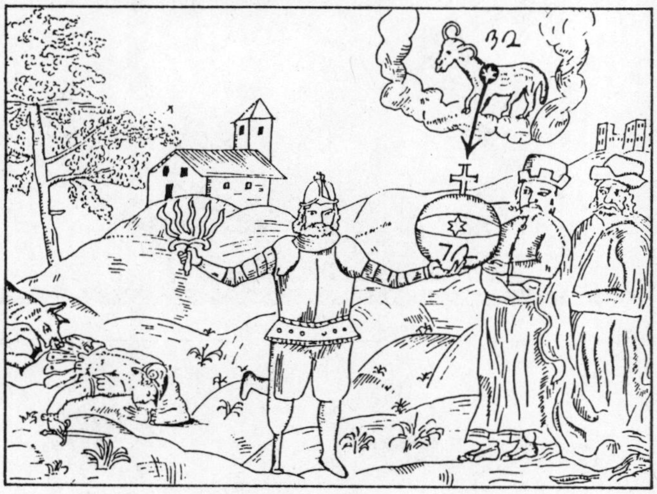

Obtaining the Materia Prima

The work was begun only when the horoscope was favorable, under the signs of Aries. Like the Materia Prima itself, Aries represents the beginning of a new cycle.

Traditionally, the Materia Prima was called the Stone of the Philosophers and was a lump of rock obtained from a mine with an appearance similar to that of all ores. It should not be confused with an end product of the Great Work, called the Philosopher's Stone.

Once found, only this rocky substance was used; no chemicals were added although fire, water, air and earth were all involved. There is still confusion as to which rocks the alchemists used as their raw material, since they were naturally secretive.

In this illustration from the 17th century *Speculum veritatis* in the Vatican Library, Aries the ram is shown in the sky linked to the globe containing the Materia prima. The wolf devouring a person to the left of the picture indicates the first principle, that of purification.

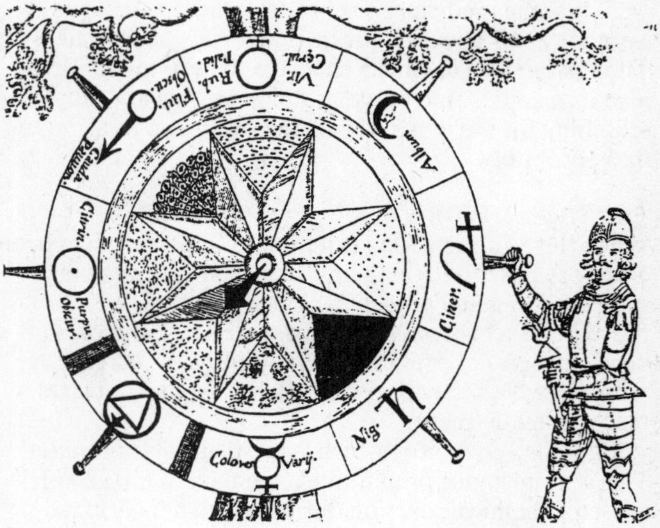

The wheel of the Great Work

The figure about to spin the wheel is Cadmus, the personification of sulfur, who carries the arrow with which he will fix what is volatile. In Greek mythology, Cadmus killed the serpent that guarded the Castalian Spring and sowed the teeth of the serpent which grew as armed men.

The wheel represents the eight main stages of the Great Work. The symbols of substances and processes in this diagram are the same as the symbols for some of the planets. Between the eight points of the star are indicated the appearance of the eight stages. For example, the black stage and the stage of the peacock's tail are easy to recognize. All stages are illustrated and described on the next page.

The imagery of alchemy

The ultimate aim of the early alchemists was to find the Elixir of Life, a universal medicine to heal all ills and create youthful immortality.

The first task was to carry out the Great Work of making the Philosopher's Stone. This substance was believed to be the universal magical substance that could be used to carry out various transmutations, such as metals into gold and liquids into the Elixir of Life.

The alchemist who achieved the goal of the Philosopher's Stone would become an Adept, meaning he who has attained the gift of God, and would join the Brotherhood of Light.

There are fascinating connections between alchemy, religious rituals, the development of Masonry and the process of human sexual intercourse and creation. Some of these links are evident in the symbolic imagery used by the alchemists in their pictorial recordings, examples of which are shown on this page.

During the Renaissance in Europe, many alchemists were making medicines to cure specific diseases, yet even they still searched for the universal cure for all ills. Though modern chemists have given up trying to turn lead into gold, some of today's pharmacists are still searching for the elusive elixir that will keep us all young into perpetuity.

THE GREAT WORK

When the Materia Prima (unique raw material) had been found, as described on the previous page, it was then subjected to many processes. Understanding these processes is a task only for the devoted researcher because their descriptions are labyrinths of secret symbolism that the apprentice alchemist had to travel to reach enlightenment.

First the secret fire "which is not flames" is prepared. This is a substance prepared from cream of tartar which causes a chemical reaction during which heat is made.

The Materia Prima is cleaned and placed in an agate mortar. It is ground with a pestle and mixed with the secret fire and morning dew. The resulting mixture is placed in an hermetically sealed vessel, known as the Philosopher's Egg. The Egg is then placed inside the Athanor, or Philosopher's furnace which keeps the Egg at a constant temperature for a long period of time. The fire in the furnace stimulates the inner fire in the mixture and is likened by alchemists to a hen sitting on her eggs.

In the Materia Prima, the two principles of mercury (cold and female) and sulfur (hot and male) interact. This process is often described as a fight to the death of two animals, resulting in the nigredo or black stage.

This stage ends when stars appear on the surface and the volatile principle flies through the air inside the microcosm of the Philosopher's Egg. While this is happening dozens of bright colors appear, so this stage is called the peacock's tail.

Later the substance turns white and then red as the red sulfur of the wise appears out of the womb of the white rose or rosa alba. This stage may be called the album and was associated with the moon.

Eventually, after many months of patient work, the alchemist hoped to be rewarded with his Philosopher's Stone, with which he could then begin the magical work of transmutation and curing disease.

The sample illustrations

(**a**) Sublimation of the Philosopher's Egg by the secret fire in the furnace is threefold. The figure on the cloud is symbolically fertilizing the processes.

(**b**) Preparation is made to separate the light from the dark which will lead to the birth of Mercury. The small, winged figure standing on the alchemist's raised right hand is Mercury, who was the messenger of the gods and carries a caduceus with the snakes of wisdom and healing,

a

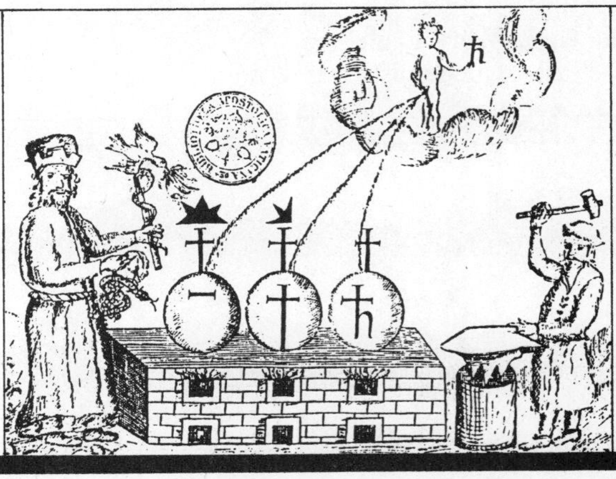

b

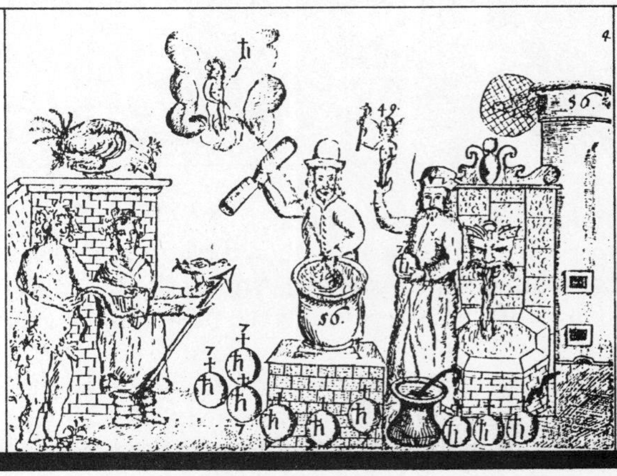

c

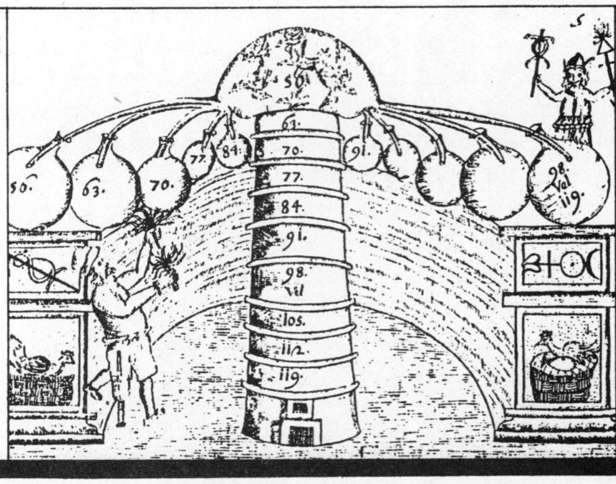

which is still used as a symbol of professionalism by some modern medical institutions.
(c) The secret fire, known as the god Vulcan, makes the birds fly, symbolizing the repeated processes in the furnace as Mercury becomes hermaphrodite by conjoining with Cadmus, who symbolizes sulfur. The alchemist is seen applying the secret fire and Mercury is top right indicating androgeny by carrying the caduceus of the female Mercury and the flaming arrowhead of the male Cadmus. The hens continue to symbolically incubate the Philosopher's Egg.
(d)-(i) In these 17th century alchemical engravings of part of the Great Work, several symbolic themes are recognizable, for example, birth, death and the joining of male and female. The serpent Ourobus, the secret fire and Mercury with his caduceus can be seen.

Sources of the illustrations
Diagrams **(a)**, **(b)** and **(c)** are from the 17th century *Speculum veritatis*, an alchemical manuscript in the Biblioteca Apostolica Vaticana. Cod.lat.7286,f.4,5. Diagrams **(d)** – **(i)** are samples of engravings of the art of alchemy to illustrate the *Philosophia reformata*, a manuscript by the German alchemist J.D.Mylius, published in 1622 in Frankfurt and now in the British Museum, London.

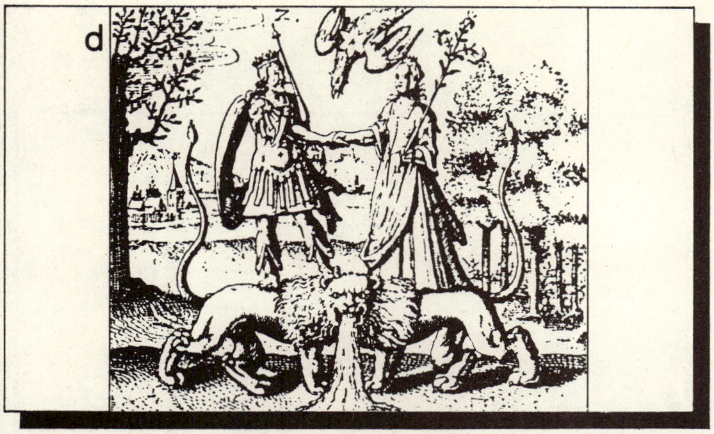

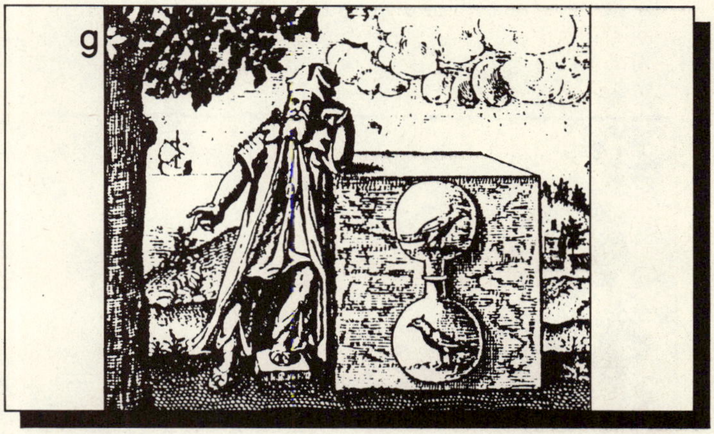

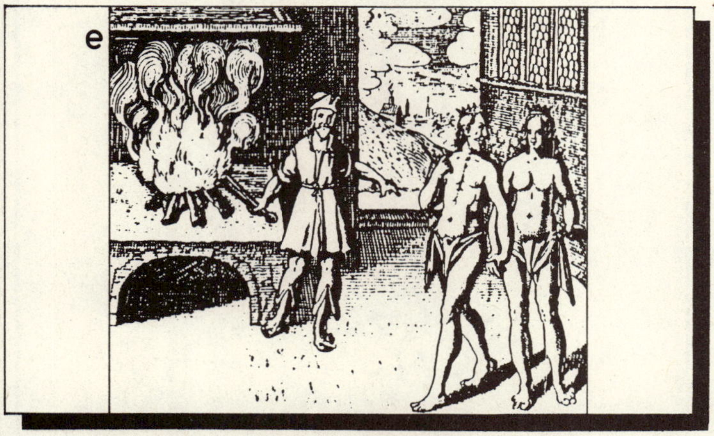

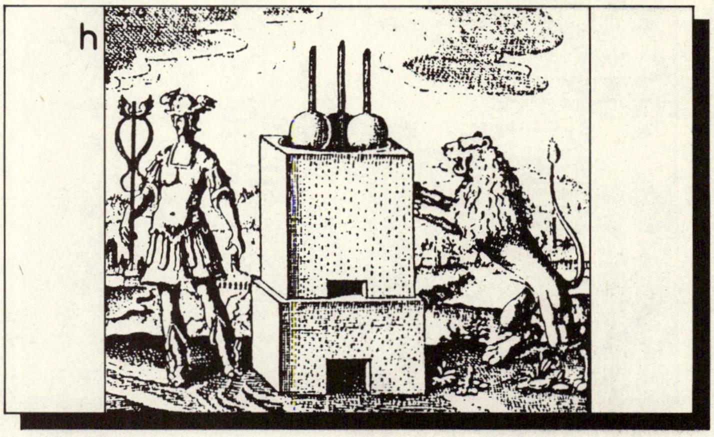

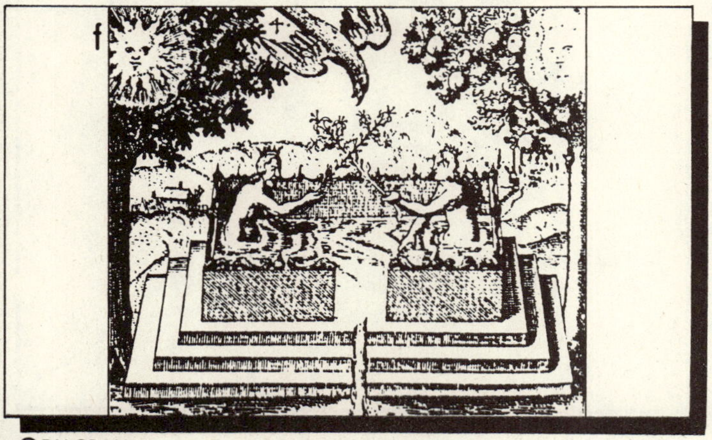

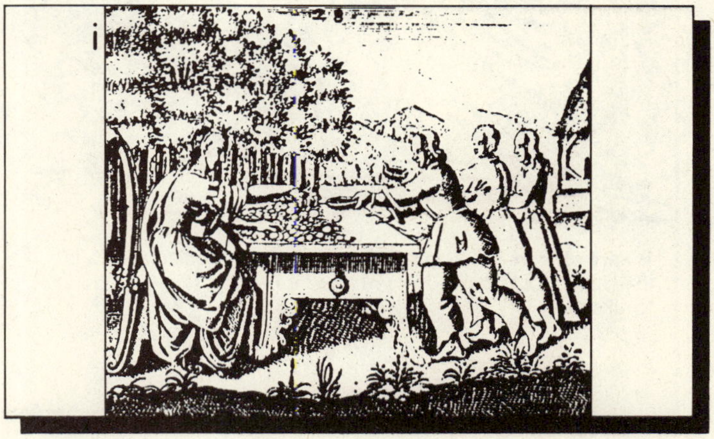

Section four

NATURE AND NURTURE

Natural methods of health care and healing include the use of diets, mineral waters and wines and some less pleasant techniques, such as blood-letting. Whatever was present in nature early man adapted for healing. Since fevers, cancers, infections and chronic problems such as rheumatism were commonplace, anything was worth trying.

In areas of the world near water, water-cures were to be found. Natural springs, geysers of hot water and deposits of kaolin and various muds were used long before the first sophisticated civilizations exploited such phenomena in spa towns and hotels. The value of salt water has long been recognized, and that other natural resource, the sun, has had its worshippers since mankind lost its animal fur.

Pregnancy, childbirth and the nurturing of infants and children provided problems for primitive people, to whom can be traced some modern alternative approaches.

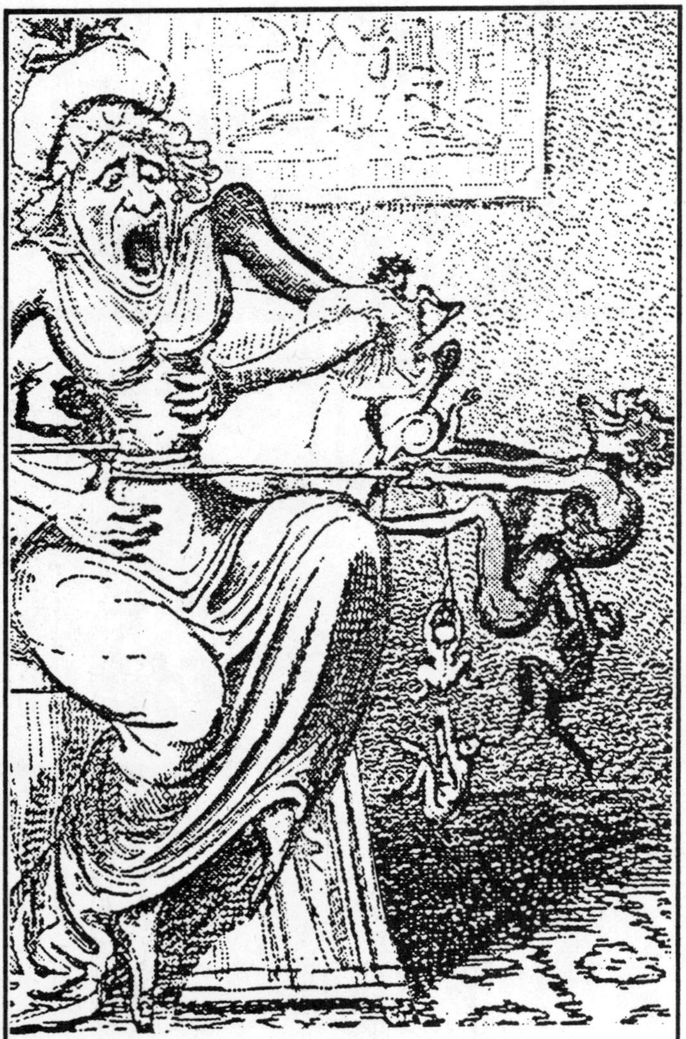

We are what we eat: Starch-leaden diets lead to constipation and ill-health. "The Cholic" by the 19th century English satirist George Cruikshank.

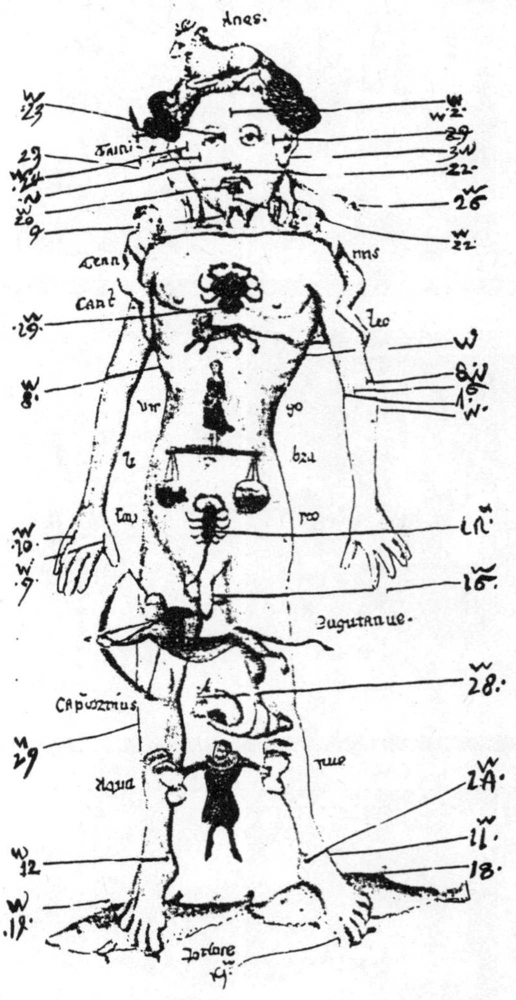

Letting blood release poisons: Medieval drawing of sites for blood-letting linked to astrological signs.

The natural substances of the body itself were often used for diagnosis and healing, especially human urine, which is still used diagnostically. Certain human tissues are now in demand for rejuvenating old or diseased parts, and organ transplantation was first tried, unsuccessfully, in some parts of the world where it was believed that the spirit of an animal remained in its organs.

Natural methods of healing included the use of natural indications, such as the correct time to pick medicinal herbs and astrological divination. In this section many of the healing properties of nature and nurture are explored. To our ancestors many of these methods must have seemed like magic, although we may have a more scientific explanation. Either way, natural healing is an area of alternative medical practice that appears to be very effective.

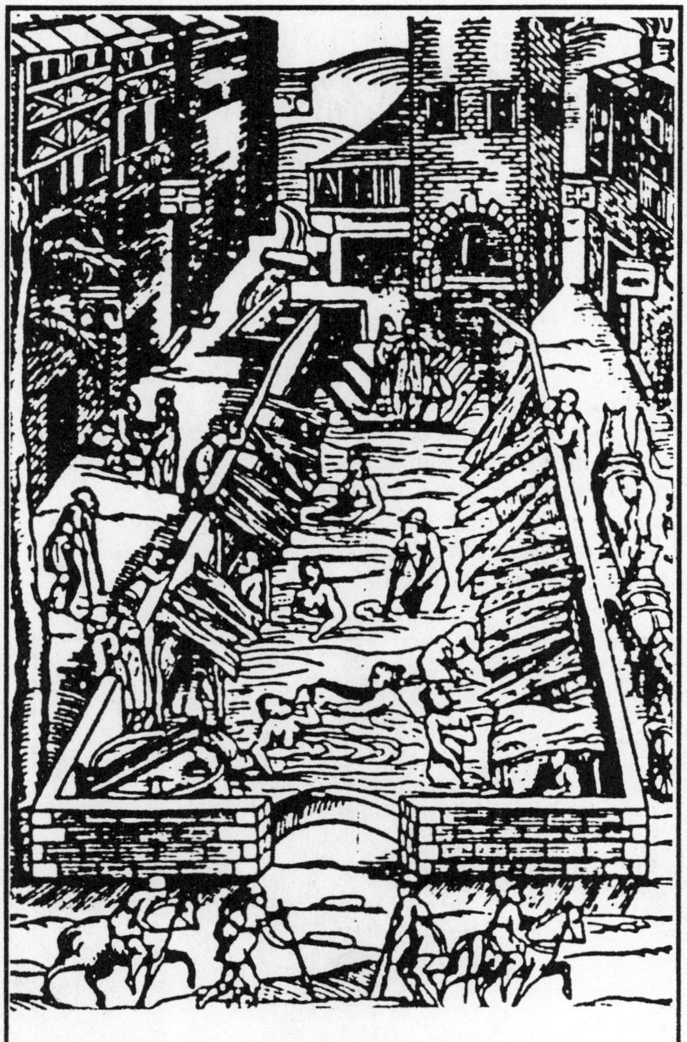

Cleanliness is next to godliness: Public baths in a 16th century health resort. This wood engraving shows sanitation was primitive.

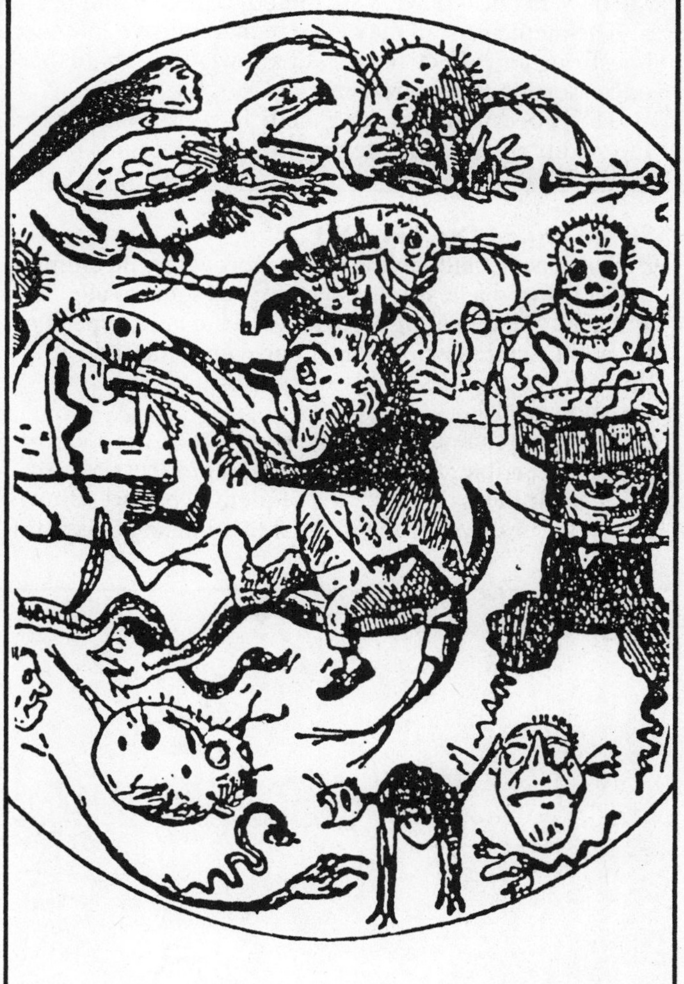

Dirt spreads disease: A Victorian cartoon depicts British politicians as germs. Comment on London's "Green Stink" of 1858 when the Thames river was choked by sewage.

The way of mother earth

Before industrialization, the nature of local environments and climate often determined which methods of healing were used. The tribal way of life, its beliefs and rituals were drawn from experiences of nature, so cultural nurturing was also influenced by mother earth. The interpretation, therefore, of what is natural varies from culture to culture, examples of which are presented here.

YORUBA HERBALISTS

The use of local plants, animals and minerals as remedies is one way in which mother earth has influenced medicine. Nowhere has the herbalist and his medicine stall been so prolific as in the Yoruba region of Nigeria, although Western medicine is becoming the normal practice in cities such as Ibadan.

The medicine stall may have a selection of seeds, roots, the fur or skins of animals, a chicken corpse, leaves, feathers and a large selection of animal parts. Most of these will be used to make medicines and will have magical powers attributed to them to aid healing.

The medicine stall may even seem repulsive, but there is a strong and effective body of knowledge behind the odd assortment of ingredients.

The processes for making medicines are complex and the acidity or alkalinity depends on which liquids were included, for example lime juice, urine or alcohol. The results may be drunk or may be used for bathing.

A popular tonic is agbo tutu, a cold medicine because heat is not used in its preparation. It is particularly effective against convulsions in small children and as a general prophylactic for anyone. It consists of green tobacco leaves marinated in either human urine (preferably of the mother) or a cow's urine. Sometimes a measure of gin is added. The medicine is, of course, a very strong solution of nicotine which in small doses stimulates the central nervous system.

A herbalist's advertisement

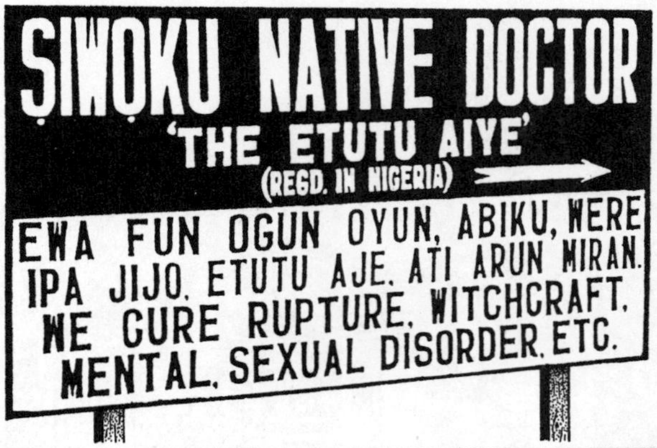

SHAMANISM IN LAPLAND

Beliefs based on terrifying encounters with wild animals have nurtured a healthy respect for the souls of all animals so that healing ceremonies were held to pacify the animal spirits whose anger had caused disease. In the 16th century, the Lapps still performed these ceremonies.

The Lapp shamans were the wise men at the court of Ivan the Terrible, who was the first tsar of Russia from 1547–1584. In this section of a sequential picture, drawn by a 17th century European artist, a reindeer (6) is eating the hallucinogenic mushroom, *Amanita muscaria*, while being hunted (6).

Three men (7) are shown drinking an infusion of the mushrooms. The one with the drum is the shaman who then goes to the reindeer (8) and they both fall down (9). The shaman then lies under his own drum (10) while the spirit of the deer communicates with souls of other animals whose anger has caused sickness or misfortune. Finally the spirit of the deer returns his drum to the shaman (11) and disappears.

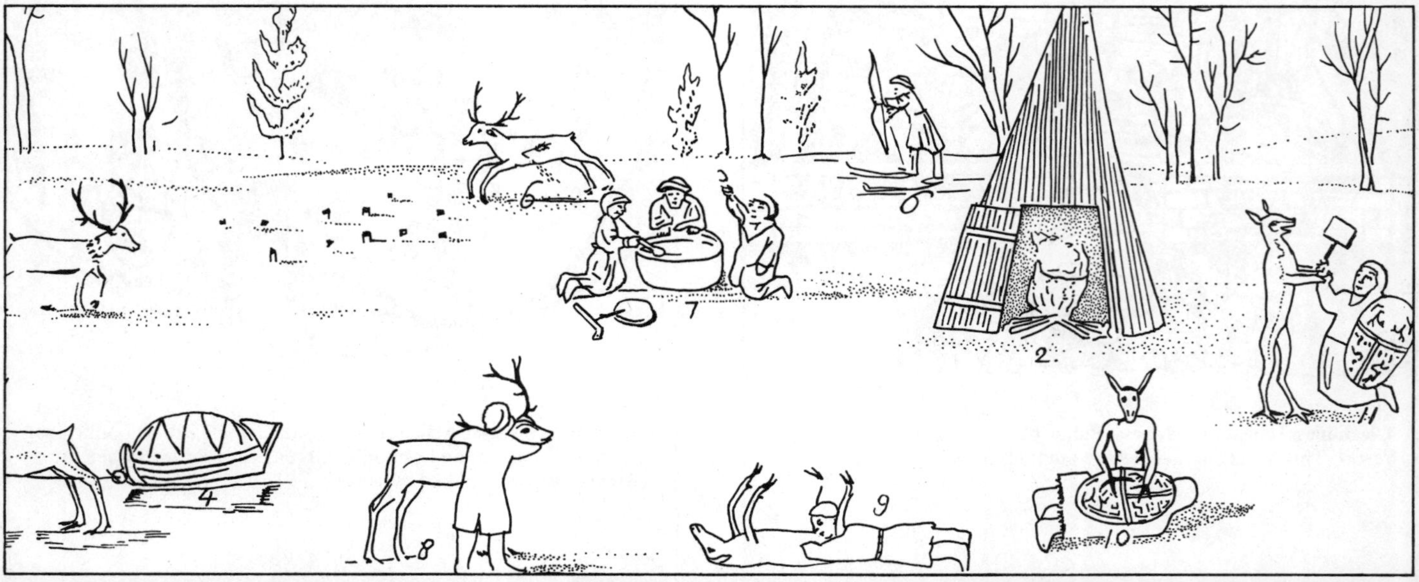

THE SEARCH FOR PEACE IN TIBET

The tough life experiences of people in the remote high mountain regions of Tibet presented them with very specific problems. Hence they evolved a practical system of medicine embracing self-reliance.

Food, for example, was classified into six tastes which would convert into three humors, or energies, responsible for digestion. Each humor could be poisoned by a mental affliction, which upset the balance of the humors and was a cause of disease.

Poisons – greed hatred secrecy;
Humors – wind bile phlegm.

Illness could also be caused by vile actions in a previous life. Either way, the individual was held responsible for attaining a peaceful mind, which would aid his return to health.

Diagnosis was done by reading the pulses, testing the urine and taking into account the age of a person and the place where he lived.

Tibetan treatment consisted of dietary and behavioral advice, pills, massage and moxabustion, which is a heat treatment of the acupuncture points with smoldering herbs. The aim was to help the patient achieve a peaceful state of mind in his social group and natural environment.

Tibetan pills were made entirely from locally available substances and often had up to 40 ingredients. However, every pill contained six superior ingredients. These were clove, greater and lesser cardomom, nutmeg, saffron and bamboo mannu, to aid the spleen, kidney, heart, liver and lungs respectively. Tibetan doctors also prescribed sweet, sour and salty foods be eaten in winter, and bitter, hot and astringent foods in summer.

Chen Ray Ze, the Buddha of peaceful mind

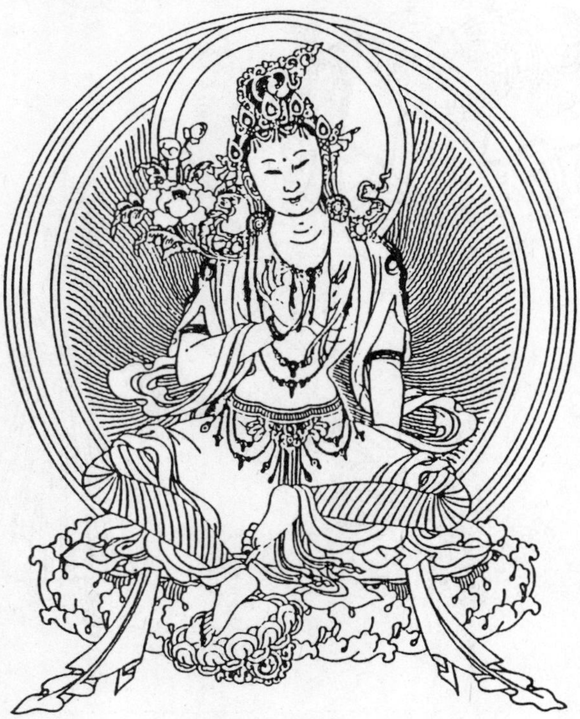

BACK TO NATURE

Even today, we are influenced by the cultural environment in which we live and many alternative medical practices are based on what is seen to be a more natural way of life.

The macrobiotic philosophy

A diet of balanced yin and yang foods is claimed to cure illnesses and keep people healthy.

Broadly speaking, yin foods correspond to the acid in food and yang to the alkaline. It is macrobiotic belief that most illness is caused by an imbalance of yin-yang in the diet. Yin foods are sweet, sour or hot foods such as fruits, drinks, and summer grown food which is soft-textured and purple, blue or green in color. Yang foods are salty, bitter, astringent foods, all those of animal origin, cereals and some vegetables. Yang foods are usually hard and red, yellow or orange in color and mature in autumn or winter.

The practice of macrobiotics varies in different regions. It is for each person to find their own macrobiotic diet from local foods and then get on with the joys of living. The correct balance of food will ensure good sleep, and freedom from illness and worry.

The macrobiotic diet has been equated with a diet exclusively of brown rice, but this is only a short-term cleansing diet. Many people who try it for ten days are surprised to find how invigorated they feel.

The basic macrobiotic diet includes 50% brown rice plus grains, such as whole wheat, rye, barley, oats, millet, buckwheat and maize. Vegetables, legumes and soy bean products, such as miso and tamari, are added. Specialties may include seaweeds, salted pickled plums which are good for digestive problems, sesame seed salt, green tea, grain coffees and mu tea, a special blend of 15 roots and herbs, including ginseng.

A Japanese hospital in Nagasaki, that used macrobiotic diets claimed that, after the atomic bomb, the low level of radiation sickness among their patients and ex-patients was due to the diet.

Animal wisdom

People who lived close to animals often followed the wisdom of animals by imitating their ways.

For example, many rural people slept with their windows firmly closed at night, contrary to some modern health care advice to keep bedroom windows open for fresh air during sleep.

Country people were aware that birds sleep with their beaks tucked into their feathers, foxes out in the open cover their noses with their tails when sleeping, and cats and dogs similarly hide their noses when asleep. Horses stand with their backs to the wind and groups of animals in open fields crowd their heads together warming the inward breath with the heat of the outward breath.

Fresh warm air seems to be what animals prefer. It has been observed that people who regularly breathe fresh warm air as they sleep, instead of cold air, rarely catch head colds.

Fertility

In almost all primitive cultures, the power of men and women to procreate was often of crucial importance to their status in the tribe and to the continuation of the tribe. Human fertility was also linked with good harvests and good fortune in battles and other situations.

A barren woman would be obliged to take all the blame for her condition and would often be rejected or even expelled from the community because it was feared her influence would ruin the crops or cause animals to die. Women were generally treated as chattels in this context.

Fertility amulets

The most common way of encouraging the spirits to bestow fertility was by wearing a charm or amulet.

In the religion of the Maoris of New Zealand, Tiki was the great Creator, and the Hei-Tiki, an amulet carved from greenstone, was very popular as a fertility charm. It is a small, round figure with an enormous head tilting to one side, thought to represent the fetus. Originally, it was said to give protection against the spirit of the unborn who was placated by being offered parents.

Among ancient Britons and in other early European settlements, mistletoe was a very powerful fertility symbol because it apparently grew without roots and flourished with green leaves and white berries throughout winter when all other things appeared to be dead. In later centuries, mistletoe was carried into homes to ensure fertility, and later still the practice of kissing under the mistletoe was supposed to bring good luck to the lovers. Sometimes the oak tree on which the mistletoe grew was also regarded as potent, and oak twigs were carried as fertility symbols.

Fertility was often thought to be contagious, so a barren woman would ask for the gift of a brooch, shawl or carved figure from a woman who had had many children in the belief that contact with the mother would result in her own conception. Some went to great lengths to weave fertility amulets from the hair of a woman who was already pregnant. Corn dollies were also woven from ripe corn and hung in the house or over the bed to encourage conception.

Rice or barley, being prolific plants, would be thrown over a couple as they retired to their marriage bed. Horse-shoes, because they had been in contact with the earth, were thought to transfer fertility. Eggs and rabbits, too, are universal symbols of fertility. Rabbits' feet were popular good luck charms. Easter bunnies mark the new life of spring time and the Christian resurrection, while Bunny girls in clubs have a more sexual nuance.

In many cultures, the fox was associated with fertility, and amulets of fox skins woud be hung in precise patterns to ensure a conception in Ancient Egypt. Foxes were also buried in vineyards or hung about the fields to propagate plants.

Some fertility rituals

Male fertility rites have included stabbing the ground with spears, a ritual common to Bronze Age people and contemporary aborigines. Many springtime festivities, such as maypole dancing, originate as fertility rituals for humans and plants. The Swedish Midsummer Festival was originally a fertility dance, the maypole representing the male and the garlands representing the female.

In 16th century Yugoslavia, there were several methods a bride could use to ensure she would have children. She could place an unlocked padlock in her bodice when dressing. Having decided how many children she wanted, she would take the same number of steps from the door of her house and then snap the padlock closed. If she was wise, she would also have a ladder ready. When her groom arrived to take her to the wedding ceremony, she would climb the same number of rungs, in case the spirits had got it wrong the first time. However, if any barley grains fell into her shoe after the ceremony, her first pregnancy would be delayed as many years as there were grains.

Fertility amulets
1 Hei-Tiki carved from greenstone
2 Hei-Tiki carved from a skull – this is an unusual carving and may also represent Tiki the Creator
3 Mistletoe growing on the trunk of an oak tree
4 A corn dolly fertility charm

1
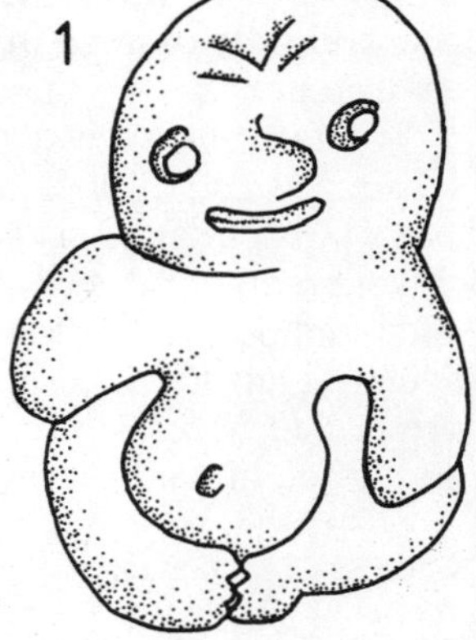

2
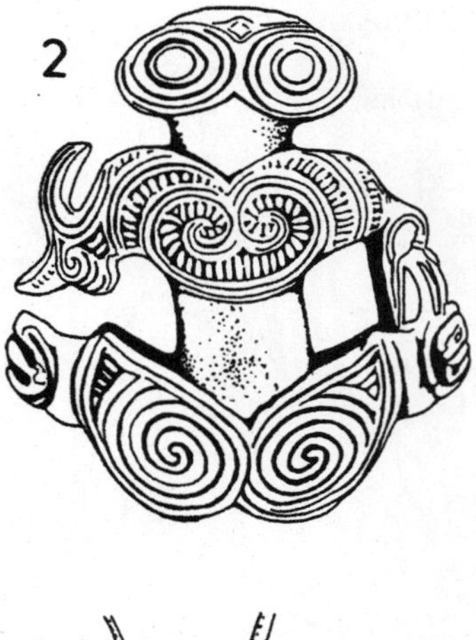

3
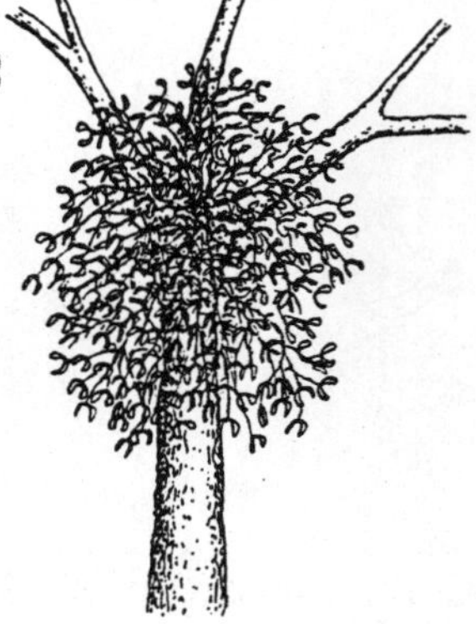

4
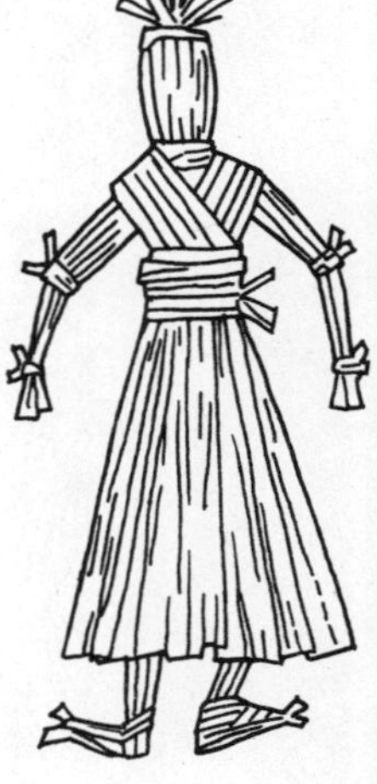

1

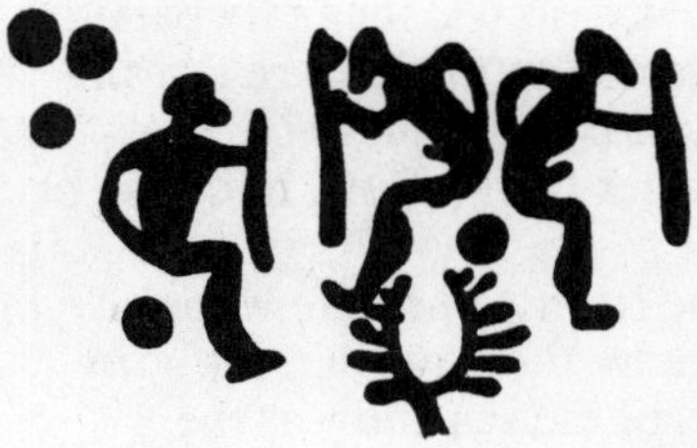

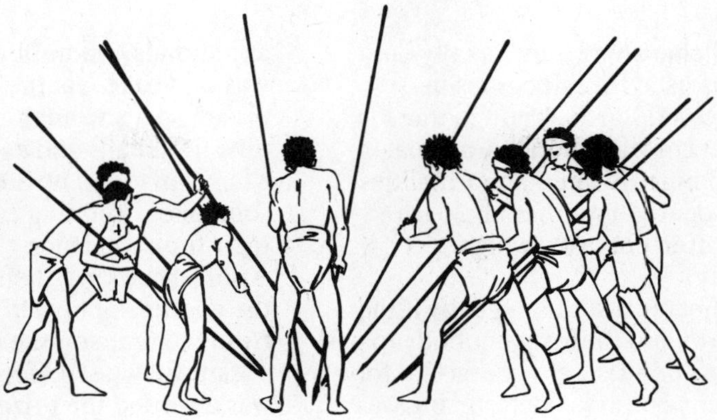

2

3

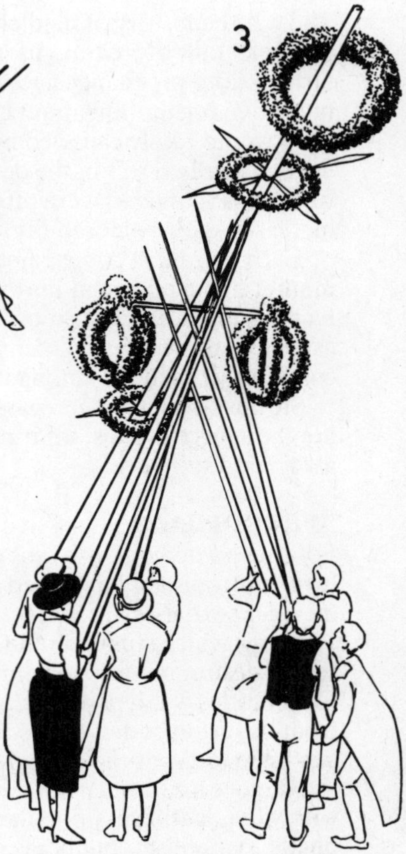

4

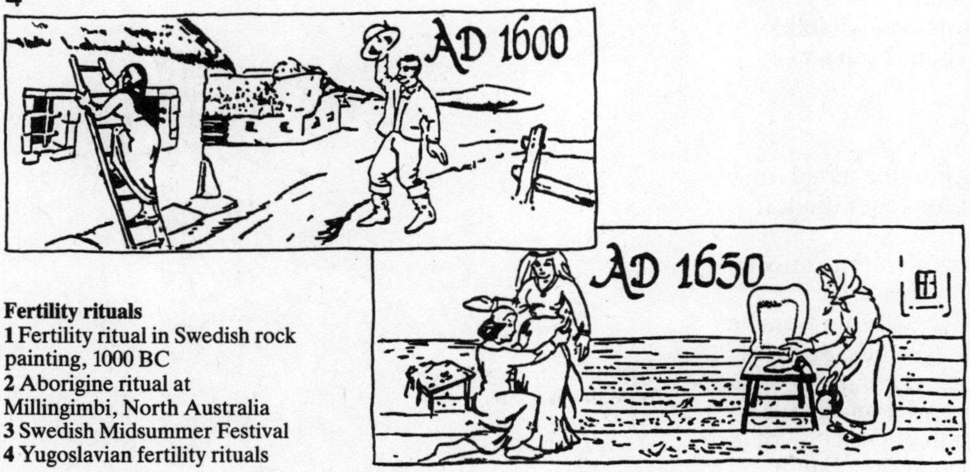

Fertility rituals
1 Fertility ritual in Swedish rock painting, 1000 BC
2 Aborigine ritual at Millingimbi, North Australia
3 Swedish Midsummer Festival
4 Yugoslavian fertility rituals

THE CELESTIAL BED

In 1780, the Scotsman James Graham opened an elegant "Temple of Health" in a fashionable London house. Here Graham treated his wealthy clients to the ultimate in health-care quackery. Modeled on the Greek temples of Aesculapius, the "Temple of Health" relied on the power of suggestion for its successes.

The ancient Aesculapian temples were built in quiet, secluded places, and the sick would arrive after a lengthy journey eager to recuperate, They would first pass through a purification ritual and were then taken by nubile virgins to rest on a large bed. During the night, the sick person would be visited by a god or his messenger who would cure the patient as he thought fit.

Graham's "Temple of Health" combined nature cure methods, such as massage, diet and rest, with the suggestion of magic being at work; however, his magic was very powerfully presented and designed primarily to help married couples conceive.

After their purification ritual of hydrotherapy and massage, attended by attractive young women in semi-transparent finery, the couple would enter the inner sanctum, where an enormous bed awaited them.

The bed itself was a masterpiece of persuasion. Twelve feet by nine feet and supported by 40 exquisitely carved glass pillars in rainbow colors, it was a luxurious environment designed to lure the couples eventually into more relaxed love-making than they had ever known. Over the bed was a large dome of mirrors, and the whole area was filled with the aroma of exotic herbs and spices.

With music playing softly, the "patients" lay in this "Celestial Bed" and were subjected to the immense pleasure of "exhilarating electrical forces" from some 15 hundredweights of magnets placed around the bed. Magnetism was the magic each couple believed would cure their infertility… and Graham was reported to have an outstanding success rate, even at £50 a night.

Some people accused him of using the "Temple of Health" as a front for prostitution. This is unlikely, as James Graham was more interested in biology than in the passions of sex, and health was his own driving interest. Furthermore, there were many alternative houses in London where the wealthy could satisfy sexual passion at a cheaper price, such as Mrs Cornelys's Pantheon, where Casanova paid 6 guineas for a night of amorous delights.

Childbirth

The written history of medicine almost universally omits to give details of treatments used for difficulties in fertilization, pregnancy and childbirth although there is much documentation about contraception. A normal birth would rarely cause comment, while abnormalities would usually result in the death of mother and baby. Those who survived were often outcasts, which increased their vulnerability.

Early primitive tribes rejected a surviving baby if the mother had died in childbirth and there was nobody to feed the child. Because most infants were breast-fed for as long as three years in many cultures, wet-nursing was commonly practiced among large family groups.

Stories that have been passed down through folklore are the source of most information about birth and its associated subjects.

APHRODISIACS

For those who had problems getting into the mood for love, aphrodisiacs have been sought for generations to increase sexual desire.

Drugs which stimulate the pituitary gland can affect sexual desire, but also may increase aggression. Cantharides was a popular aphrodisiac, which was made from the dried bodies of the Spanish fly beetle. It is still available today as the dangerous drug, cantharidin.

Rhinoceros horn, ground into a powder and supped with wine, is still very popular, presumably because of its phallic symbolism, but it has no effect on the pituitary gland at all.

Alcohol and cannabis have always been consumed in large quantities by those who hoped to sexually arouse their partners and themselves by reducing inhibitions, but the total effect of both substances is to make a person's autonomic responses more inhibited in the long run.

Love potions

In many parts of the world, to make a boy fall in love with her, a girl would soak her nail clippings in the favorite drink of the boy of her choice. Some of the most potent love potions were said to contain the blood of the lover.

An old German belief instructs a man to cut his little finger and let some of his blood drop into the woman's drink. As for women, they had only to add a few drops of menstrual blood to their lover's drink to ensure fertilization. Since blame for lack of offspring, or even for the lack of a male heir, was almost always attributed to the woman, many a wife under threat of desertion must have resorted to this superstition.

Forecasting future outcomes has always been popular, ranging from ancient rituals performed at full moon to the reading of crystal balls, palms and tea-leaves. Love potions have included bat's blood, the powdered feet of mice and dust obtained from dry-baking doves, but the most common love potion still in use in the Western world is marzipan.

A paste made from butter, sugar and ground nuts such as almonds, walnuts, hazel nuts and nutmeg, marzipan was said to reveal the identity of a future husband in a dream. All a woman had to do was roll the marzipan into nine little balls and eat them one by one before retiring. Many girls (and boys) still sleep with a piece of someone's wedding cake under their pillow, to dream of their future partner.

Aphrodisiacs got their name from Aphrodite who was the goddess of love in Greek mythology. She was born from the foam on the waves of the sea and was the unfaithful wife of Hephaestus. The mother of Eros, she was awarded the prize for beauty in a contest judged by Paris.

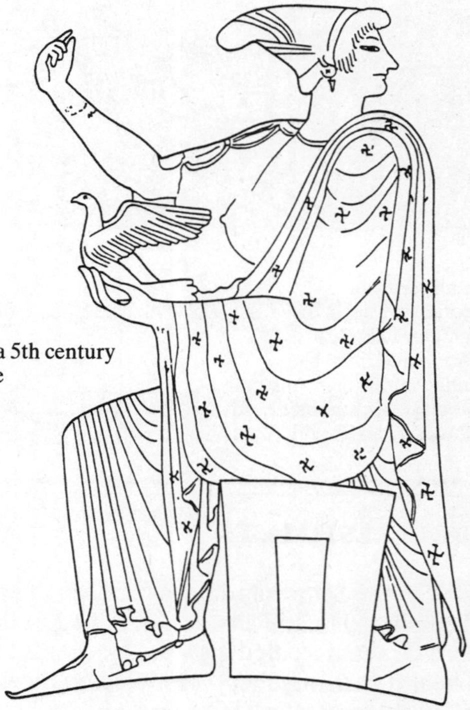

Aphrodite, from a 5th century BC Athenian vase

THE CHILD-BEARER

Sometimes women have been revered, but often they have been regarded as dangerous, for example, menstruating women, pregnant women and women who had recently given birth were often temporary outcasts from their community. Frequently orthodox religions perpetuated these inhuman attitudes, some of which still exist today, even among civilized nations.

It is a Christian belief that Jesus Christ was conceived to a virgin by the Holy Ghost or spirit of God. The subsequent adoration of the virgin mother has made it clear to generations of girls that having sex makes a woman unclean. Boys have been given a double message: the most desirable wife is a virgin and yet it is boys who despoil the virgin's purity.

In the past in most tribes, women were regarded as the possessions of men. Hence the chastity belt was devised to protect the man's property (i.e. his wife's vagina) in his absence. Made of animal skin, bark or metal, some women were locked inside these unhygienic devices for months and many died from painful infections.

Sexual impotence in either sex was said to be cured by eating the kidneys of a rabbit. Since rabbits breed vigorously, this was a cure by sympathetic magic.

The fox has been associated with fertility by the ancient Egyptians and many other cultures. Amulets of fox skin were worn by both men and women. Modern fox tails and furs are still associated with sexuality.

Some old folk beliefs from Southern India

A menstruating woman could not take part in family rituals in case she passed her supposed impurity to the whole family. Women "in pollution" were isolated, fed separately and worked alone for three days. However, paradoxically, it was believed that a barren woman would become fertile if she touched a child during her menstruation. The problem would be to get near enough to touch. The woman would also be blamed if anyone in the child's family then fell sick!

Childbirth

There is no evidence to show that labor and childbirth was any easier or harder than it can be today. There were some painkillers but the agony of a lengthy, unproductive labor was usually relieved only by screaming and pulling on the arms of helpers.

A Cesarean section is birth through an incision in the wall of the abdomen and is believed to be the way Julius Caesar was born. Many women gave birth this way without painkillers. Many also died through shock, loss of blood or infection.

To give birth, a woman would generally be supported by other women as she sat in a crouching position. In some parts of the world a birth stool would be used. Giving birth in water was also popular where there was warm, clear water available. Whatever the method, the mother would be quickly on her feet again.

In the West, among some natural childbirth groups, there is a move to resurrect this method, using a large plastic or wooden tub erected in the family home, filled with warm water.

THE NEW BABY

Although ancient superstitions are being replaced by the latest fads about modern babycare, older members of some families may still remember some of these superstitions.

It is unwise to weigh a baby too soon after birth and it would be fatal (to the baby) to show it to a mirror before the first birthday.

The spirituality of a male child should be carefully nurtured, as he will carry the family name. Blue is the color of the spirit, so a boy should be wrapped in a blue cloth. Pink for a girl was an afterthought.

A baby should be carried upwards, for example upstairs, before it is carried downwards or bad luck will befall it and it will never rise in the world. (It should be remembered that most babies would be born at ground level in the distant past.) In New Guinea, some tribes never allowed a child to touch the earth until it was two years old, to avoid it being taken over by the evil spirits that live in the earth.

To prevent stammering, babies should not be tickled, some say under the chin, others say under the feet.

A baby's nails and hair should not be cut until the first birthday. Some say if the nails are cut too soon, the child will become a thief. (This belief was linked with the idea that the soul of a person could be lost by throwing away parts of the body.)

In New England, it used to be said that a child would grow up to be ignorant unless it had fallen out of bed three times before its first birthday.

The first person to kiss a baby, apart from its mother, must be chosen with great care, because that person will give the child its temperament for life.

Clothes handed down from older children were considered to be lucky (a very practical idea) and a child should never be called an angel, because this would be tempting fate.

Nine strands of red silk, knotted nine times and hung round a child's neck would ease teething pains. Any tooth lost naturally, or later by extraction or accident, should be preserved or buried in a special place, to avoid any evil influence.

CONTRACEPTION

Ancient texts do not always distinguish between contraception and abortion. The earliest text is the Egyptian Petri papyrus from 1850 BC which recommended plugging the vagina with a mixture of honey and natron (native sodium carbonate). Another contraceptive was a pessary made from crocodile dung.

Sheaths were in common use across the globe from earliest times, to protect a man from insect bites, infection and injury. They were only used as condoms later when finer materials were used. The ancient Egyptians also practiced their own version of vasectomy for men and ovariotomy for women. Swallowing castor oil seeds was a common contraceptive for women and coitus interruptus was a well-known method used by men.

A contraceptive lint tampon, for use by women, was described in the Ebers papyrus: lint was to be moistened with acacia and honey. Tips of the acacia shrub contain gum arabic, which when dissolved in water and fermented produce lactic acid, which was used in early 20th century spermicides.

For diseases of the genitals, such as thrush and gonorrhea, the ancient Egyptians recommended fumigation with peppermint and a medicine made from alum, garden crocus and the gum of the Alexandrian *Spina Aegypta*.

Natural sponges were popular during menstruation and were also thought to act as a contraceptive, by soaking up the sperm fluid. The leaves of a willow tree, rennet from a hare and Cedar gum have also been favored as contraceptives throughout the ages.

What's in a diet?

A diet is the combination of foods eaten regularly by a person. Special diets may be designed for specific reasons, such as low fat diets for people with gall bladder troubles, muscle-building diets for athletes, controlled carbohydrate levels for people who suffer from insulin-dependent diabetes and a whole plethora of diets for reducing weight.

When selecting a diet it is as well to remember the old adage: what is one man's meat is another man's poison. Diet must take into account individual factors such as upbringing and metabolism.

NATUROPATHIC DIETS

Naturopathy is a system of maintaining health and treating ailments which is based on the understanding that the body contains its own curative forces.

The Greek philosopher Hippocrates stated that good health depended upon keeping these curative forces vitalized by achieving the correct balance of rest and exercise, a stable emotional life and adequate nourishment.

Many of those who have put this philosophy into practice in the past have been farmers and other rural people. Nutrition therapy has become a fundamental part of naturopathy, and psychodietetics is the use of diet to cure emotional and other psychological disorders.

CAN DIET CURE DISEASE?

In February 1953 multiple sclerosis was diagnosed for Roger McDowell, a British writer. A few years later he was virtually paralyzed, couldn't speak properly and was almost blind. He experimented throughout his illness with different diets, which at first stabilized his condition. Fifteen years later his symptoms began to disappear and he could see, speak and walk again. By the time he reached his sixties, he was living a normal active life.

He aimed to find a diet that restored the chemical imbalance he assumed had caused his body's inability to build replacement tissue for the myelin sheaths of the nerves. His diet excluded all gluten, which is found in wheat, rye, barley and oats, and was low in sugars and animal fats. It was high in unsaturated fats, vegetables and fresh fish and fruits. He also devised his own vitamin

THE PRIMITIVE DIET

The health and longevity of some primitive communities has been studied in depth, especially in relation to the claims that animal fats have a debilitating effect on humn circulation. Some early studies produced some conflicting results. (Refer to **Section Six: Natural remedies** pp.138–139) Some tribes ate large quantities of animal meat, yet remained healthy and free from circulation problems.

Further studies during the 1980s of healthy tribes such as the Masai and Eskimos who had not become westernized, showed that while both tribes ate more meat than the average Westerner, the proportion of polyunsaturated to saturated fats eaten was three times greater than the average Westerner. The primitive diets were also ten times richer in vitamin C than recommended standard intakes in the West.

It was also discovered that the meat of wild animals eaten by these tribes contained eight times less fat than the average farm animal and contained the important fatty acid, eicosapentanoic acid (EPA).

EPA protects against the dangerous over-production of the saturated acids in the system. It has also been suggested that EPA itself is involved in the prevention of malignancies and arthritis as well as cardiovascular conditions. EPA is present in fish oil and in the meat of wild animals, but not in the meat of the farm-bred animals.

Are fats part of the solution?

Doctors such as R. C. Atkins in America and R. Mackarness in Britain have promoted high protein/low carbohydrate diets, similar to the primitive diet, for weight loss, high energy and the reduction of excessive cholesterol levels in the blood. They have encouraged patients to disregard the calorie count but to limit carbohydrates on average to 30g or 1oz, depending on personal metabolism. High carbohydrate levels are found in grains, cereals, pasta, sugar, syrups and fruits.

Dieting on fatty meat, fish, fowl, butter, cream, eggs and small amounts of green salad and green vegetables may seem like a contradiction, but results have shown it to be an effective diet for many people providing they supplement it with B, C and E vitamins under the supervision of a doctor. Providing the proportion of one part fat to three parts protein is kept, the obese patient can eat as much as he likes and will lose weight despite eating as much as 3000 calories a day.

Atkins, Mackarness and other doctors have suggested that it is the combination of fats with carbohydrates that is unhealthy, not the fats in themselves.

Primitive diets

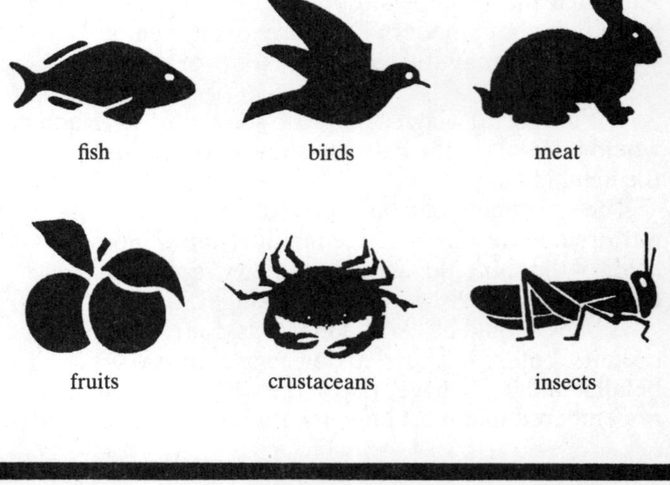

supplements. He never claimed a cure, only that the diet controlled the disease.

Dr Joseph Evers, the West German doctor who specialized in treating multiple sclerosis, also devised special diets, which are not gluten-free but include much raw food, such as raw vegetables, sprouted seeds, fruit, milk, eggs, rolled oats, honey and plenty of water. He also included some fermented food.

Many clinics now use diets to help those suffering from cancer, some of which claim excellent results. It would appear, however, that precisely the same diet does not have the same effect for different people, so personal adjustments have to be made. Many naturopathic practitioners are convinced that the correct diet is crucial to good health. Nobody yet agrees what is a correct diet, except that fresh fruit and vegetables are better than large quantities of refined, sugary food.

Allergens

A whole list of disturbances have been connected with food allergies, for example sensitivity to preservatives and colorants. In a large proportion of people, asthma, migraine, colitis, obesity, headaches, eczema and hyperactivity in children have been treated successfully by the elimination of food additives. However, it is not yet clear whether the cure is because of the removal of additives and empty calories or because food without additives is naturally more nutritious.

NUTRITION IN SEAWEED

Many ocean plants are highly nutritious. The ocean plant, *Macrocystis pyrifera*, commonly called kelp or the sea vegetable, contains combinations of minerals and vitamins that are essential to humans. It is probable that when humans spent part of their evolution living at the edge of the sea, kelp first became popular as it could be easily harvested by hand.

The sea covers about 71% of the earth and is estimated to have an average depth of 2.38 miles. Every metal and mineral compound has been drained into the oceans from the land and from the skies over millions of years. The sea is a rich food resource for many living creatures and sea kelp is a testimony to its richness.

Kelp grows best in six to ten fathoms of water on a rocky bottom. It anchors itself to the rocks and grows fifty feet a year up to about seven hundred feet long, feeding entirely off the water around it. Olive brown, the kelp has a thick trunk from which grow files of six or eight long, tapering leaves regularly on either side.

Edible seaweeds are popular in several maritime communities and the Japanese take kelp regularly. Many sailors used to keep pieces of dried kelp to chew during their journeys.

Kelp grows in great abundance off the coast of California and is harvested, dried and turned into tablets, granules or powder to be used as a food mineral supplement for both animals and humans.

Kelp used inland

The late Dr W. A. Price of Cleveland, Ohio studied people living in remote areas to try and determine the cause of tooth decay. He discovered Peruvians who normally lived at altitudes from 12,000 to 16,000 feet carried small bags containing dried kelp which they chewed from time to time. When he enquired why the people traveled so far down to the shoreline to collect the kelp two or three times a year, they said they needed it to "guard the heart."

The composition of kelp

It has been suggested that the composition of the human body and the composition of seven gallons of sea water are the same. It would therefore seem sensible to make use of the excellent nutrition available in the sea by eating fish, seafood, edible mosses and seaweeds, of which kelp is probably the richest and cheapest. The blue-green algae, known as spirulina, that is found on remote freshwater alkaline desert lakes is also a food resource packed with vitamins and minerals.

Kelp analysis produced by G. W. Cavanaugh, the late Professor of Agricultural Chemistry at Cornell University. All figures are percentages:

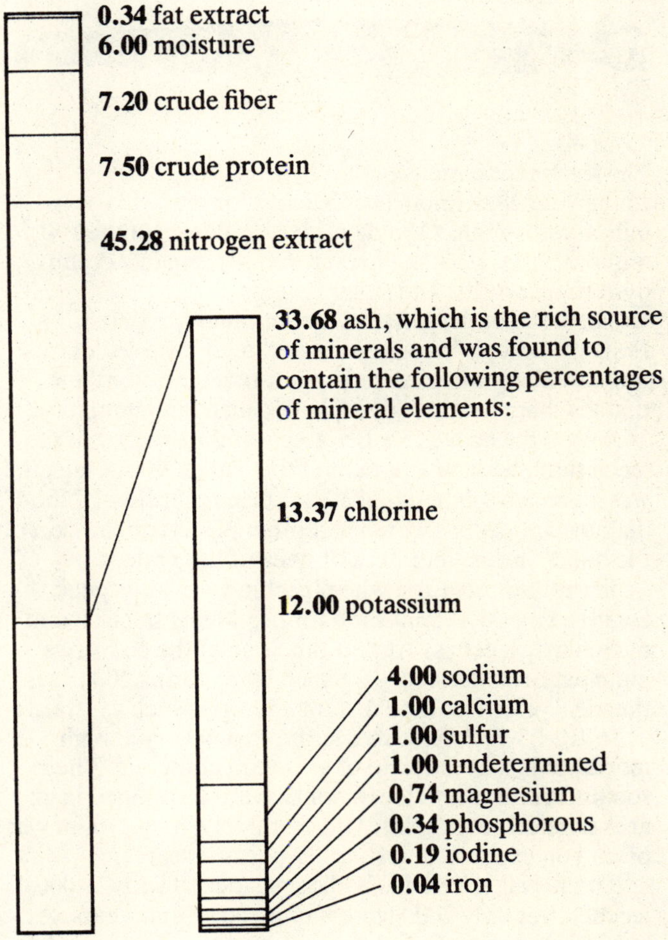

©DIAGRAM

Good red blood

Blood-letting was a standard procedure in many parts of the primitive world, ranging from pricking warts and cutting boils to more magical actions such as scoring the skin of the head to let out the spirits of madness.

Hirudo medicinalis, the grey, German variety and the most common leech, is an aquatic blood-sucking worm which has been used for 2000 years to suck "bad blood" from people with severe fevers. It became so popular in Europe in the early 19th century that its price rose, and it became an endangered species. Now the leech is proving useful once more in certain kinds of modern microsurgery. Although the Hirudines were the most popular, other parasitic species were sometimes used, such as the *Haementeria costata*; however, these were not as effective. When supplies of the *Hirudo medicinalis* ran short, the Hungarian variety, *Hirudo officinalis*, was used.

a The *Hirudo medicinalis* or common leech
b The smaller *Haementaria costata*

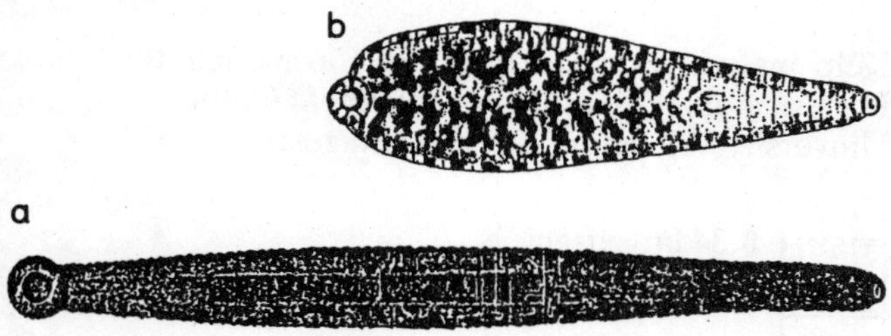

THE LEECH AND LEECHCRAFT
In the 5th century in Europe and Asia, a leech was a physician and leechcraft was the art of healing. Since the parasitic leech had long been in use in India and Egypt, it was named the healer for good reason.

The underside of the leech is grey with black spots, and topside it is black with yellow stripes. It attaches itself with three sharp teeth, which very gently prick the skin. It then secretes a saliva which contains hirudin, a powerful anticoagulant. It takes about half an hour to gorge itself with blood (about a teaspoonful). The leech then detaches itself, or it can be persuaded to leave earlier by rubbing salt on its back.

Bleeding with leeches from a 19th century engraving

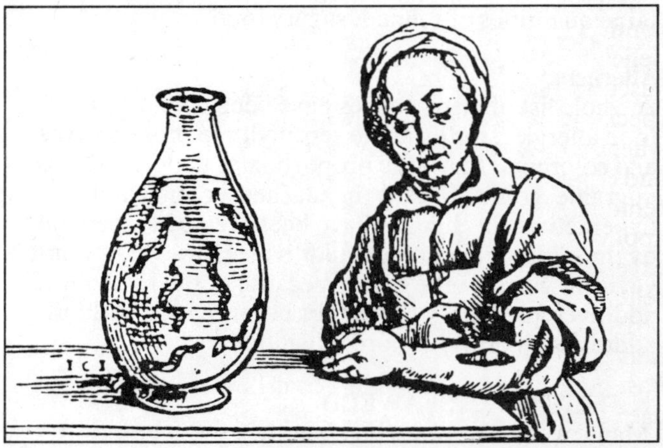

The leech economy
In the year 1827 imports of leeches for medical use in the military hospital at Val de Grâce, in Paris, totalled 30 million. They were the main treatment against typhus, dysentry, enteritis and other fevers.

The head of the hospital was military physician François Joseph Victor Broussais, who believed that these diseases were caused by internal irritations and that leeching would reduce the localized inflammation.

So convinced was Dr Broussais of the efficacy of the leech that every new patient at the Val de Grâce hospital was given a fresh batch of 30 leeches, regardless of the diagnosis. Leeches were most often placed on the skin of the hands, arms, feet, legs or neck of the patient.

In the 19th century, when leeching was at its peak, Sweden gained a reputation for producing the best and most hardy leeches. At that time one of the country's main exports was leeches, which would bring 100 times the local price if sold to distant countries such as Brazil.

In 1834 Swedish leeches suffered a period of high mortality just at the time of a cholera epidemic. Their stocks dwindled and leech ponds were developed in an area outside Stockholm. Unfortunately, no restraint was placed on exports, and supplies became scarcer.

The new leech ponds had been stocked with 25,000 leeches, yet only 2000 were harvested in four years. At that time it was not known that leeches only reach sexual maturity after seven or eight years. A few years later a national inventory of leech stocks was introduced to control exports and prevent another economic disaster.

National stocks went for use by the rich and for export. Local village supplies continued to thrive, as it was cheaper for the poor to buy their leeches from the women who went out to gather them.

Sweden exported a million leeches a year, and countries such as England and Germany would often have to import 100 times more than they could produce themselves. In the 19th century the leech economy was big business in Europe, and the pirating of leech supplies was fairly common. Theft of Swedish leeches by Norwegian pirates strained relationships between the two countries for many years.

The leech-gatherers walked into shallow ponds, pulling the leeches off their legs before they had a chance to get attached. The leeches were then stored under water in batches of 100 in small barrels the women strapped to their waists (see engraving on opposite page).

The first records of the medical use of leeches was in the Benares area of India. Leeches were popular in Ancient Egypt and were mentioned in Greek, Roman and Arabic medical texts. Translations filtered into Europe during the Middle Ages.

In 16th century Europe, the leech had been abandoned in favor of mechanical blood-letting with lancets and artificial leeching tools known as bdellometers, from the Greek *bdella* meaning leech. By the 18th century blood-letting was so common that English physicians were called "leeches," and the word began to acquire its derogatory meaning: physicians charged very high fees for draining a person's blood. How ironic that the common name for this "little healer," the leech, should have come to mean something so despicable.

Many prominent physicians, however, preferred to continue using live leeches because they were more delicate, took less blood and never caused infections or vascular damage. They also learnt how to apply them to specific areas by using a leech-glass to control exactly where the leech would suck. Leechs were very popular and effective for reducing the swelling of black eyes, removing tooth abcesses and many other small applications where the removal of inflammation, pus and excess fluid were indicated. They were invaluable for the relief of pressure after delicate eye operations.

Both rich and poor, the famous and the infamous were familiar with the leech. The French chemist Louis Pasteur (1822–95), who had a brain hemorrhage at the age of 40, was treated by the application of 16 leeches behind one ear. He recovered from the hemorrhage but was paralyzed on his left side.

Today, leeches are being used again by some doctors on bruises and to reduce swelling after delicate microsurgery. For example, in the UK, a London man had his finger re-attached after an accident, and leeches were used to control the build-up of fluids which would otherwise have destroyed the work. In modern surgery, leeches are used only once for one patient and then destroyed, to prevent any infection.

A leech pot for storage

In the Museum for the History of Medicine in Copenhagen, a leech pot can be seen that was still in use in the 1930s.

There was a layer of sand in the bottom of the pot which was filled with water in which the leeches could be stored in a cool cellar for up to six or seven years. A gauze covered the top of the jar, protecting it from ammonia, tobacco smoke and camphor, all of which would affect the leeches adversely. It was the job of the apprentice pharmacists to keep the leeches well-fed . . . by dipping their big toes into the water once a day.

The value of the leech

Why was the leech so popular for so long? It was not only its delicacy and blood-letting efficiency that proved to be so useful. Leeches secrete hirudin, the most potent anticoagulant known to science. Their saliva has also been found to contain 10 other pharmacologically active substances, including hyaluronidase and collagenase, two connective tissue enzymes.

Hirudin itself is a potent antithrombin, inhibiting the enzyme thrombin, so central to the clotting of blood. Thus it has great value as a drug for the treatment of blood disorders where clotting is a danger. As there are no acute side-effects, hirudin has some advantages over heparin, which is currently used to prevent clotting, for example of blood samples.

Unfortunately, there is now a great shortage of medicinal leeches, so a process for cloning hirudin by means of a synthetic gene is under investigation, but this would not be as rich a substance as the naturally occurring hirudin with its 10 other pharmacologically active substances. Consequently, leech-farms have been set up. One in Wales breeds on a large scale and is expected to produce enough natural hirudin to combine with the use of cloned hirudin.

Yorkshire women gather leeches, 1814

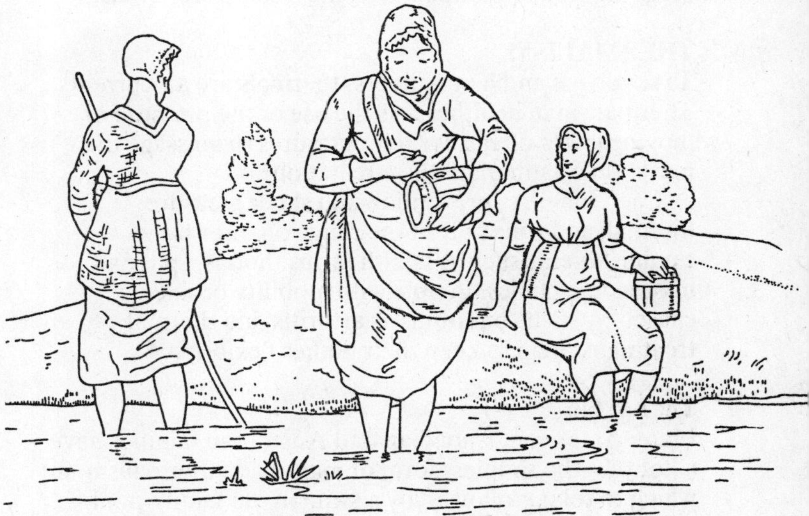

Sweat it out

Most primitive communities took part in communal sweats for cleansing and healing, for spiritual fitness and for sheer pleasure. The North American Indian sweat lodge, the Roman sudatorium, the Ethiopian felwaha, the Turkish hamman and the Finnish sauna, were all designed to raise a sweat.

COMMUNAL SWEATING

The sweat lodge

This was a closed tepee with a central pile of pre-heated stones round which crowded anything from 20 to 100 people. The more people there were, the hotter the lodge would become, since the heat-power of an average human being is half a kilowatt. After an hour or two in the sweat lodge, during which some swaying and chanting would take place, there would be a quick dip in a nearby lake or stream, or even a roll in dew-laden grass, followed by a vigorous rub-down.

The sudatorium

The Romans were fond of luxuriating in communal bathing pools. Lined with attractive tiles and filled with running water from a local spring, the pool was surrounded by a colonnade and high wall for privacy and shelter from the hot sun.

Sudatoria were smaller, fully enclosed, baths of water kept hot by an underfloor heating system. Steam was produced by pouring water over heated stones. After the sweat, people would plunge into the larger pool. The Turkish bath was designed in a similar way.

The sauna

This is an old Finnish ritual during which a few people sit naked in a wooden bath-house, built on the edge of a lake.

Steam at 212°F (100°C) is made by throwing cold water over the heated stones. After a good sweat has been raised, circulation is also stimulated by beating the skin with birch twigs and finally there is a plunge into the icy waters of the lake. The original sauna was a much more vigorous treatment than the other sweat baths.

THERMALISM

To skydivers and hang-gliders, thermals are air currents. Thermalism in healthcare is the use of the pressure of moving water of various temperatures to massage the muscles and stimulate the circulation.

Used for cure, prevention and sheer pleasure, thermalism forms part of the range on offer by establishments such as health farms, hotels, spas and nature cure clinics. People with mobility problems caused by such conditions as arthritis find thermal treatments help to keep their bodies flexible.

The hot tub

Many American, Canadian and Australian families have a hot tub, the simplest form of man-made thermalism, in which to relax, followed by a swim in the family pool. Located indoors or outdoors, a wooden tub is part filled with water maintained at a level above body temperature. Several people can sit on an underwater bench and relax. Often the water is circulated through underwater jets which gently massage the body. Many baths and tubs use water jets and swirls, such as the Jacuzzi and the whirlpool.

Balneology

This the therapeutic use of natural spring waters or mineral waters, so-called because they contain inorganic salts such as chlorides and carbonates. Spring water may be naturally hot or cold.

European spa towns are those that were developed where natural springs were available. The ancient city of Bath, in England, has had public mineral baths since Roman times. Research has shown that it is probable that some minerals can be absorbed directly through the skin. Visitors would also drink the mineral water while relaxing after bathing.

Hungarian spas

In Hungary there are more than 450 thermal springs many of which are very hot, even in winter. For example, the hot lake at Héviz is usually above 75°F (24°C) in the coldest winter. The waters of this lake are renewed every twenty-four hours directly from a powerful natural spring. The slightly radioactive and sulfurous water is enjoyed by many who stay at expensive health hotels. It is also commonplace to see ordinary people relaxing in public spa baths, playing chess on a floating cork board.

THERMALISM IN ETHIOPIA

Ethiopia is situated in the African Rift Valley, an area of historic volcanic activity that now has some of the world's most spectacular hot springs.

Traditional Ethiopian medicine included herbalism, bleeding, cupping, cautery and a variety of thermal cures using these volcanic springs. Rheumatism, skin diseases, leprosy and venereal diseases were all said to be cured by regular thermal bathing.

It was also a belief that spring water was of divine origin, so miracle cures for serious terminal conditions were sought. The outstanding feature of all thermal baths in Ethiopia was their high temperature. They were known as felwaha meaning boiling water. Anything from 120 to 140°F (49 to 60°C) was common.

Patients used to stay at the baths for several days, drinking the spring water mixed with honey and linseed, which produced copious sweating, an important aspect of the treatment.

People with different diseases were segregated: there was the leprosy pool, the scrofula pool, the rheumatism pool and there was always a pool reserved for ordinary, healthy bathers.

Most of the treatment pools were covered with straw and bamboo thatch, which protected the bathers from too much direct sunlight and enclosed the heat, producing steam which also induced sweating.

A European 19th century traveler once described his first experience of entering a thermal bath as ". . . a plunge into darkness and a cauldron of almost boiling water." He describes how he gasped, partly from the shock of the heat and partly from the steamy, sulfurous fumes. After a while he felt very relaxed and was able to become completely submerged.

The baths were pools about ten feet in diameter and 2½ feet deep, surrounded by straw seats just above the water level where people could sit and sweat. The aim was to remain there for at least an hour. As many as 40 people could be crowded into one bath and there would be a queue of hundreds waiting outside.

The Emperor Tewodros II (1855–1868) had a large thermal pool built at Wanzagay which was supplied by a strongly gushing jet of sulfurous hot water. The pool, about 30 feet in diameter and four feet deep, was used daily by Tewodros' successor, Yohannes IV, to relieve the rheumatism from which he suffered.

THALASSOTHERAPY

From the Greek word, *thalassa*, meaning sea, thalassotherapy is the tonic effect of time spent in the sea or in sea water.

External sores, wounds, skin burns and skin ulcers all benefit from regular bathing in the sea, providing the seawater is not seriously polluted. The combined effect of water massage and the salt and other minerals is most beneficial.

Many seaside towns built hotels where people could take treatments using sea water. The Dead Sea has such a high concentration of salt that it is possible to sit in it. Some of the most modern thalassotherapy centers have recently been built along the French coast and are spreading across the Atlantic.

Offering a biomarine fitness course, there are such delights as the "douche affusion," a warm, seawater shower and combined almond oil hand massage done while the client lies on a white waterproof mattress.

Bathing in a brown algae bath of bubbling hot water and hosepipe massages are encouraged daily. Foot care includes walking in pools lined with tiny pebbles and the main pool is like a slice of the sea itself, except that it is filtered seawater pumped from a mile out and kept at a constant warm temperature. The waves are strong enough to swim against to improve cardio-respiratory capacity.

Aquatic exercises, open-air hot pools, several Jacuzzi, a high-tech gym and jogging on the beach leave clients with healthy appetites which are fed with French health food of the highest class. Our ancestors who splashed in jungle pools, mountain lakes, mud-lined rivers and coastal seas had all the benefits of thalassotherapy, without the cost, although they faced some natural dangers.

MUD BATHS

The modern mud bath involves being covered all over with a layer of hot, grey sea mud, brown river mud or even being painted with a koalin paste, and then being wrapped to gently "cook" in aluminum or tin foil. As a skin cleanser, there is nothing like it.

Cosmetic mud face-packs that come in a packet are mild compared with complete body bath of hot mud, as fashionable ladies were aware in the 18th and 19th centuries. Dr James Graham, who invented the "Celestial Bed" for infertile couples, also did a brisk in mud baths. The bath-house was kept warm while several ladies stood in holes in the ground, which were lined with tiles. Hot mud was then dropped into the hole. Some holes contained seats so that the clients could sit down and be covered to the shoulders in the mud.

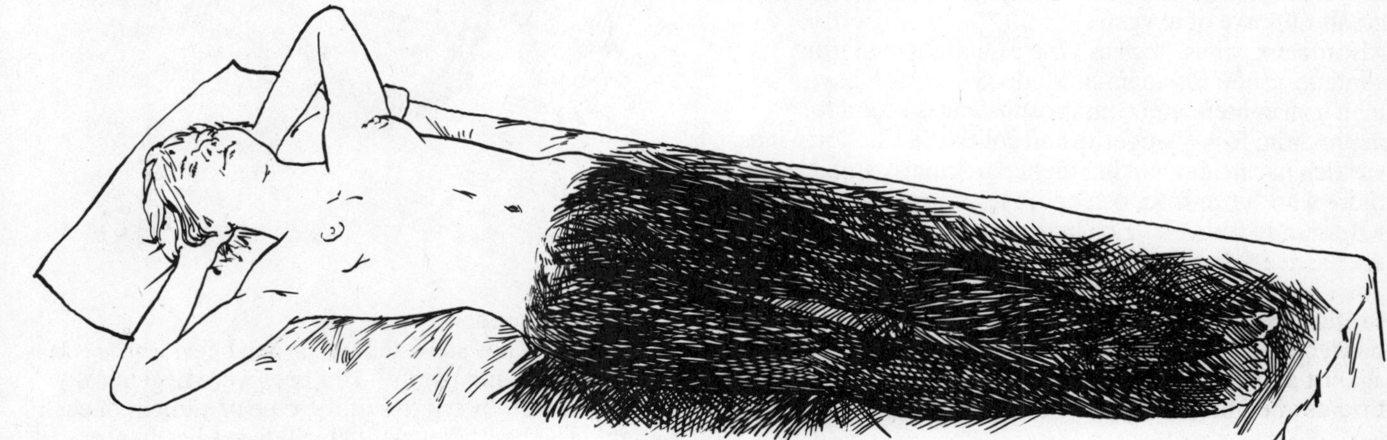

Nectar of the gods

In Greek and Roman myths, nectar was the name given to wines drunk by the immortals. It is also the sweet substance collected by bees from flowers to make honey. Wine, honey and other food and drink have been used throughout the ages as pleasurable tonics to ensure continued health or therapeutic remedies when illness struck. Most often they were only available to people in the higher social orders, which may have contributed to their image as something exotic and even magical.

HONEY

Manufactured by bees who are very selective about the flowers they use, honey is recommended in place of refined sugars and maple syrup. Honey contains traces of elements we need in small quantities, such as copper, manganese, silica and aluminum. Being partly pre-digested by the bee, honey is excellent for digestive problems and is an instant energy source. Some pollen honey contains vitamin C and other vitamins.

Many bacteria cannot live in the presence of honey because the potassium contained in it dries out moisture from them and they die. This may be why honey has been used, for at least 2000 years, as a salve for wounds, particularly for skin ulcers that are vulnerable to infection and harsh antiseptics.

WINES

The disciples of the Greek medical philosopher Hippocrates regarded wines as the first medical aid and many 17th century French hospitals, such as Trousseau and Dieu, gave their names to the wines they had produced for medication. Wine was also used to sterilize wounds. Whisky and rum have been put to similar uses.

Grapes and their wines

In general the grape contains 80% water, a quantity of grape sugars and many minerals such as magnesium, calcium, sodium, potassium, glucides, phosphates, proteins, tannoids, phenols, some vitamins and various anti-bacterial substances. Wine is a food, a medicine and a pleasure. Some examples of French wines are given here.

- Champagnes contain potassium tartrate which aids the suppleness of the muscles. Champagne also enables a greater uptake of oxygen.
- Bordeaux wines, such as Graves, have a high iron content, useful for anemia. Médoc wines also have a high iron content and contain substances useful for depression, loss of appetite and colitis. St Emilion wines are rich in calcium making them particularly suitable for those who suffer from osteoporosis or brittle bones.
- Burgundy wines are rich in iron and other minerals and are particularly recommended for older people. Their potassium content is good for low blood pressure and cardiac insufficiency. High in calories, they help to put on weight. The tannin in young Beaujolais is useful against diarrhea and its antibiotic effect is good for sore throats and mild chest colds.

The grape cure

Mono-diets are an alternative to total fasting and the grape cure is an example of one of them. First recommended by Dr Johannes Budwig in South Africa, where grapes grow in abundance, the grape diet was used by a colleague, Basil Shackleton, who lived on it for over 50 days. His experience was described in a Californian publication in 1971. He tells of how an abscess on his only kidney came away spontaneously after only 23 days on an exclusive diet of grapes. The problem was one that conventional medicine had failed to solve. In his case the grape cure was life-saving, as he had already lost his other kidney.

MEDICATED BEE VENOM THERAPY

Another treatment available primarily to the rich and famous in more modern times was a therapy that involved injections of medicated bee venom, the injection being given by the bee sting.

Until the late 1980s, Dr Julia Owen had a private medical practice in Kent, England treating people very successfully with the bee venom from specially bred strains of bee.

Dr Owen inherited the knowledge and skills of medicated bee venom therapy through six generations of doctors in her Austrian family and improved upon the techniques, as had those before her.

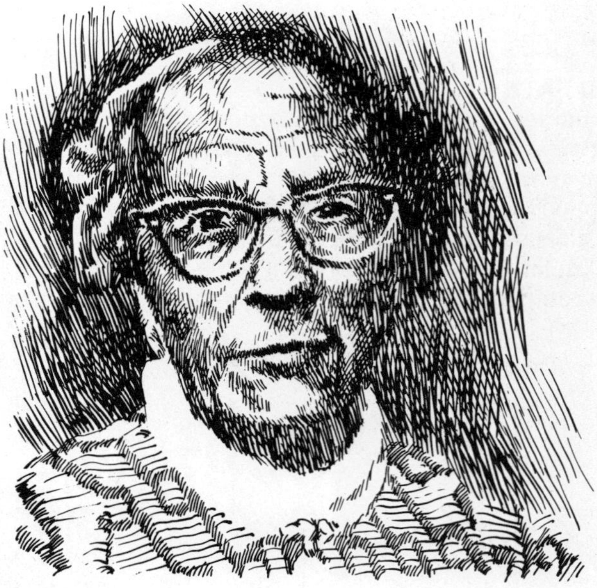

Dr Julia Owen

Preparing the venom

Dr Owen did not use ordinary garden bees, whose stings are dangerous and painful. Her bees were hygienically bred and carefully fed to suit the type of ailment of each patient. The bee's diet would include medicaments

GINSENG
Ginseng grows in Korea and Eastern Asia, and similar varieties grow in Japan, Nepal, the Himalayas of India and in North America. *Panax ginseng* is a rare shrub of the *Araliaceae* family that grows in secluded forests; the root takes four to seven years to mature. The branched, fleshy white root, covered with fibrous tendrils often looks like a person with arms and legs, hence the Chinese name for it means man-plant.

History of ginseng
Three thousand years ago the Chinese regarded the root of *Panax ginseng* as a magical healer. Emperor Shen Nung first wrote about its medicinal uses in his *Materia Medica* and he placed it as the most important potent herb. He claimed it as a tonic for the five viscera that quietened the animal spirits, strengthened the soul, dispelled fears, expelled evil, brightened the eyes, opened the heart and brought understanding. Taken over a long period, it would also stimulate the body and lengthen life; hence ginseng is often called the root of life.

So powerful was the effect of ginseng that the Chinese and the Tartars fought wars over the territory where it grew. There is a long mythology about ginseng, such as the story of the Jesuit missionary, Father Jartoux, who, fatigued and at death's door in 1714, was given a root of ginseng to suck and within an hour was fit to travel again. American ginseng is a herb of the same species, *Panax quinquefolium*, the five-fingered root.

Ginseng today
Modern research has found ginseng to have a positive effect upon the cerebral cortex of the central nervous system. It has a cumulative effect and is excellent to fight fatigue, depression and general debilitation at any age. Tests have not found any harmful effects.

Ginseng is available as tablets, in powder form and as root pieces. Its price depends on its size, age and shape. A gram twice a day for a month is the usual dose as a tonic for the over 40s. A half to one gram a day could be taken over a much longer period to combat fatigue in older people.

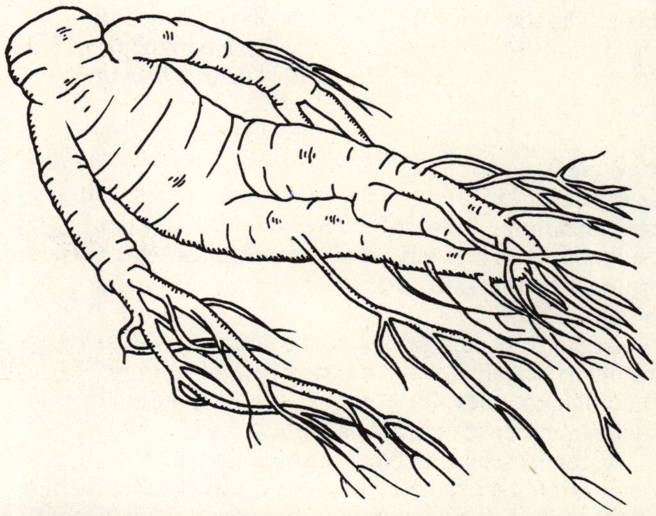

about which she would never reveal any details, except that she would ferment the feeds into a liquid form.

Since each patient was treated with bee stings from bees specially fed, the treatments, which could last from between three weeks to three years, required a large number of bees.

The bees she used did not produce honey or large colonies and selection for therapeutic use had to be done carefully so as not to frighten each colony from which perhaps a thousand bees would be used. Alarm among the bees would lead to their killing the queen bee in their efforts to protect her. Loss of the queen would have meant loss of the bee strain.

Giving the therapy
The bee sting was applied by pinching the bee behind its head, to control it as it was applied to the patient. It stung the patient who would feel very little pain and the bee would die immediately after losing its sting.

Dr Owen treated several famous people including the King of Italy, Professor Pirani the electronics expert, Rigo Tovar, member of one of Mexico's leading pop groups, and Professor, later President, Benes of Czechoslovakia.

She treated ankylosis, osteo- and rheumatoid arthritis, asthma, dermatitis, diabetes, eczema, psoriasis and was especially successful treating deafness and blindness due to retinal degeneration or resulting from childhood scarlet fever or measles. Retinitis pigmentosa, a chronic hereditary complaint common in Latin America, was also responsive.

Standard diagnostic techniques were used, such as blood and urine tests and X-rays when appropriate. The demands made on Dr Owen became so great that she had to restrict her work to those suffering from asthma, deafness and blindness, which she chose because she was able to cure these ailments completely.

A GENERAL TONIC
Popular among medieval kings and later among people who worked in hot, humid conditions in factories in the late 19th and early 20th centuries, this recipe is still drunk as a tonic.
1 pint port wine
1 pint old beer
1 pint black beer (stout)
1 pint boiling water
1lb brown sugar
Mix together and bottle.
Drink a glass when you feel fatigued.

New life for old

The Ancient Egyptians mummified their kings and queens, and placed them inside tombs together with supplies of gold, jewelry, tools, linen and such personal effects as they would need in the next life.

The belief in another life to be enjoyed after death was common among ancient civilizations and some form of reincarnation or spiritual life after death is the belief basic to almost all the world's religious systems. A modern atheist, lacking any such belief, may arrange to have his ailing body packed away in the deep freeze of a cryonic institute, awaiting a future when medical science has found a cure.

However, rejuvenation in this life has always been the hope of most people. Above the entrance to their hospitals, the Ancient Greeks displayed words of inspiration which, translated, read: "No man leaves here except that he is cured." No doubt incurables were never admitted.

New parts

A rejuvenating effect has been claimed for the cell revitalization therapy of the Swiss researcher Paul Neihams, which involves the transplantation of cells from newborn lambs to intra-muscular sites in the human body.

Organ transplantations, while giving new life to the receiver, usually depend on the death of a donor, although a kidney, for example, can be donated from a living member of a patient's family.

Recent research in burns units and surgical departments specializing in skin-grafting has found that severe burns and other wounds, such as varicose ulcers, so deep that they are resistant to grafting, were able to grow new skin when treated with tissue from an afterbirth. This does no harm to anyone and makes use of tissue that is usually thrown away after the umbilical cord has been cut.

It is perhaps not surprising to discover that good use of the afterbirth has been made by several primitive societies, sometimes to eat, sometimes in medicines, but more often as a temporary poultice for open wounds. Here are some more examples of attempts to rejuvenate by natural methods.

LET THERE BE LIGHT

Water, air, fire (warmth and light) and earth (food) have long been the four basic elements regarded as vital to life. Color therapists have always promoted light, not only as a cure but as an essential to good health and there is some evidence that sun-worshippers of the ancient world knew that certain rays of the sun were more beneficial than others for some conditions.

Now the scientific world has caught up with magical primitive and alternative methods. At the 1990 meeting of the American Association for the Advancement of Science, neurological researchers at the University of Texas Health Science Center announced that light, in particular from the blue end of the spectrum, can heal a range of conditions, such as depression, loss of sex drive, low sperm count, jet lag, anorexia nervosa, poor ovulation and myalgic encephalomyelitis (ME) and other conditions affecting the immune system.

NATURAL VISION THERAPY

Dr William H. Bates (1860–1931) was a prominent New York eye specialist who taught in the Post Graduate Medical School when the current theory was that vision defects were caused by deterioration of the lens and were therefore irreversible.

Bates concluded from his examinations of thousands of eyes that accommodation, i.e. the ability to focus near or far, was not a function of the lens but of the eye muscles and he believed that, like any other muscle, they could be retrained.

The methods Bates used began with relaxation and his results showed that the exercises corrected or partly eased the following defects:

myopia, having difficuty with distant vision;
hypermetropia, difficulty with near and far vision;
astigmatism, distorted vision;
strabismus, squinting;
presbyopia, near-sight difficulties in old age.

Some of the basic Bates exercises

1 Palming: placing the palms over the closed eyes to exclude all light, without pressure, or an eye-mask can be used. This rests and relaxes the eyes.
2 Swinging: to counteract staring, which puts enormous strain on the eyes. Swinging the whole body by partly rotating from side to side is the most effective. The aim is to allow the eyes to remain still and the focus to relax and sweep across the scene without stopping and staring.
3 Blinking: this clarifies vision. The normal eye blinks frequently and gently, so the habit of blinking is encouraged.
4 Sunlight: two or three minutes spent lying in the sun with eyes closed and head slowly moving from side to side. Never look directly at the sun, nor lie with head still. After, spend some time palming. If you intend to continue sunbathing, cover the eyes completely with anything that totally excludes light and is cool. Use sunglasses that have a proper filter.
5 Imagination: Bates encouraged all his patients to practice using their imagination and their memory, since impairment of either adds imperfections to the visual image.

Time and patience are required to gain benefit from Bates' methods. One famous patient was Aldous Huxley, whose sight had been so defective in his first twenty-five years that he could hardly read, even with spectacles. Using the Bates method, he regained his sight and dispensed with spectacles.

Head of the research team, Professor Russel Reiter, claimed that his team had already had success in treating people, using the simple device of a powerful lamp that can be plugged into an electrical circuit and used to sit under for a while.

It has been found that the level of the light-sensitive hormone melatonin in the body is directly related to health. Produced by the pineal gland, high levels of melatonin are produced in darkness, and melatonin has a depressive effect on body functions. When there is exposure to good light, the melatonin levels drop and the body functions improve. Reiter claims that conditions have improved after a few days treatment with the lamp.

GENETIC ENGINEERING

Mention should be made of the techniques that are about to make the human race face the possibility of having a designer-body. When the thousands of human characteristics have all been correctly matched with their genetic position on the DNA protein chains that make up the human chromosomes, it may become possible to select exactly which characteristics are desired.

While the possibility of saving a fertilized egg, and therefore the future fully-grown person, from a deforming or debilitating gene, seems desirable, the question of eugenics raises its potentially ugly head once more. The super-pig and the designer-cow are already with us; so are all the problems they are bringing with them. Do we want a world full of supermen and superwomen who all behave predictably and are perfect in every respect?

The possibility of cloning, i.e. reproducing an exact copy of a living entity by asexual reproduction is commonplace in the world of horticulture. The idea of a human clone, not an identical twin, but an exact repeat of a person may have some attraction to those who would have liked there to be another Elvis. Whether or not it is natural or sensible to engineer genetic clones or genetic perfections are matters to be examined carefully.

JOGGING AND FLOGGING

In 1976 Larry Lewis, a retired waiter, celebrated his 106th birthday by jogging as usual. His daily run was the 6.7 miles around the Golden Gate Park in San Francisco. Jogging has been a life-saver for many people who suffered from heart attacks. The regular exercise has rebuilt the strength and suppleness of cardiac muscles and contributed to general rejuvenation. One of the original promoters of jogging was Arthur Lydiard, the New Zealander who used to run in marathons. He claimed that jogging also reduced fat deposits in the blood and was one of the best forms of relaxed, unpaced running. For those who suffer from knee problems due to too much heavy jogging on hard pavements, regular swimming has a similar rejuvenating effect.

A good beating

In some medieval communities, flogging was part of the curative process. Used on younger people who suffered from chronic diseases or incapacitating ailments, the patient was first submerged in a nearby river, then chased, to make him run, and beaten with twigs by several adults. The dipping, running and flogging was repeated several times, until the patient was exhausted. Then he was rubbed all over, wrapped in warm, clean cloths and carried back to his bed to rest and finally recuperate from the illness. The intention during this ritual was to chase away the evil spirits that were causing the illness.

THE SNAKE OF LIFE

The life-creating sexual energy, called the Kundalini in Indian Tantric religion, is always represented as two intertwined snakes that make the continuous figure of eight.

The snake on the caduceus carried by the mythical Greek god, Mercury, is the symbol of life-saving medicine, but there is an older legend that tells why the snake is the symbol of life.

A child was ill and weak with a fever. A bowl of fresh goat's milk was brought to tempt the child to drink but he refused. While the bowl was standing a snake came and drank from it. The doctor, desperate to seize any opportunity to raise the parents' flagging faith, told them it was an omen. If the gods were pleased with them, the snake's milk mixed with the goat's milk would cure their child.

Whatever the reason, the child recovered shortly after drinking the milk and thereafter the snake became a symbol of life-giving medicine.

It is human contrariness that the snake also has acquired wicked, though not always evil, associations.

The Kundalini snake symbol

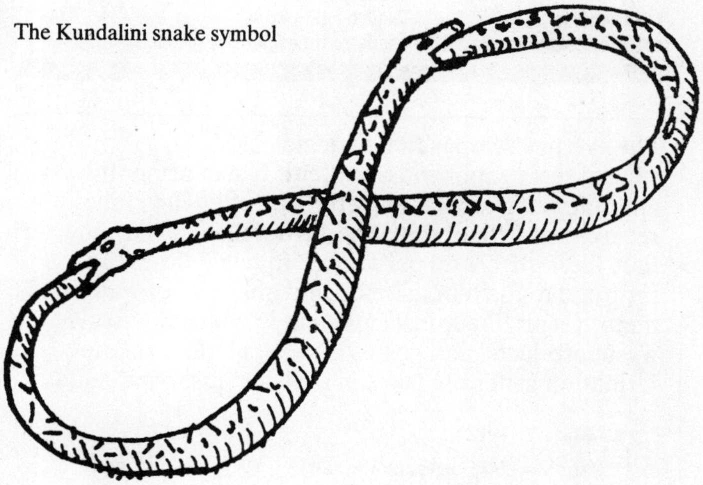

REFERENCE: See **Section Seven: The best of both worlds** (pp.152–153) for more information about ME, which is also known as Chronic Fatigue syndrome or Seasonal Affective Disorder.

Water of life

Water is as crucial to life as oxygen: 70% of the normal body weight is made up of water which is lost during urination, excretion, breathing and sweating and is replaced by drinks and food containing water. If the volume of water lost during one day was not replaced, the body would be in trouble and after three days without water most people would die.

The body's water supply

An area in the central base of the brain known as the hypothalamus controls the supply of water and several other body functions, such as appetite, sex drive, aggression and body temperature. The hypothalamus monitors conditions in the body and stimulates the nearby pituitary gland to produce hormonal messengers to correct any imbalances.

For example, when the water content of the body falls, the hypothalamus registers an increased salt concentration, resulting in thirst, and the kidneys are also instructed to reabsorb water that would otherwise be evacuated as urine. When the body is accumulating too much water, the hypothalamus registers a reduced salt level and the kidneys begin to send more urine to the bladder.

Distribution of water as body fluid

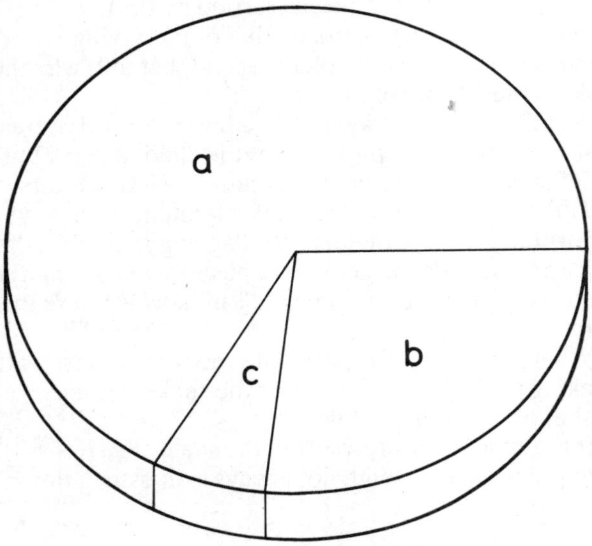

Total water content 45 liters (9.9 gallons)
a Cells contain 30 litres (6.6 gallons)
b 12 liters in between the cells (2.64 gallons)
c 3 liters circulating in the bloodstream as plasma (0.66 gallons)

Water leaving the body

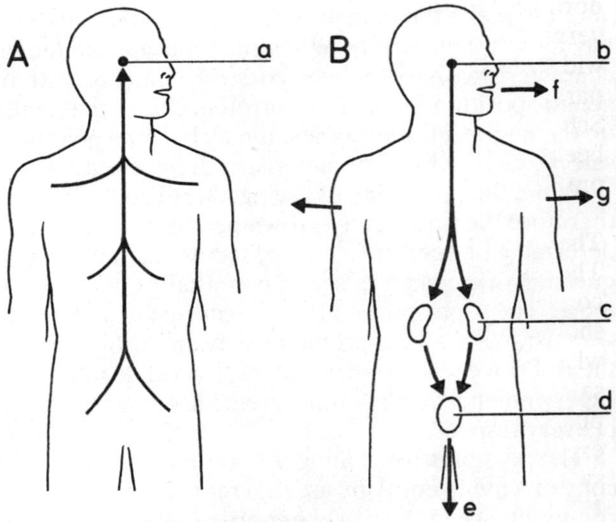

A Hypothalamus monitors body fluids
a Hypothalamus
B Water loss from body
b Pituitary stimulated by hypothalamus
c Kidneys instructed by pituitary
d Bladder stores urine
e Urination **f** Breathing out **g** Sweating

The average composition of urine

The largest proportion of water is lost in urine, the actual amount being regulated by the kidneys. The kidneys receive one fifth of the output from the heart from which they filter off 120 ml per minute for cleaning; 119 ml is returned to the bloodstream and only 1 ml of water per minute is retained, just sufficient in which to dissolve the waste products, and passes into the bladder as urine. Urination generally takes place when just over half a liter (1 pint) of urine has collected in the bladder.

Except for the urine, which is normally acidic, the body fluids are slightly alkaline. It is another job of the kidneys to adjust this acid/alkaline balance. One of the first indications of excessive stress, ill-health or a lack of the essential tissue salts is when the acidity of the urine changes and remains alkaline for long periods, particularly first thing in a morning and before meals.

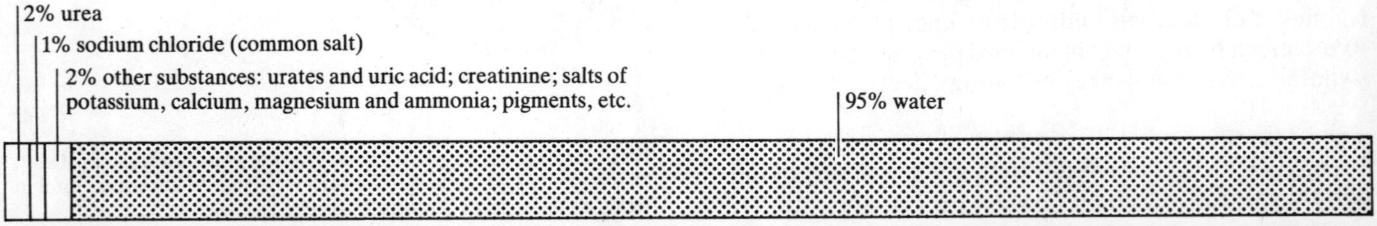

BIOCHEMICS

In the mid-19th century, the German Dr Wilhelm H. Schuessler devised a system of treatment using the discovery that twelve chemical salts (electrolytes) were common to all cremated bodies. It is a property of electrolytes that they do not burn or melt.

Schuessler set about discovering which salt was essential to the maintenance of which life process. He claimed that every disease-state could be attacked by the use of the appropriate tissue salt. It has since been confirmed by modern scientific research that these tissue salts do exist in the living body and are essential to its well-being.

In many ways Biochemics is a branch of homeopathy, since the salts are prepared in ways similar to homeopathic medicines and are taken in similar doses to normalize the imbalances in the body. However, they are very commonly taken as symptom-relievers and are widely available in America, Europe and many other parts of the world as first-aid home remedies. Since Scheussler's time, some thirty other trace elements have been identified and are also used by contemporary practitioners.

The twelve Biochemic tissue salts

The numbers and abbreviated names are those in common use. The main function of each tissue salt is shown, followed by some examples of symptoms for which it might be used. Anyone wishing to use tissue salts should refer to the full instructions enclosed with purchases. For serious disorders and in case of doubt, an experienced practitioner should be consulted as similar symptoms often have different causes.

1 Calcium fluoride CALC.FLUOR.
Maintains elasticity of tissues. Good for bad circulation, varicose veins, piles, tooth enamel.

2 Calcium phosphate CALC.PHOS.
Essential to the formation of bones, teeth and gastric juices. Good for indigestion, chilblains and teething.

3 Calcium sulfate CALC.SULF.
Purifies the blood. Good for acne, pimples, sores, wounds that are slow to heal and catarrh.

4 Iron phosphate FERR.PHOS.
Essential to the oxygenation of the blood. Good for coughs, colds, fevers, congestion and inflammation.

5 Potassium chloride KALI. MUR.
Keeps the blood in good condition. Good for coughs, colds, bronchitis, tonsilitis, measles and chickenpox.

6 Potassium phosphate KALI.PHOS.
Nutrient essential to nerves. Good for stress, worry, headaches, nervous indigestion and nervous headaches.

7 Potassium sulfate KALI. SULF.
Oxygenates tissue cells. Good for skin complaints, catarrh, loss of hair, poor nails and stuffiness.

8 Magnesium phosphate MAG.PHOS.
The nerve stabilizer. Good for cramp, neuralgia, sharp pains, sciatica, spasms, hiccups and menstrual pains.

9 Sodium chloride NAT.MUR.
Distributor of water. Good for loss of taste or smell, tears, constipation, drowsiness, muscular weakness.

10 Sodium phosphate NAT.PHOS.
Acid neutralizer. Good for acidity of blood, gastric problems, heartburn, rheumatism, lumbago, fibrositis.

11 Sodium sulfate NAT.SULPH.
Eliminator of excess water. Good for liver problems, biliousness, influenza, problems during humid weather.

12 Silicic oxide SILICA
Conditioner, cleanser and stimulator. Good for brittle nails, dull hair, bad cases of body odor and boils.

Combination remedies

There are 18 combination remedies consisting of three to five of the tissue salts. These are likely to be more useful, since none of the tissue salts operates in isolation in the body. The combination remedies are lettered from A to S and are sold for very specific ailments, for example,
for migraine and nervous headaches: Combination 'F'
for backache and allied pains: Combination 'G'
for hayfever: Combination 'H'
for infant's teething pains: Combination 'R'
for stomach upsets: Combination 'S'

Electrolytes

The body fluid contains many electrolytes. These are salts which, when dissolved in water, split into their constituent ions, each with a positive or a negative charge. Sodium, potassium, calcium, phosphate, chloride and bicarbonate are the ions found in largest quantities in the body fluids, both in the cells and outside them.

Ions form when elements combine. For example, when the sodium element combines with the chlorine element to form sodium chloride, sodium loses an electron to chlorine, leaving the sodium ion with a positive charge and the chlorine ion with a negative charge. Electrolytes are, therefore, good conductors of electricity.

Ions can move freely in or out of the cells, depending on the concentration of ions already present. In normal circumstances, for example, there is a higher concentration of potassium ions inside the cells and of sodium ions outside the cells.

The body contains a large number of electrolytes, sometimes called tissue salts or minerals. The Biochemic method of treating disease is based on the use of the twelve most common tissue salts.

REFERENCE. For more information about acid/alkaline balance, refer to **Section Six: Natural remedies** (pp.138–139). For information about homeopathy, see **Section Six: Homeopathic remedies** (pp.134–135).

Inheritance or environment?

It has long been known that certain disabilities and physical strengths and weaknesses are inherited but the idea that there may be other predisposing factors to diseases is growing.

Disposition factors

The most obvious predisposition toward any disease is through genetic inheritance. For example, hemophilia, a condition in which the blood cannot clot, is carried genetically through females from one generation to the next and affects only male offspring.

Other disposition factors are due to upbringing (e.g. poor nutrition), conditions in the environment (e.g. long-term pollution) and the outlook of the person concerned.

Indirect pollution

The effect of long-term direct contact with pollutants such as gasoline fumes, cigarette smoking or skin contact with certain chemicals has always been of concern. However, the effects of indirect contact are coming to light, for example, the effect of pesticides on the food chain, of animal feeds and animal antibiotics on meat and of chemical waste on fish.

Inherited pollution

Recent studies in several countries have revealed that the children of some radiation workers have a greater risk of contracting leukemia than do children in the population at large. The parents involved are men who have received what has been called an "acceptable level" of radiation over a period of time. It has also been found that the risk is lower for men who have been exposed to a high dose, but only over a very short time.

Optimism is a healer

In the 1960s, Maxwell Maltz, an American skin-graft surgeon, was puzzled as to why some of the people who had suffered great disfigurement in accidents recovered quickly and others didn't.

He found that patients behaved according to what they believed to be true. Badly disfigured people who believed in themselves and were optimistic about their future were successful, and people who had no self-respect and only wanted to cling to things as they used to be before the accident, failed to recover, even when no disfigurement remained.

THE INVADERS

Foreign substances entering the body are greeted with a variety of responses from the body. Most foods are welcomed, digested and used. The reaction to some drugs, such as alcohol, throws the body temporarily off-balance, and it takes some time to recover.

The invasion of foreign proteins, such as the young tissues from animals introduced during the cellular therapy developed by the Swiss doctor Paul Niehans in the 1960s, causes the body's connective tissues to react. These tissues, known as the reticuloendothelial system (RES), act as a protective lining, attack invaders and stimulate the body's growth and anti-growth systems which in turn keep the aging process at bay.

Keeping the connective tissues in good shape is therefore important. Movement and exercise are essential for this, since when the body is in action, the small blood capillaries that serve these tissues are kept active. When the body is inactive, these small capillaries tend to shrivel and become useless, affecting the blood supply to the tissues and the skin.

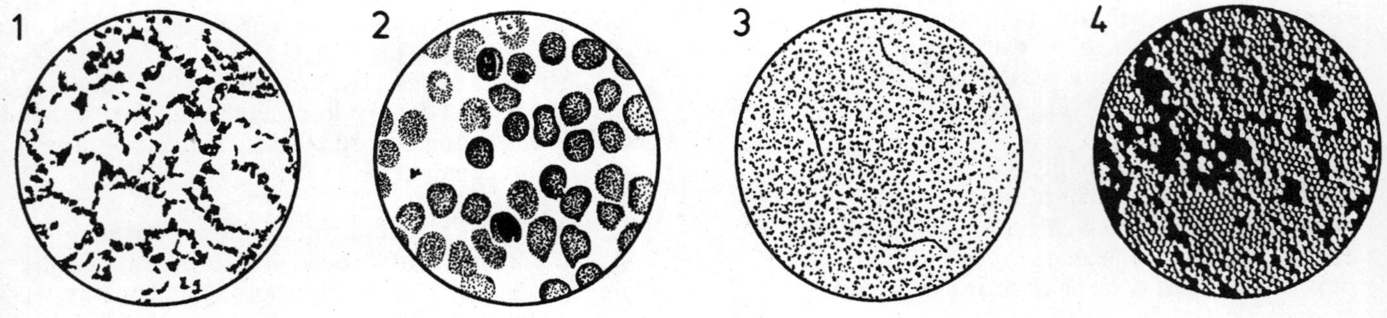

VISUALIZATION

The purpose is to train the brain to want to stimulate the body into postive action.

Like riding a bicycle, visualizations should be of actions that have a pleasurable direction. An immobile bicycle cannot even stand up for itself, but a bicycle in action keeps its balance by moving forwards.

Without a rider, a bicycle can move forwards, keeping its balance without falling over. A rider who believes he is going to fall off will do so. So the patient is asked to push his brain into action and let it keep its own balance.

Visualization of direct attack

Patients are asked to close their eyes and imagine the scene inside their bodies. The diseased situation is described and they have to imagine, for example, their own cells fighting the virus invaders and destroying them.

Visualization of the end result

People are encouraged to imagine what they will do when they are better and to imagine themselves feeling full of energy, singing, dancing or climbing a hill without any problem. Imagining the wind in their hair, the sun on their faces and the glow of their own bodies as they actively take part in their favorite activity helps the person to believe in himself and his own future. Looking forward, not backwards, is encouraged.

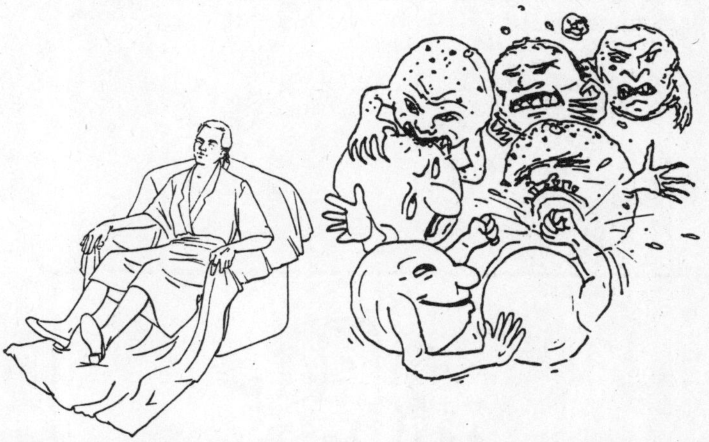

A patient visualizes the battle with virus invaders

The invading viruses

A virus is a submicroscopic organism that consists of a central core of nucleic acids enclosed in a shell-like protein. In this state it remains inert and can exist in animals, plants and the human body for years.

If a weakness enables one virus to invade a cell, then it will disrupt the cell's DNA, and use this genetic protein to reproduce itself.

A healthy body reacts with a sequence of responses, including producing an anti-viral protein known as interferon, which prevents the viral growth from spreading. If a person has inherited genetic tendency toward a particular disease, it may still be avoided by healthy living and a positive, optimistic outlook. Then, even if the virus does get a hold, the recovery is more likely to be quick and complete.

Viruses cause many diseases, including influenza, the common cold, chickenpox, hepatitis, herpes, shingles, measles, mumps, smallpox, typhus, yellow fever and several forms of cancer.

The attempt to synthesize effective anti-viral drugs has so far evaded the allopathic drug industry. Anything that destroys a virus will also destroy the cell tissue. It may be that instead of trying to treat only part of the problem, i.e. the virus, a more holistic approach will have to be made to help the whole body, which, after all, is fitted to attack all invaders.

There are already indications that some conventional Western doctors are beginning to look for ways in which the whole body can be stimulated to protect itself more efficiently against an increasing variety of viruses. Exercise and a correct diet are being advocated, which are the bastions of holistic naturopathy, and another approach is to encourage people to use visualization and imagination to aid prevention and the healing process.

5

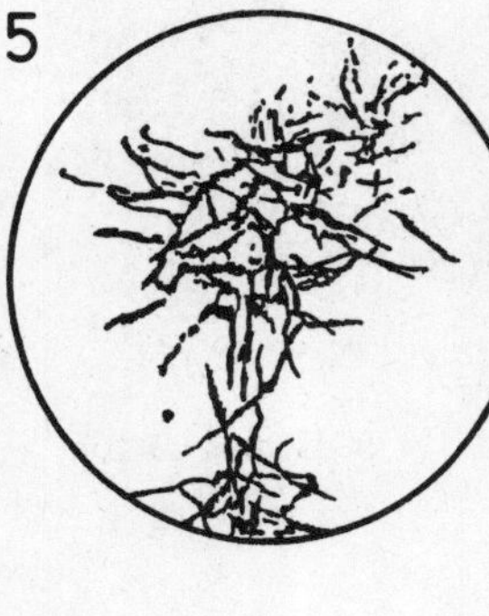

6

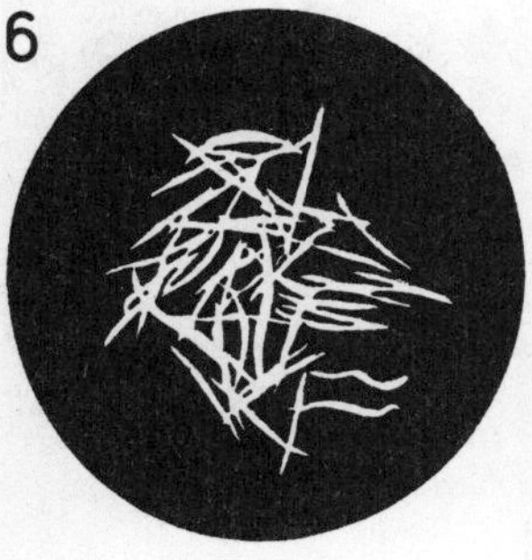

Six disease-bearing organisms (much magnified)
1 Staphylococcus aureus: boils and food poisoning
2 Plasmodium malariae: malaria parasite
3 Treponema pallidum: syphilis
4 Poliomyelitis virus: polio
5 Trichophyton violaceum: scalp ringworm
6 Enterobius vermicularis: intestinal pinworm

Section five

RELAXING INTO FAITH

Belief is at the root of most of the faith healing methods that have been used over the centuries. The belief may have its source in a particular religion or simply in the magic and rituals of the culture in which a person was raised.

Having faith means allowing forces that are beyond personal control to take over. Often the processes involved a symbolic journey, like the religious journey of *Pilgrim's Progress*. Sometimes the patient had to allow himself to be put through processes that were not always pleasant and, as in the case of many shamanistic practices, lasted many days.

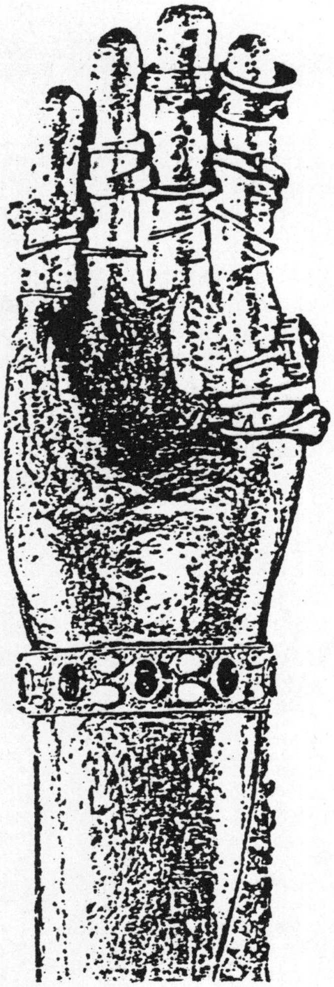

Healing powers of objects: Preserved hand of St Blaise encased in an 11th century German reliquary of gold and precious stones. It was believed to transmit miraculous cures.

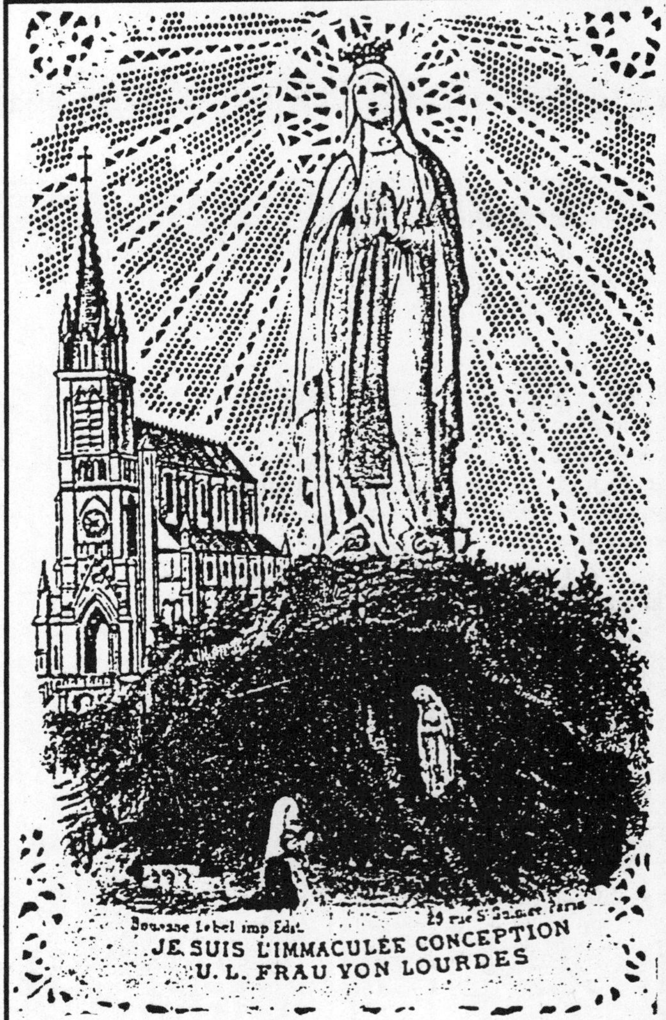

Healing powers of places: An 1867 postcard of the Roman Catholic shrine of Our Lady of Lourdes in SW France.

The use of light, color, sound, heat, rhythm, chants and visual symbols was commonplace. Belief in the power of artifacts and rituals was strong, but the greatest faith was placed in the healer. It is sometimes difficult to distinguish between psychological suggestion and wholehearted faith. Perhaps many of the methods were successful due to a combination of both.

Along with faith in the doctor and faith in the method, many of the approaches described in this section depended also upon a belief in the structure and function of the human body. Some believe in body electricity, others believe in energy centers known as chakras. Having faith also implies believing in oneself and the power of one's own body to heal itself.

From shamans to black boxes, relaxing into faith can promote healing to a remarkable degree.

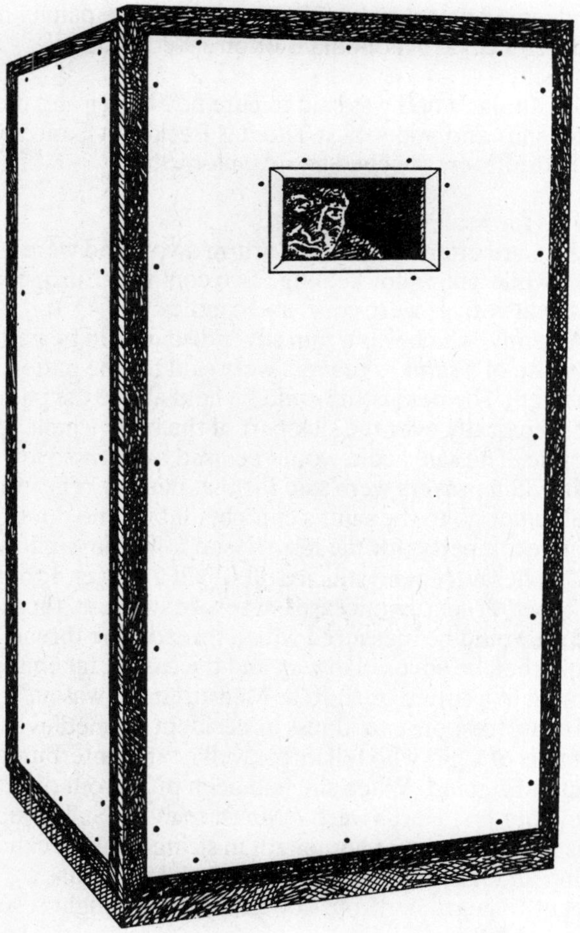

Healing powers of energy rays: Dr William Reich's orgone box or energy accumulator in which patients were said to experience mysterious healing rays trapped by the metal-lined wooden box.

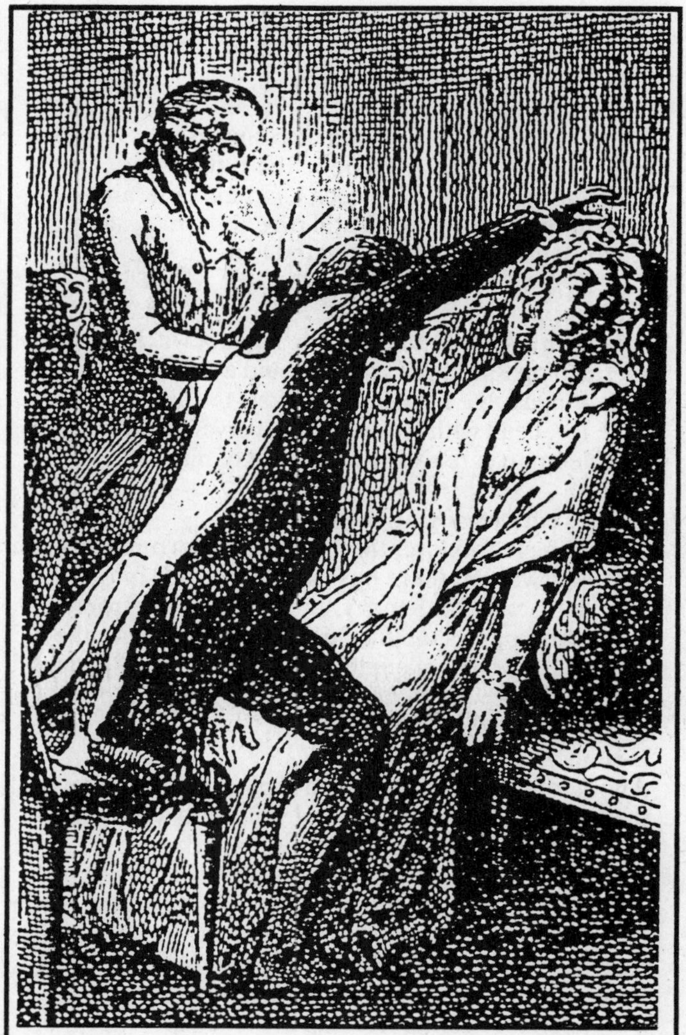

Healing powers of magnetism: Franz Mesmer treating an invalid by transmitting animal magnetism. An 1784 investigating commission found his cures depended on the individual's imagination.

The way of the believer

Religion and healing have always had a close relationship and the miracle of healing has often enhanced the power of religious beliefs. Believers have turned to their prophets, saints and icons when praying for relief from disease and disability.

The way of the believer is healing by no other means than the power of God, which can act either directly or through the medium of a special place or person, such as a shrine, a holy well, a church or at the hand of a saint or his remains.

What may be called a superstitious act by some usually has its source in stories about the life of the prophet, for example Jesus Christ. The use of the cross as a symbol for healing, or healing by touching something used by a saint, both have their origins in stories about the life of Christ. The cross on which he was crucified is a holy symbol used to ward off evil and being healed by touching a holy article originates from the story of the woman who was healed when she touched the hem of Christ's garment.

SOME CHRISTIAN BELIEFS

Healing by making crosses

There are many stories about crossing used as a cure in folk medicine in England up to the 19th century. Crossing one finger from each hand for general protection from disease is still practiced today as are adjacent crossed fingers for good luck.

A cross on:

- rising bread protected it from being bewitched;
- a sleeping foot, with saliva, would awaken it;
- the tongue, the head and the chest to cure fever;
- the forehead with balsam, and every limb with petroleum to cure a man who is out of his wits.

Crosses cure whooping cough

According to folklore, the mark of a cross on the back of a donkey was left there by Christ as he rode into Jerusalem on Palm Sunday. A child suffering from whooping cough should be tied to a donkey with the cross in its fur and taken to a crossroad and walked up and down each road until the child is cured.

Healing from ablutions

Another medieval cure for whooping cough was to drink the ablution, i.e. the water and wine with which the chalice is cleansed after the priest has taken communion. A common practice was to wash out the mouth of a baptized child with the holy water, to prevent the child from suffering toothache. Holy water was also used to wash the eyes of anyone who had seen a ghost, so as to prevent repetition of the unnerving event.

A person suffering from severe fevers or possession was advised to drink a mixture of herbs, garlic, holy water and ale from a church bell, while mass was said over it seven times.

Healing by touching holy artifacts

Wearing a heart made from church metal was a very common form of protection against disease. For example, a cure for sore breasts was to be found by going to a church at midnight, taking a little lead from every diamond-shaped window and making a heart to be worn in a bag hung round the neck.

In about 316 St Blaise, the Bishop of St Sebaste, is said to have brought back to life a boy who was choked by a fishbone. Ever since then, St Blaise has been asked to cure sore throats, thorn pricks and all forms of choking and suffocation. A reliquary in gold and precious stones was made in Germany in the 11th century, said to contain the arm of St Blaise, and is touched by pilgrims.

The Roman Tribune, Quirinus, claimed that his daughter was cured of a disease of the throat after she kissed the chains that had held St Peter.

St Apollonia, who was martyred in Alexandria under Emperor Philip, had her teeth beaten out for her Christian beliefs. According to legend, she was standing at the gate of heaven when the Virgin Mary passed by and decreed that she should never again have pain in her teeth. Hence, St Apollonia is often asked to heal toothache.

St Guthlac's belt was said to cure headaches and the knife, shirt and boots of St Thomas Becket in Canterbury Cathedral, were touched to aid childbirth.

Votives for healing

Votives are offerings made to affirm a vow and were given while asking for healing. Two common European medieval votives were coins and candles.

A penny, which was a thin silver disc, would be bent in the name of a saint as prayers were said for the patient in a sickbed. The bent coin would be held above the patient and specifically over the sick part of the body whenever possible. The same coin would be used over and over again when prayers were said for that patient. The coin would later go to the saint's church, and was no doubt some recompense for the loss of lead from the windows.

Candles were, and still are, lit to aid a prayer. From at least the 6th century, in cases of severe sickness, the patient would be measured with a thread. The thread would then be covered in wax and the candle taken for burning to a shrine or church. Measurement was an automatic response to illness or accident. A medieval text tells of a girl who fell into a well near Canterbury, Kent in England. When she had been pulled out of the water, her first words were, "Measure me to St Thomas." This meant, measure her length in string, make a candle with it and take it to Canterbury to ask St Thomas à Becket to guard her from any sickness that might result from her fall.

In many churches today, every candle is a prayer.

Wells and holy water

Springs and wells associated with saints have always

been places where the sick have sought to be cured. There was a curious connection between the head and the well in Great Britain, in particular in Scotland.

The early Celtic dwellers of Scotland were head-hunters at one time in their development. Later the head became associated with the soul and was of such importance that even after death the head was often kept. Legends tell of heads that ate at feasts and gave advice.

The places where decapitated heads rested were often regarded as holy places and, according to legend, many springs appeared where such heads had fallen. The water from those springs was believed to be holy water that could cure the sick. Quite often a skull would be placed in or near the well so the water could be drunk from it using the skull. Measles, whooping cough and epilepsy were the most common diseases for which a cure was sought.

Coventina's Well

One of the best known holy wells in Great Britain is Coventina's Well, which is near Hadrian's Wall in Northumberland, close to the border between Scotland and England. In the 1870s three bronze heads and a real human skull were found in the well, together with huge quantities of brooches, coins and broken pottery, thrown in as votives or gifts for prayers answered, or to ensure a prayer for healing would more likely be answered. There are the remains of several Celtic altars nearby, some dedicated to the Celtic goddess, Coventina.

Well of the Heads

There are several sites known as Tobar nan Ceann (Well of the Heads) in the islands and on the mainland of Scotland.

One of these wells is quite close to the modern road that runs between Inverness and Fort William at Glengarry. It is marked by an obelisk topped with carvings of seven heads. In common with many "Wells of the Heads" it was believed that drinking some water from this well before sunrise on the first Sunday in May would protect the drinker from all harm for a full year.

Holy water amulets

A less pleasant but religiously more potent use of water for healing was the practice of washing the remains of 'saints' clothing, possessions and even the dead body, and retaining the water in a phial around the neck to protect the wearer.

The severely sick would drink some of the water, which was often stored locked up in churches, since the supply of such water was limited. There are few records of what actual effect these practices had, but it is clear that many people fervently believed in their efficacy. The fear of disease would be extreme in those early times, shortly after the death of Christ, when there was little hope for a cure by any other means.

MAZDAZNAN

This is a practice of healing based on the philosophy of two great prophets and of the Ahura Mazda, the Creative Intelligence of ancient Middle Eastern thought. The prophetess Ainyahita, 9600 BC, and the prophet Zarathustra, 6900 BC, were Iranian sages who both preached a belief in one God and a philosophy of right living, now adapted into Mazdaznan.

The modern Mazdaznan Association was founded in 1902 by Dr Otoman Zar-Adusht Ha'nish (1844–1936), who spent his youth in a remote community in Iran, where he overcame a heart complaint using breathing techniques. He studied medicine in Europe and lectured on healing in Europe and America, translating the philosophies of the prophets into a viable modern New Thought movement, known as the Mazdaznan or Master Thought. In practice there are five linked areas.

Mazdaznan breathing

The function of breathing is to maintain physical and spiritual life. There are exercises to develop the twelve senses, including extra-sensory perception and spiritual inspiration.

Deep, rhythmical breathing is taught to improve general health and intelligence. The aim is to achieve inhalation and exhalation that lasts for seven seconds each, with a pause of one second between. This is said to calm, slow down and steady the heart beat.

Mazdaznan dietetics

Raw, lacto-vegetarian foods form the basic diet and such cooking as is needed is done in ways designed to preserve the vitamin and mineral content. In many ways, Mazdaznan methods are naturopathic, making use of fasting for inner cleansing, bathing and herbal remedies.

The amounts of different types of food are carefully balanced according to individual body types.

Mazdaznan personal diagnosis

Self-understanding is encouraged through a very complex form of personality-typing, taking account of body- and head-shape, thought modes, strengths and weaknesses and family background.

Glandular science

Endocrine function is regarded as vital to intelligence and spirituality. The thymus and the pineal gland are given particular attention. Slow exercises, rhythm breathing and humming are performed daily in the belief that they will improve glandular functions.

Eugenics

The study of the regeneration of the individual and the procreation of children is the fifth area in which Master Thought is practiced, mainly as education of the young and of young parents. Much attention is given to choosing compatible partners who are then encouraged to build a strong family unit on which a Mazdaznan civilization can be perpetuated.

The tree of life

Trees have always symbolized the journey a seeker must make to attain knowledge. In the Garden of Eden, the tree is the source of knowledge, while the mystical knowledge of Judaism is the Kabbalistic tree of life, often given form as the Menorah, the branched candlestick used by every Jewish family.

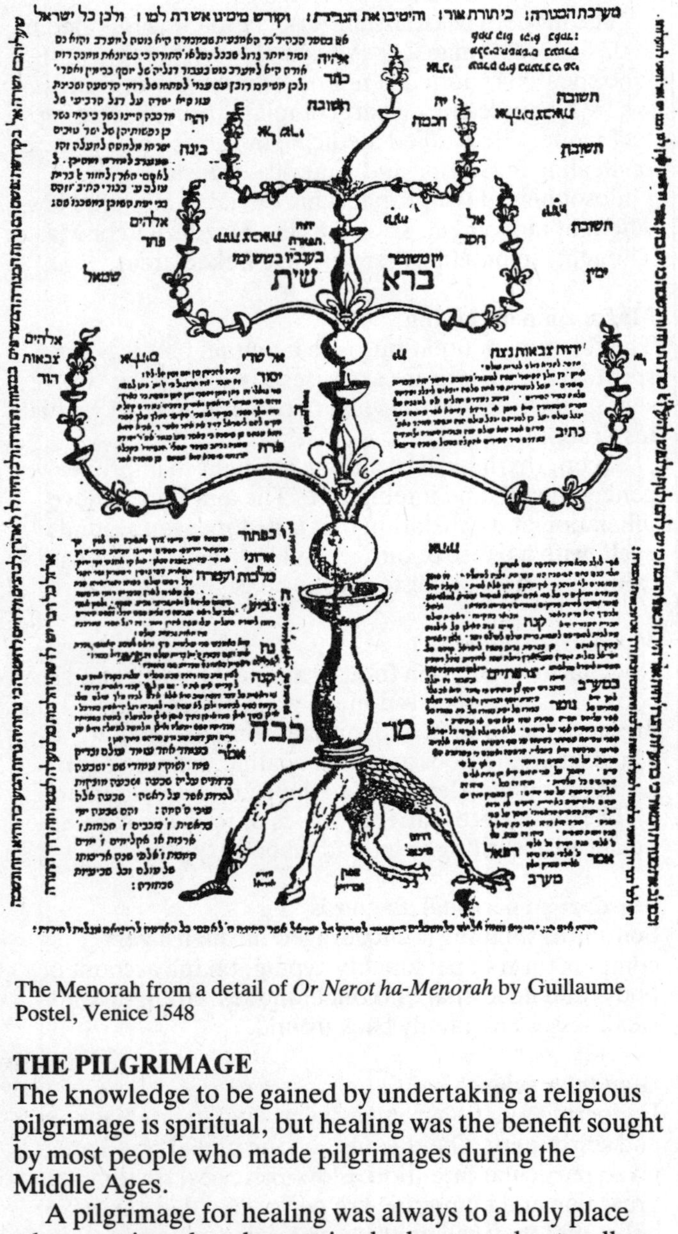

The Menorah from a detail of *Or Nerot ha-Menorah* by Guillaume Postel, Venice 1548

THE PILGRIMAGE

The knowledge to be gained by undertaking a religious pilgrimage is spiritual, but healing was the benefit sought by most people who made pilgrimages during the Middle Ages.

A pilgrimage for healing was always to a holy place where a miraculous happening had occurred naturally. The journey often represented the journey to heaven or to paradise that would, hopefully, be made one day, so the pilgrimage fulfilled many of the believer's needs

The healing shrines

Sick people often made annual pilgrimages to a favored shrine. Many visited one shrine after another, casting lots to decide which one to visit next, believing that the hand of God was directing even random choices. Their journeys branched from home like the branches of a tree. They returned home after each pilgrimage before embarking on the next, although a round trip might often have been shorter and less tiring in the long run.

One medieval European text, a medical journal of the time, records a person making pilgrimages for 14 years before a partial cure was granted and another who visited 84 shrines, collapsing with exhaustion at the last, where he died.

Belief in the healing power of the pilgrimage to a shrine is strong, despite the very small numbers of actual cures that have been claimed and recognized. For example, in 1929, 800,000 people visited the grave of an American priest, seeking cures, yet only 100 claimed any kind of relief. Over 3 million people visit the Christian shrine of Lourdes every year, yet of the 5000 who have claimed to be cured there during the last 120 years, the church has officially accepted less than 100 as miracles of healing.

Two English shrines

Perhaps the best known place of pilgrimage is to the tomb of St Thomas Becket in Canterbury Cathedral in Kent, where he was murdered in 1170. *The Canterbury Tales*, written by Geoffrey Chaucer (c1340-1400), are a collection of stories told by a group of pilgrims.

The shrine of Bishop St Thomas Cantelupe

A less well known shrine was that of Thomas Cantelupe at Hereford Cathedral, where, in the years around 1290, hundreds of suffering, crippled pilgrims would make their way. Some would be carried on litters, paying a penny to be brought from nearby villages, while one person is recorded as traveling from London in a wheelbarrow, pushed by family and friends for over 100 miles.

Miracles of healing had occured at Cantelupe's tomb and people gave offerings both in hope and in gratitude. At its height, Cantelupe's shrine had a reputation that had spread all over England and beyond, because papal records show an enormous hoard of offerings had already accumulated only twenty years after his death.

Papal commissioners went to make an inventory at the shrine on 29 August 1307. This is what they found:
170 silver ships
129 silver images of diverse human limbs
436 wax images of men
1,200 wax images of parts of the body and limbs
77 wax figures of horses and other animals
large numbers of wax ears, eyes, breasts, teeth etc.
95 children's shifts (dresses)
108 walking sticks for cripples
10 candles as large as a man
38 cloths of silk and gold with many girdles (belts)
520 gold or silver rings
96 gold or silver brooches and pins
plus diverse precious stones, lances, swords and spears, iron chains offered by prisoners and uncountable numbers of coins and candles.

While the poor made wax images, the rich fashioned their images from precious metals to represent the part of the body that needed healing. When the image was of a whole person, the pilgrim was either sick all over or taking precautions against the spread of the disease.

The clothes and jewelry would be from the sick person and the walking sticks indicated that some who had arrived needing a crutch, had left able to walk again. Sick prisoners had only their chains to give and the weapons came not only from soldiers but also from the common man who necessarily carried a weapon for protection on any journey.

The commissioners stayed at Hereford for 78 days, noting that in the two months of September and October 1307, 86 more images, three more ships, two more children's shifts and hundreds more coins and candles were added to the collection.

The very existence of so many offerings would be taken as proof by some people of the miraculous powers of the dead Thomas Cantelupe, who was not canonized until 1320. Since Hereford is a long way inland, the reputation of the shrine must have spread far, as the presence of the images of ships indicated that sea-going families from coastal settlements had also made a pilgrimage there.

At the shrine

Most pilgrims sat or lay in the church, or in the shrine itself, waiting to be healed. Often they had dreams or visions during which they were visited by angels or the saints.

Sometimes women had to wait outside the shrine or even outside the church. For example, in the 12th century, St Cuthbert of Durham was reputed to be a misogynist who punished females who dared to enter his church. People often sang or prayed aloud and when the crowd was gripped by hysterical fervor, people were knocked down or crushed.

It is a belief in both Christianity and Islam that by making a journey to a distant holy place one can acquire the grace of God, symbolized in the tree of life. This belief is still firmly held by thousands of people who undertake modern pilgrimages, such as to the shrine of Our Lady of Lourdes in France.

The miracle of Lourdes

In 1844, mill worker François Soubirous and his wife had their first child whom they named Bernadette.

Times were hard in the village of Lourdes and became harder for the family when Soubirous lost the use of an eye and was sacked from his job. By then there were other children to feed and an outbreak of cholera had almost claimed the life of Bernadette, leaving her asthmatic.

Due to a famine, Bernadette went away to work as a nanny for a while until January 1858, when, aged 14, she returned to Lourdes and went to the free school run by the Sisters of Charity.

Three weeks after her return, she was out early with her sister and a friend, collecting firewood as usual. In a grotto in the rocks, above a rose bush at Massabielle, she saw a glow of light and the vision of a beautiful woman she later referred to as *Aquero*, meaning 'that one' in her local dialect.

Her claims to have seen a vision of the Virgin Mary on two occasions drew public disapproval, but one properous woman thought the vision must have been the ghost of a pious child who had died the previous year and took Bernadette back to the grotto, where she saw the vision again.

Between 18 February and 4 March Bernadette saw the vison of *Aquero*, or Our Lady, 13 times and her audience grew from a few local villagers to a crowd of 8000. *Aquero*, it is claimed, told her secrets, showed her the sacred spring in the grotto and carried out several healing miracles. Political and religious problems arose and there were increasing battles between the authorities.

On Easter Wednesday, 7 April, Bernadette saw the vision again, burning her hands in a candle flame in her ecstasy. Afterwards her hands were examined by a doctor, Pierre Dozous, who was present throughout, and declared her hands unharmed.

She last saw the vision on 16 July and at the age of 22 became a nun in the town of Nevers. She died at the age of 35 after long illnesses in 1879.

After her death, Lourdes' reputation grew as a healing shrine. It is interesting to note that in the region around Lourdes were at least four other places where shrines had been dedicated to Our Lady. The stories were similar; at one, a shepherdess had seen a vision of a Lady that led to a cult following, a chapel being built and the appearance of a spring of holy water. Our Lady of Lourdes and Our Lady of Garaison, of Poëylanun, of Héas and of Piétat are all shrines within the Lourdes area of the Pyrenees where miraculous healing is said to have taken place.

Pilgrims at Lourdes waiting for Mass in the Grotto

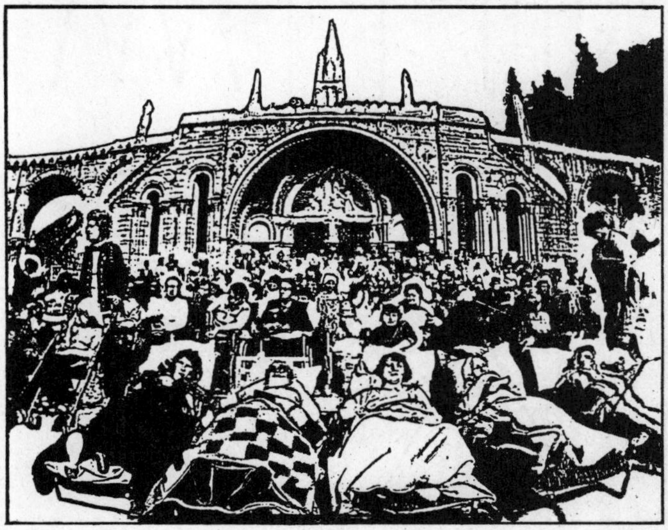

©DIAGRAM

Hidden patterns

Certain shapes, proportions and positions have a positive influence on the well-being of people. This fact has been known to ancient peoples and is used to advantage by some artists, graphic designers, architects, fashion houses and choreographers. Patterning has also been used by some healers to aid the healing process.

Archetypal patterns

During the 1950s Dr T.A. Westlake, an English psionic doctor, claimed 300 cures by patterning homeopathic remedies. He and his colleagues devised a series of two-dimensional patterns and three-dimensional shapes and tested them by matching them with homeopathic and herbal remedies.

A small phial of the remedy was placed on the pattern or within the three-dimensional model and transmitted mentally to the patient. With the correct pattern, the remedy was effective. With the wrong pattern, the same remedy was ineffective. Once the correct pattern had been established, it was discovered that in some cases it was only necessary to write the name of the remedy on the pattern. Dr Westlake suggested that all patterns are forces in their own right, just as the nature of an atom or molecule is related to its shape.

His propositions have been followed up by Malcolm Rae, an Englishman who works in the field of radionic therapy. He has researched the archetypes of

PATTERNS AND SHAPES

In pictures, things on the left are interpreted by the imaginative, emotional right brain and things on the right are interpreted by the logical, dogmatic left brain. This fact is often put to good use in films, for example, in the film *Casablanca*, when in many of their scenes together Humphrey Bogart was right of center and Ingrid Bergman left of center.

The shape of a container is known to have an effect on its contents. The bacterial action that makes tasty yogurt is said to increase when it is in a conical container, and the taste of beer in rectangular barrels is different from the taste when it is stored in cylindrical barrels. Sick mice living in spherical cages heal more quickly than those living in any other shape.

a Vertical lines are dynamic and rousing
b Horizontal lines are passive and restful
c A triangle on its base is stable and secure
d A triangle on its point is unstable and stimulating

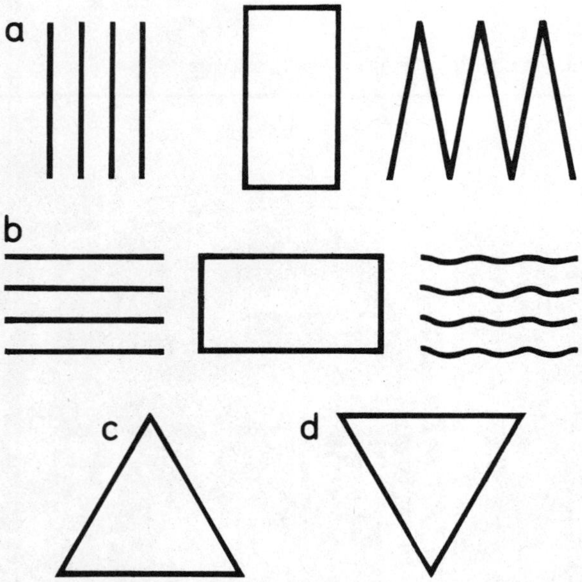

Pyramids

The pyramid is probably the one shape that has caused most interest since the 1930s, when Antoine Bovis, a Frenchman, was on holiday in Egypt. He observed that small animals that had died inside the Great Pyramid had not decomposed but had become mummified.

In the late 1940s, a Czechoslovak radio technician called Karl Drbal patented a cardboard pyramid that could prolong the life of a razor-blade by up to four months. It took ten years to discover how the pyramid razor-blade "sharpener" worked. Water reduces the strength of steel by up to 20%. Used razor blades retain tiny droplets of water along the cutting edges, even when wiped dry. This dampness further reduces the sharpness of a blade. By placing it in the pyramid, with both blade and pyramid aligned north–south, the residual dampness completely dried out. Scientists speculated that some kind of electro-magnetic force field was sufficiently concentrated inside the pyramid to dehydrate the blade.

Pyramid healing

Pyramid shapes, constructed of cardboard, have had many claims made for them. It is said they enhance sleeping, delay aging processes and heal minor wounds more quickly than normal.

Recent experiments in the US by Kathy Coggin and Bill Kerrell have shown that the taste of food improves when it is stored under pyramids. Coffee is less bitter, the acidity of fruit is lowered, wine improves and frozen foods regain their natural flavor. Food is said to keep fresher longer in pyramid storage.

Biofeedback experiments have shown that trained meditators, who can control their brain wave patterns, were affected by an open pyramid being lowered over their heads. Their *alpha* and *theta* brain waves were doubled in amplitude, and they reported feeling a greater sense of warmth, tranquility and weightlessness and had visions; some even experienced clairvoyance and clairaudience.

homeopathic remedies and devised a way of imprinting them on water or lactose tablets using electromagnetism. This method of preparing homeopathic remedies is now in common use.

The golden ratio
The shape of a building affects its occupants, and when the design of a building is based on the ratio 1 to 1.618 it makes a harmonious spatial relationship. Known as the golden ratio, it is present in paintings, designs and buildings both ancient and modern.

A is to B as A+B is to A. When B is 1, A is 1.61803398... (a number with an unending decimal expansion, known as an irrational number). This number is known by the Greek letter *phi* and should not be confused with the other irrational number known as *pi*, which is the ratio of the circumference of a circle to its diameter.

The golden series
The ratio can be expressed as an infinite series, the previous two numbers being added to find the next in sequence. Approximations are shown in the series below; the greater the number, the closer it is to the exact ratio.

1:2:3:5:8:13:21:34:55:89:144:233:377:610, and so on.

The golden ratio is not an accidental ratio chosen by ancient people, although it may have been used intuitively long before people realized that many living structures conform to it. The *phi* ratio appears many times in nature and is especially elegant in the logarithmic spiral, the structure of many shells.

The logarithmic spiral built on whirling squares
Starting at the center, the side of each square is the sum of the sides of the two previous squares. C=A+B; D=B+C; E=C+D, and so on.

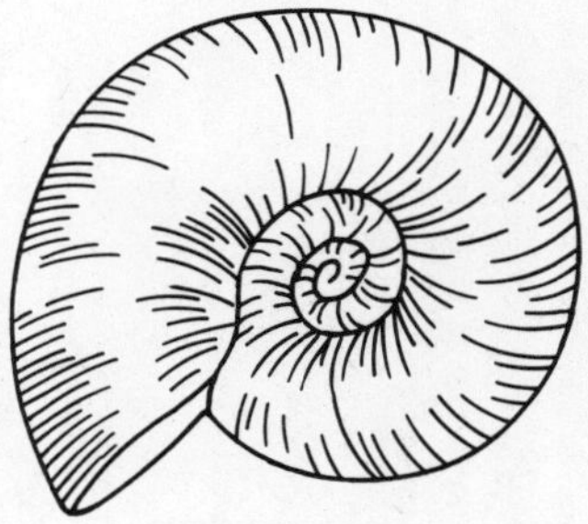

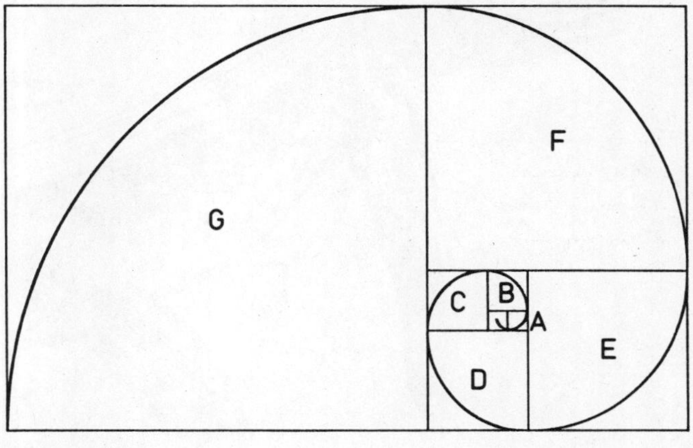

REFERENCE: For more about radionics and psionic medicine, refer to **Section Five: A little black box** (pp. 106–107) and **The mystical senses** (pp. 108–109) and **Section Six: Homeopathic remedies** (pp. 134–135).

Exactly how the pyramid works is not yet understood. It appears to concentrate certain energies, not all magnetic. It is also thought that the shape may enhance the ionization balance in the air which has a healing effect.

The proportions of the Great Pyramid
The Great Pyramid in Egypt is aligned to magnetic north and is a geometric and geographic wonder. The basic proportions are used to construct open-sided healing pyramids.

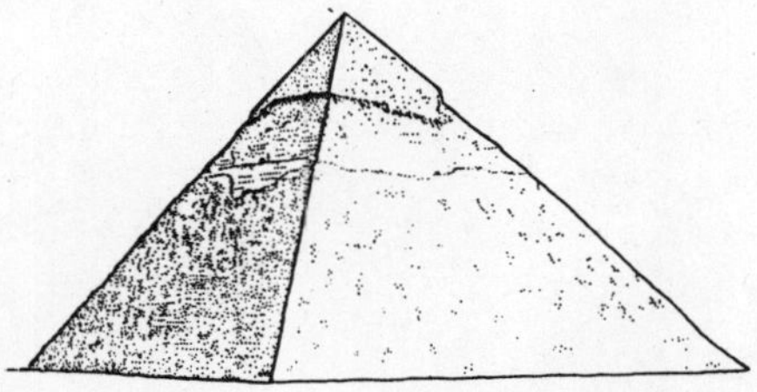

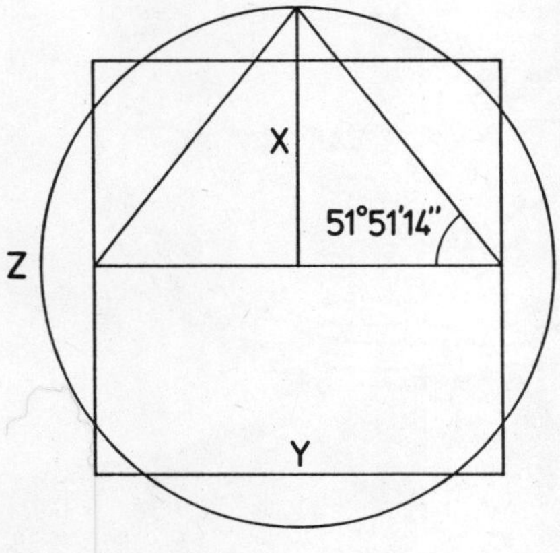

The height, X, is the radius of the circle, Z. The square base of the pyramid, Y, has the same circumference as the circle. The angle of each side of the pyramid to the base is as shown on the diagram above.

Shamanism

The shaman was the central figure in a primitive religious system which developed in pre-Bronze Age times in the far north of Asia. Even up to the 19th century, classical shamanism was still practiced in remote communities. The shaman was a person of great power in what was originally a classless society.

It is interesting to note that the United Nations World Health Organization has a policy of encouraging traditional healers to continue using certain herbal and shamanic cures while training them in hygiene and midwifery.

A modernized form of shamanism is found among the Khanty of Siberia, who still regard sickness as an indication of a lost or stolen soul. Although the term shaman is often loosely applied to the medicine-man or witchdoctor of other aboriginal cultures, Asiatic shamanism developed within a distinctive view of the universe.

SHAMANISTIC VIEW OF THE UNIVERSE

There are three worlds controlled by spirits. Ulgen is the benevolent deity of the upper world. On earth, the central world, 55 of his sons and daughters live in the west and are good spirits. The other 44 are wicked spirits, led by Erlen Khan, who live in the east. The earth is disc-shaped, held together by a great belt and supported on the back of a sea monster. When the monster swims it causes earthquakes, and holes appear in the earth leading to the lower world.

The soul of the shaman is reared in a nest in the cosmic tree, which grows from the navel of the earth. If the nest is high in the tree, he will be a great and powerful shaman; if low down, he will be a small shaman with only minor powers. Otherwise he will be an intermediate shaman.

A Vaults of the upper world
B Cosmic tree
C Pillar of the world
D Hole to lower world
E Belt of the earth
F Monster
G Cosmic sea

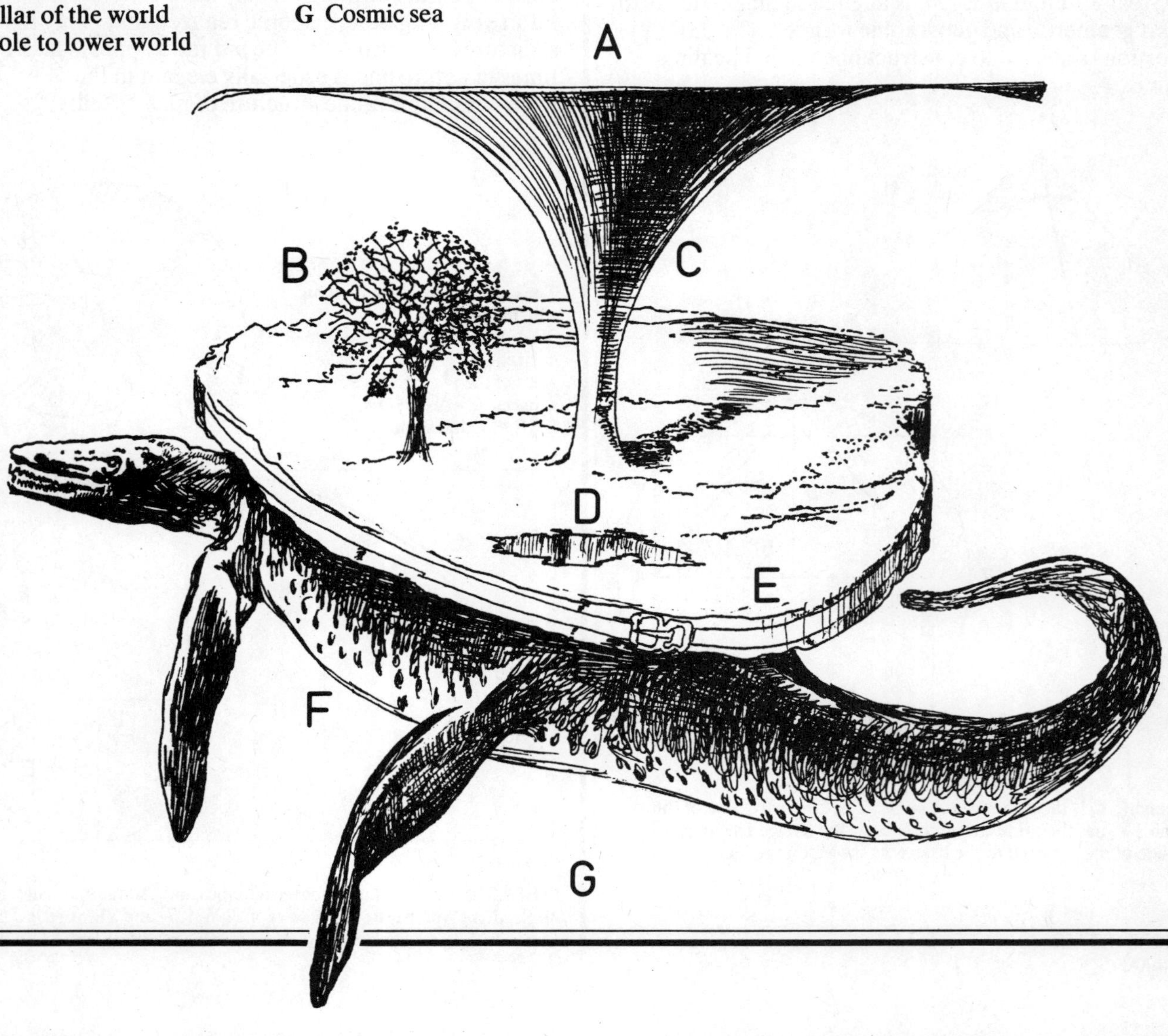

Who is the shaman?

The noun, shaman, derives fom the Tunguso-Manchurian word *saman*, meaning "he who knows." Familiar with the spirit world, which he enters while in an ecstatic trance, he is a healer, a diviner and a psychopomp, i.e. an escort of souls into the spirit world.

The true shaman is called by the spirits to his vocation before birth, inheriting the soul of a dead shaman. He is recognized at birth, usually by a physical sign, such as an extra tooth, and grows up aware of the suffering he will have to endure.

His initiation occurs at adolescence, when he may be tortured for days or even months. It was a common practice to make cuts all over the body to discover any extra bones, another proof of shaman inheritance. During the torture, he cries out in agony, faints, becomes hysterical, has visions and generally resists his calling, which is said to cause the shaman sickness of mind from which he must cure himself. When he finally capitulates and accepts his vocation, he falls into a lengthy sleep, after which he awakens as the shaman.

Some modern anthropologists think the shaman was a psychopath; others regard him as a wounded healer who healed himself. In the 1960s, the French scientist and writer Claude Lévi-Strauss tried to expose shamanic activities among Eskimos as quakery and ended by becoming a successful shaman himself.

The characteristics of a true shaman

1 Inherited vocation.
2 Physical and/or mental abnormality.
3 Goes into ecstasy at will by beating a drum made from the skin of the animal his soul rides during ecstasy.
4 Calls spirits to work for him and appeases local spirits, such as those of the polar bear and walrus.
5 Wears a ritual gown and headdress.
6 Sings, dances and performs a drama to bring about healing and appease the spirits.
7 Uses massage, Arctic herbalism and simple surgery.

Eskimo shaman with the drum used to induce the trance state

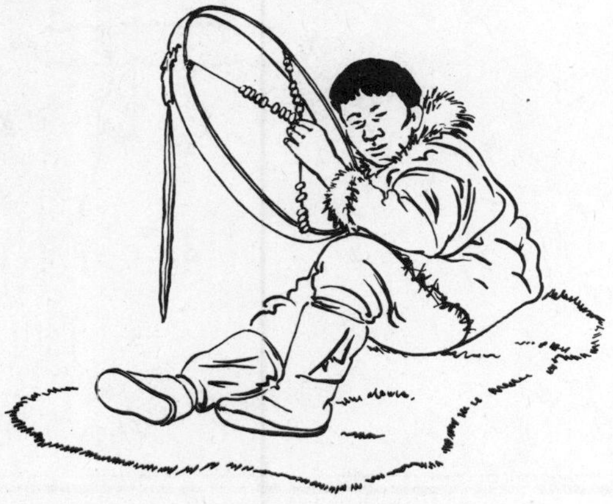

A shamanic healing ceremony

This description is adapted from a report made by an American medical anthropologist, Joan Halifax, who was studying the Cayapa tribe in the remote jungle of north Ecuador in the 1980s.

All day sick people came from near and far to the Cayapa shaman's jungle home. They sat and lay on the split bamboo floor. As evening approached, candles were lit and the ceremony began. Drumming, singing, whistling and the rattling of dried leaves were carried out by the shaman and his helpers. They had drunk infusions of sacred plants that would help them to visit the spirits and invoke their powers. Everyone became involved in drumming, singing and dancing.

At the height of his great frenzy the shaman went into a trance, and the candles were extinguished. Everyone fell to the ground, exhausted but exhilarated.

Throughout the darkness of the night the shaman worked with each sick person in turn. He sucked pebbles, spat them out, blew smoke, exhorted, persuaded and cajoled the spirits to leave and take their sickness away, sometimes offering them repose in objects such as sticks or even a dog. By morning, many were healed and all felt renewed. The anthropologist was amazed by the immense sense of compassion she experienced when the shaman had worked with her.

Why so many were cured remains a mystery. Were they really ill? Did the intensity of the communal activity give everyone a boost in self-confidence, which always assists healing? Or perhaps many were cured because they believed in the power of the shaman. Certainly abreaction and transference form part of the psychology of healing.

It is now thought that the ritual drumming, dancing, shouting and singing may induce the production of pain-relieving chemicals in the brain, such as endorphins. This may also be true of modern psychological rituals such as abreaction exercises in group encounter work.

Tulayev, shaman of the Karagas, Siberia, in 1927

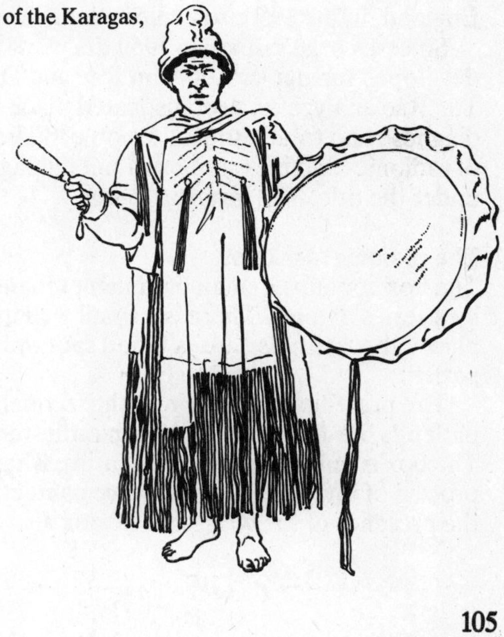

A little black box

One of the most mysterious and intriguing methods of healing is radionics, which is mental diagnosis and treatment at a distance through the medium of an instrument in a little black box, utilizing what is called the radiesthesthetic faculty of the doctor or other practitioner.

The growth of radionics

While its antecedents, psychic and absent healing, have been practiced for thousands of years, modern radionics grew from an observation made by an American professor of pathology at the turn of the century. Dr Albert Abrams noticed that the resonance of abdominal percussion changed when a patient was facing a different direction. Assuming this was an electro-magnetic factor, he devised a way of measuring resonances and kept records from his examinations of patients with identifiable diseases, taking care to have them all face the same direction. He discovered, for example, that tuberculosis reacted at 15 ohms, syphilis at 20 ohms and carcinoma at 50 ohms.

He did hundreds of tests and found he got the same results using spots of blood. By comparing his results with healthy persons he determined measurements for a range of diseases. When he published his results the medical world was very hostile. However, in 1924, the year of his death, a medical committee ran a series of tests under controlled conditions; the results confirmed Dr Abrams' findings, to its astonishment.

Few allopathic doctors would risk their reputations using such an unorthodox method, but in the 1930s Ruth Drown, an American chiropractor, pioneered radionics as an alternative to the use of drugs and surgery. Later an Englishman, Dr Guyon Richards, measured the auras of people, visible on a Kilner screen, and correctly diagnosed diseases radionically long before they became clinically detectable.

It was George de la Warr and his wife who initiated a new phase in the growth of radionic practice and instrumentation. They and their assistants set up the Radionic and Magnetic Centre Organization at Oxford, England, in the 1950s to explore the radionic field.

Since George's death in 1969 the work has been developed further by Malcolm Rae and David Tansley. The Rae analyzer is a sophisticated black box used to diagnose and treat patients. Psionic medicine is a branch of radionics and is described in full on pages 108 and 109 under the title: **The mystical senses**.

The radionic black box

The box contains a small bar magnet that can be rotated by a series of dials. There is a small well in which is placed the "witness," i.e. a blood spot or hair from the patient.

The practitioner tunes in to the frequency of the patient's life-fields using his own radiesthesthetic ability. The box is only to focus and measure what is, in reality, a process of invisible, long-distance contact facilitated by the presence of the witness. The box also has a small membrane, that is touched as a series of questions are asked about the disease. A positive answer is indicated when the practitioner's fingers stick to the membrane, due to changes in his nervous system and radiesthesthetic ability. The deviation from a healthy norm is recorded on a diagnostic chart.

THE LIFE-FIELDS

Radionics is based on the idea that a whole person has three parts: spirit, soul and form. Form consists of the physical body, the etheric body (aura or bioplasma), the emotional body and the mental body, each of which emanates a life-energy field which can tune in to the energy fields of other people, animals and plants.

Radiesthesthetics is the ability to tune in to other life-fields, using one's own life-fields. For example, thought transfer is tuning in on a mental level. Disease is said to be caused by miasmas, which are emanations from left-over vestiges of previously acute conditions, such as childhood measles, or by toxins from current conditions, such as influenza or a period of worry or grief.

Toxins and miasmas interfere with the life-fields of the organs and chakras and cause congestion and lack of coordination between the parts of the body form. The aim of radionics is to identify these causes and stimulate the energies that will eliminate them.

The form body
a Mental life-field
b Emotional life-field
c Etheric body or aura
d Physical body

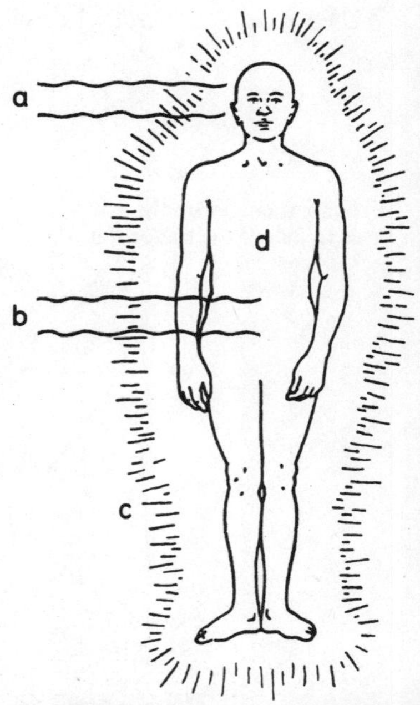

Radionic treatment

If radiesthesthetic diagnosis is mysterious, then the treatment appears to be pure magic. The main method is radiesthesthetic, i.e. life-fields are influenced at a distance by the practitioner who again uses the black box as a means of measuring the effect. Treatment also may include homeopathic, herbal and dietary remedies, vitamins, minerals and color therapy. Manipulative therapies may also be recommended.

Moderate success has been achieved with people, and radionics has proved excellent for pain and chronic conditions. It should be remembered that most people only go to an alternative practitioner when all other methods have failed. Radionics, however, has been extremely successful in affecting animal health and crop yields.

A radionic diagnostic chart

The upper chart indicates the deviation from optimum health of the organs and functions of the body. The lower one charts the condition of the seven chakras, which are the locations of concentrated life energy. Having pin-pointed affected areas, such as respiration and the throat chakra, causative miasmas and toxins are sought, and the general condition of the whole person is noted.

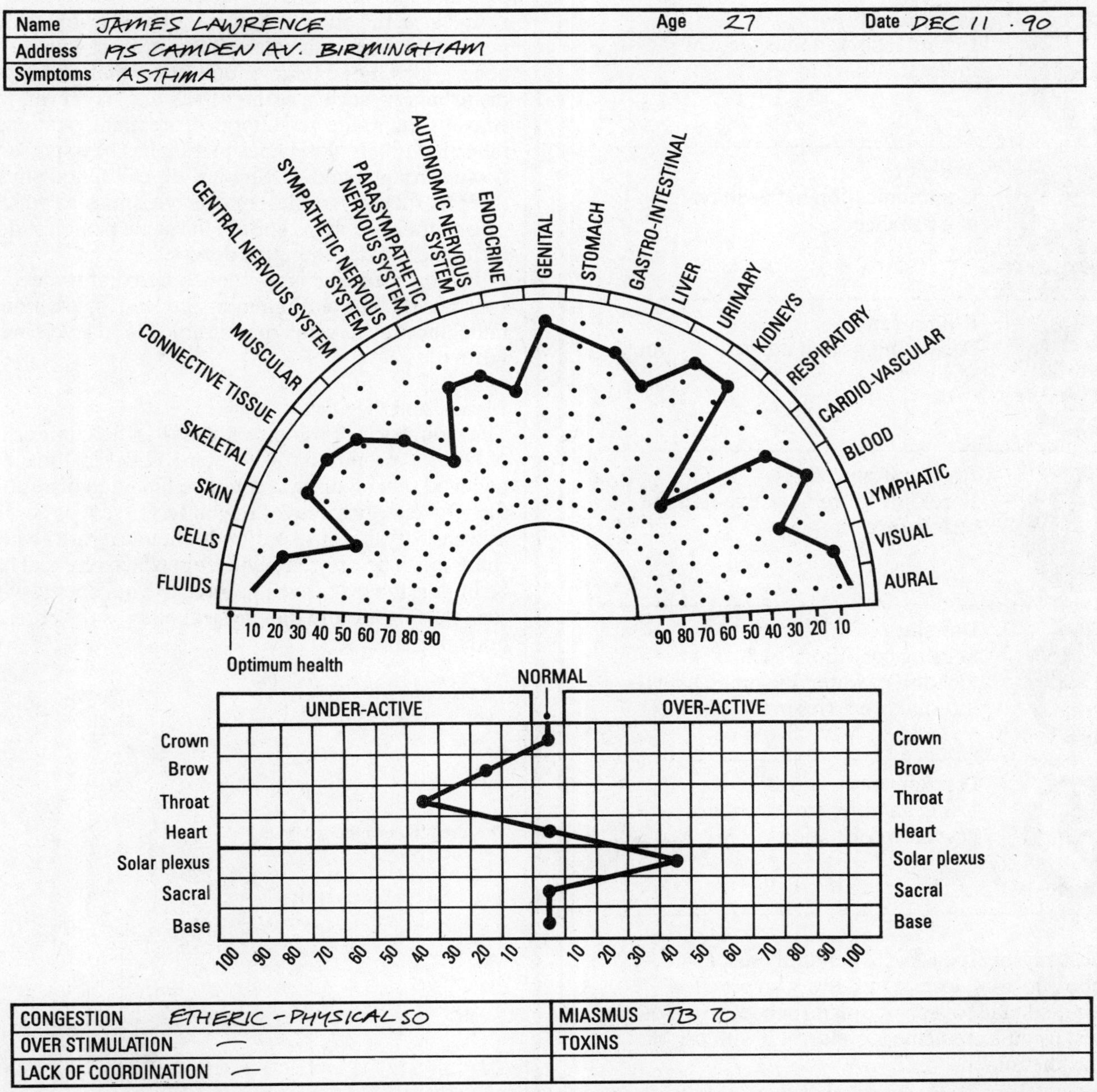

The mystical senses

The five senses of sight, hearing, touch, taste and smell are used through specific organs, i.e. the eyes, ears, skin, tongue and nose. However, they are not our only way of gathering information from the outside world. The kinesthetic sense, operating through the muscles, reveals spatial position, and the sense of balance is adjusted from minute fluctuations in the fluid inside the semicircular canals of the inner ear.

The degree of sensitivity varies among people, and cultural upbringing may ignore some senses and develop others. Some people are able to detect fractional changes in shades of colors, while others are color blind and cannot distinguish between greens and reds. Sometimes a link in the brain is formed between two senses; consequently some people can "hear" colors, for example, or "taste" sounds.

THE MYSTICAL SENSES

These are psychic or extra-sensory perceptions, outside the normal five senses but which may be interpreted in the brain visually or aurally, etc.

Intuition
Instant, spontaneous recognition or understanding.

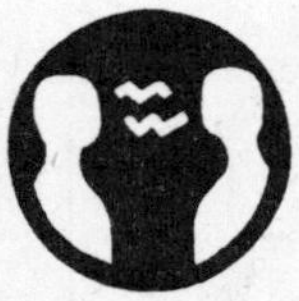

Telepathy
Communication between two minds at a distance.

Clairvoyance
Seeing things that are actually out of sight.

Precognition
Foreknowledge of an event in the near future.

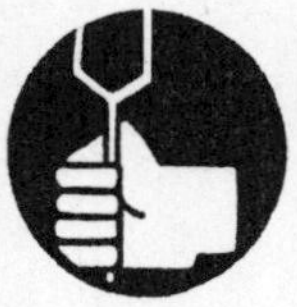

Dowsing
Sensing conditions such as the location of water, magnetic fields or internal processes in the body.

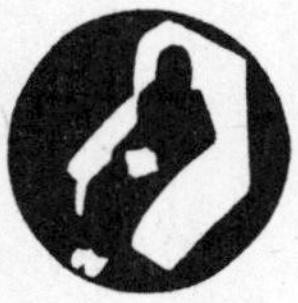

Psychometry
Using an object to tune in to psychic information.

These mystical senses are generally suspected by orthodox doctors, except by a few who practice psionic medicine for specific disturbances. As its name implies, psionic medicine is concerned with psi, or psychic phenomena.

PSIONIC MEDICINE

This is a branch of radionics developed in England by Dr George Lawrence and applied by some orthodox doctors who use orthodox methods for the physical body and psionic methods for the etheric body, when it is disturbed by a miasma. Miasmas are memories of old sicknesses.

Because the etheric body is timeless, psionic doctors believe that miasmas cause illness in successive generations. For example, they claim that many modern disturbances, such as asthma, eczema, hay fever, sinusitis, migraine and allergies, are manifestations of an inherited tuberculosis miasma that has been passed down through families. Similarly, a childhood physical disease, such as measles, may leave a miasma which can cause other problems later in the same person's life, including the degenerative diseases.

Psionic medicine is also concerned that some substances, such as aluminum and lead, cause etheric imbalances even when measurable blood levels are normal.

Disease and the aura

The main basis of psionic medicine is the Unitary Theory of Disease proposed by surgeon J.E.R.McDonagh, who believed that all disease could be linked to disruptions in the vital energy forces of the body. He saw physical life as transitory, because our body chemicals are always changing. The only baseline from which physical life can be built is the primitive life force or vital energy which is seen pulsing around the physical body as the etheric body or aura.

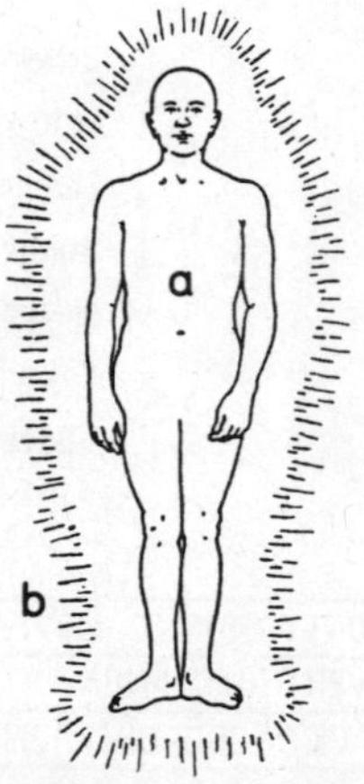

The physical and etheric bodies
a Physical body
b Etheric body or aura (pulsation of life energy)

Perception of mystical, supersensible forces is a largely neglected human ability. Those people who are psychic or clairvoyant, or who are able to see auras and communicate telepathically, are either treated as rare mystics or dismissed as charlatans. Intuition is often regarded as a suspect sense, although everyone uses it, and sensitive people are tolerated but given little respect in a world that is devoted to logic and the scientific proof of cause and effect. But without moments of irrational inspiration the world would be an even poorer place.

McDonagh's cycles of life activity
Primitive energy forming the aura.
First cycle: sub-atomic particles, such as electrons, are constantly being replenished.
Second cycle : groups of atoms are formed.
Third cycle: atoms link to make molecules.
Fourth cycle: building of proteins from molecules. An imbalance is the result if the aura is disturbed. McDonagh saw all disease as a degree of protein disturbance, cancer, for example, being a serious imbalance of protein production.
Fifth cycle: structuring body organs. At this stage, traditional symptoms of disease are clearly manifested if there has been a protein imbalance.
Sixth cycle: building the whole physical body.

Diagnosis and treatment
Any disturbance in the primitive energy force will affect the first three cycles and result in a protein imbalance. Psionic doctors claim that the potential sickness can be detected in the aura by psychic sensing (dowsing is the preferred method) before the damage has begun to be manifest in any of the levels and long before the physical symptoms can be detected, when it is often too late to prevent the physical damage we call disease.

To detect irregularities in the aura, psionic doctors use their intuition combined with a series of questions asked of a pendulum during dowsing. Treatment is given both psychically by thought transference and homeopathically. Color therapy is also used; disturbances of the aura are often manifested as a change of color from a brilliant blue to a dull and dirty yellow.

Dowsing by pendulum
Swinging a pendulum is the most popular way of tuning in to the mystical senses that can detect changes in the human aura. A small ball or crystal is hung from a fine, strong thread which is held in one hand. Questions are asked and answered yes or no by the swings of the pendulum (see also p.149).

REFERENCE: For more information about radionics and about color therapy, refer to **Section Five: A little black box** (pp.106–107) and **Rainbow health** (pp.118–119).

The six cycles

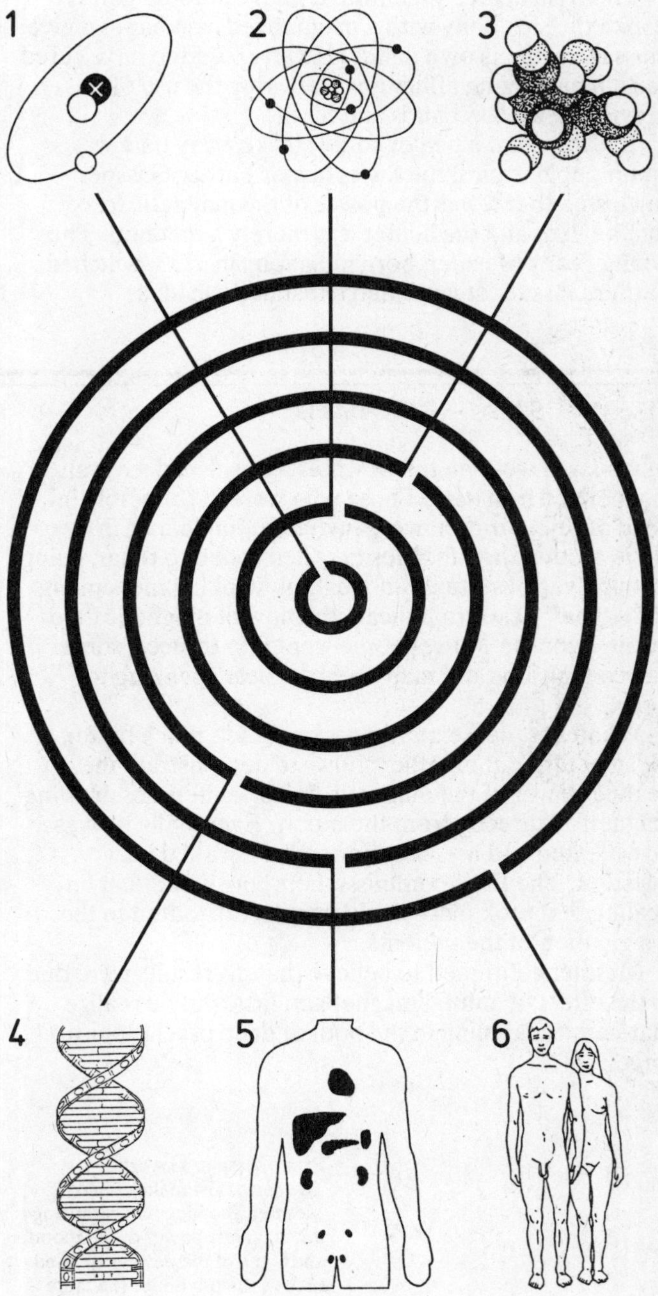

A healthy charge

The use of a magnetic charge for healing is an ancient treatment that was revived by Paracelsus, who was born Theophrastus Bombast von Hohenheim in Zurich in 1493. He took the name Paracelsus and many of his ideas from the Roman physician Celsus, some of whose writings had been discovered 50 years earlier. Paracelsus developed his own ideas and is thought to have tried to use the magnetic forces of magnets to heal illnesses of the mind.

The full exploitation of magnetism began in the 17th century, when many magnetic healers worked with the sick and were often given full recognition.

The Irish healer Valentine Greatriks would gently stroke the sick body with a magnetized iron bar and give massage with his own hands. He is reputed to have cured certain paralyzing afflictions, restoring the use of previously useless hands and feet.

The idea that a healer could stroke away pain was commonplace until the Swiss healer Father Gassner suggested that it was the power of the magnetic force that healed, and the healer was merely a medium. The young Franz Mesmer, born in Saxony in 1733, watched Father Gassner at work and expanded the idea.

Mesmerism

Mesmer was convinced that the healing element was animal magnetism which, like mineral magnetism, could be stored in iron bars. He worked in Vienna, where he was a close friend of Mozart. A girl musician who had been struck blind had been taken under the wing of the court, and through Mozart Mesmer contacted her and offered her treatment. She went to live in Mesmer's house, and after several sessions her sight began to be restored. The girl was delighted, but others were not so happy. Local doctors were jealous and tried to descredit Mesmer. Then the girl's parents were worried they might lose their daughter's pension, which had been granted by the Empress. They took her away from Mesmer and her sight deteriorated . . . but they retained their income.

Mesmer was angry and decided to leave Austria and settle in Paris. There he tried new methods and his magnetic bath became the talk of Paris society.

MESMER'S MAGNETIC BATH

Into a large wooden tub of water were placed several magnetized iron bars. Those who were ill or merely in need of revitalization were invited to join hands in a circle around the tub. Mesmer then spoke to them, going through various rituals and making stroking movements above their heads to indicate the flow of magnetic fluid through the air. Many people went into trances, some had convulsions and many heard voices speaking to them.

Whatever their experiences, most felt much better. Mesmer also put on other shows to demonstrate the healing power of the magnetic fluids, sometimes drawing magnetism directly from the moon. Eventually he was investigated and his "mesmerism" was called into question. The Paris commissioners concluded that any healing that took place could only be attributed to the imagination of the patients.

Mesmer continued to believe that his results were due to the effect of animal magnetism; little did he realize that he was dabbling in the pool of deep psychological forces.

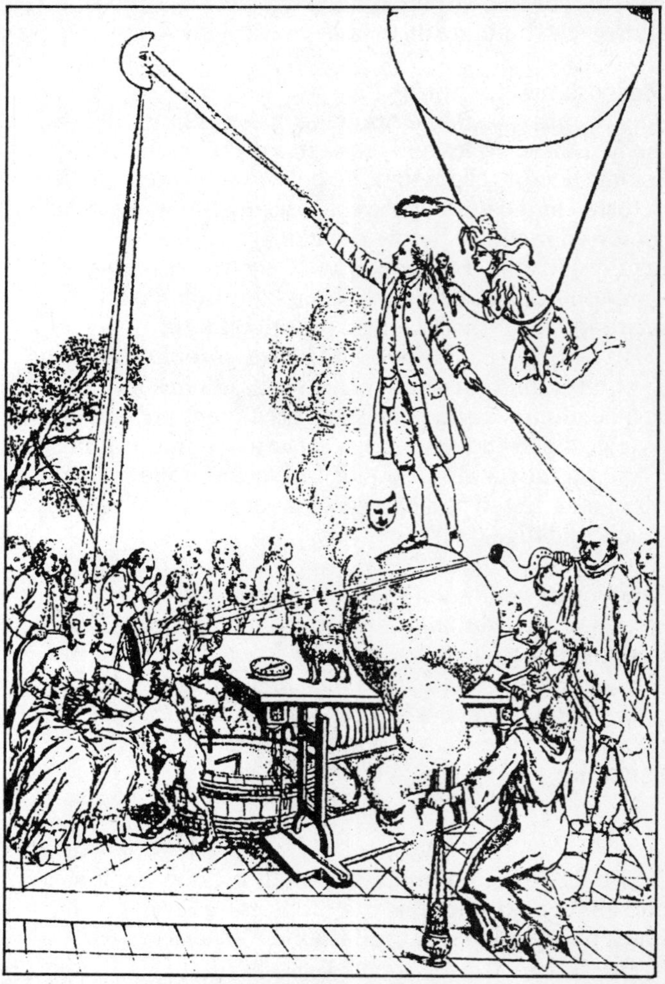

Franz Mesmer at work
The cartoonist makes fun of Mesmer, showing him capturing the magnetic power of the moon and some of the devices he used, such as the tub under the table

Convulsive seizures

The induction of some kind of brief convulsion or fit seems to give people a sense of well-being, although it may be temporary. Methods from all over the world and at all times in history for inducing a fit encompass shock treatments.

The electric eel used in Roman times was placed on the head and gave the patient a high voltage shock. Modern electro-convulsive therapy used for psychiatric disorders may be under greater control but is, in effect, the same as electric eel treatment.

Conversion sessions that take place during evangelical meetings involve self-induced convulsions, usually in a trance state. The process is similar in voodoo dances, the Tarantella and most ritual circle dances. Modern fashions in dancing, such as disco, acid-house and all-night sessions, induce trance-like states and sometimes mini-convulsions. The use of high-volume sound and strobe lighting aids the process.

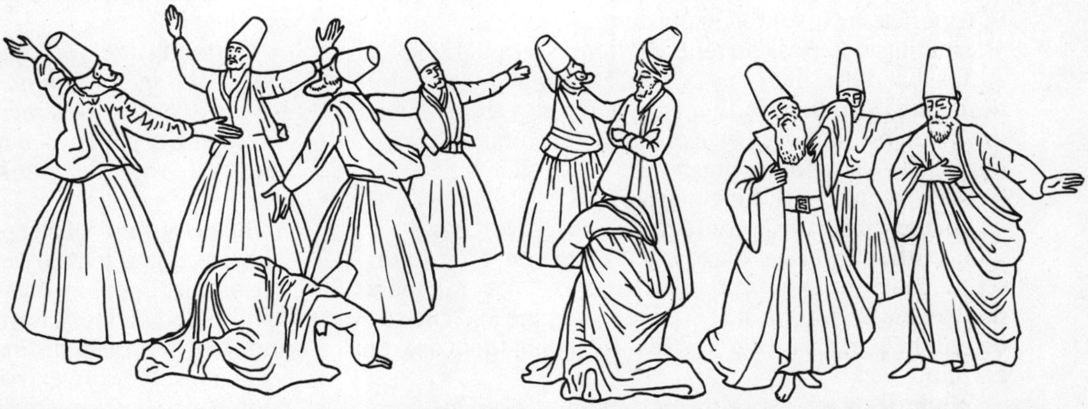

The Muslim dancing or whirling dervishes, a Sufi brotherhood founded in the 13th century

MESMERISM WAS NOT HYPNOSIS

Mesmer believed that the healing magnetic force came from the planets, and his devices were only a means of channeling the energy force. He had no knowledge of what we call hypnosis and would not have recognized the link that has been made between it and mesmerism.

Mesmer might have been more sympathetic to the idea that the natural energy life-force in humans could be enhanced by magnetism, but his own work was closer to spiritual healing than to hypnosis.

Unfortunately, after his death, egocentric individuals claimed to have personal magnetic powers, and stage shows demonstrating magnetism were born; they often discredited the work Mesmer himself achieved. The power to induce a trance state in another person was called mesmerism, but in reality that is what we now call hypnosis, a process that is discussed in **Suggestive healing** on the next page.

Mesmerism was, however, the beginning of our understanding of an important phenomenon that has been used for centuries: the power of the imagination while in a trance state.

Popular writers also discredited Mesmer's work. Here Svengali is using his evil magnetism in George du Maurier's novel *Trilby* (1894)

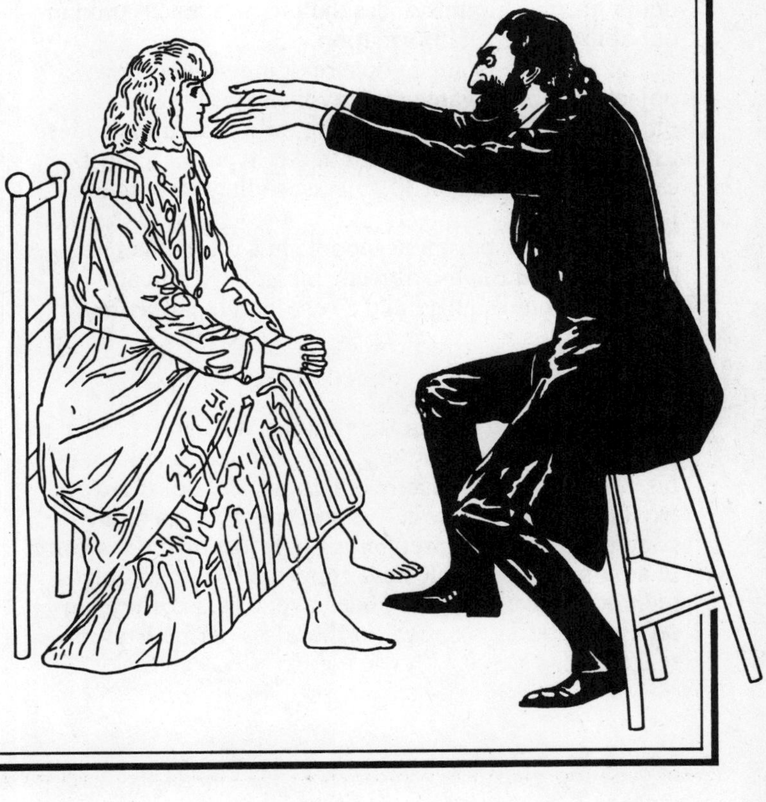

Suggestive healing

Although we may pride ourselves on our ability to stay in control of our own minds, we are all, fortunately, open to suggestive healing. Hypnotic suggestion is not, despite popular belief, available only to weak, emotional people.

Since women were supposed to be the weaker sex, most early illustrations show a male hypnotist putting a female subject into a trance, although there is no reason why it should not occur the other way around.

This biased attitude still causes people to ignore the potential of hypnotic suggestion for healing and to continue to regard hypnosis as some kind of power the strong have over the weak. Understanding how the mind works is a help in exploring the latent powers of hypnosis.

The amazing mind of Nikola Tesla
Born in Croatia, now part of Yugoslavia, in 1856, Nikola Tesla was a prodigious scientist. As an electrical engineer in America, he invented many devices, such as alternating electrical current and fluorescent lighting.

Tesla had the mind of a genius. He did all his designing in his head without any reference to written or drawn plans. He could give different machinists exact dimensions of separate machine parts, which, when finished, would all fit together perfectly.

Furthermore, Tesla could test his machines in his mind without ever having to build them first. He would set the machine in motion in his head and, several hours or even days later, would recall the machine and check out all the parts for wear and tear by taking them apart in his mind.

While Tesla was working on something else, his subconscious mind was putting the machine through its tests. It was as though Tesla had put part of his mind into a trance and it went on working, regardless of whatever else he might be doing consciously.

Accurate recall
Nikola Tesla must have had an extraordinary memory. In this respect he is not so different from other people. We all remember enormous amounts of information, yet under normal circumstances there is a wide variation in our ability to recall information.

For example, some people remember only a few objects in a party game that involves recalling 30 objects which have been seen for only 1 minute. Modern experiments have shown that under hypnosis almost everyone can recall all 30 objects, so they were not really forgotten at all.

In another experiment, people in a room filled with hundreds of unrelated objects, including a film and changing sounds, all gained a very high recall score under hypnosis.

Eidetic memory
Nikola Tesla had yet another ability. When he recalled a list of objects from memory, he would see them, not in his mind's eye, but exactly as if they were out there in front of him. This is called eidetic memory, an ability common among children but usually lost by the majority of adults. Some people have reported that their eidetic memories have returned under hypnosis, i.e. they can see remembered scenes "out there" as perfectly as the real thing.

Anesthetic hypnosis
It would appear then that the hypnotized mind can operate better in some circumstances than the conscious mind.

Certainly a relaxed, passive awareness can be most useful during operations. For example, dental patients having major work done on their teeth under hypnosis have neither pain nor anesthetic side-effects and can cooperate with the dentist.

A Japanese study of suggestion under hypnosis
The leaves of a local tree were causing severe allergic dermatitis. People with and without this condition were blindfolded and tested with leaves from the allergy tree and leaves from an ordinary chestnut tree.

The results were extraordinary. Under hypnosis, people who had previously had the allergy showed no reaction to the allergy tree leaves when told they came from the chestnut, while they reacted with skin blisters when told that the chestnut leaves were leaves from the allergy tree.

Also, several people who were not normally allergic, reacted with blistering when told they would have an allergic reaction to the leaves. Yet once out of hypnosis, they returned to normal.

Inflammation, blistering and mottled swelling are the visible signs of an allergic skin reaction. This is produced when the capillaries allow greater quantities of histamine to permeate the tissues. If under hypnosis the capillaries change their behavior and no skin reaction occurs, then bypassing the conscious and allowing the unconscious to direct events would seem to be a very valuable way of treating many disturbances. This is contrary to the belief that deliberate, conscious positive thinking is a way to cure sickness.

An 1845 subject of hypnotism glimpses his future

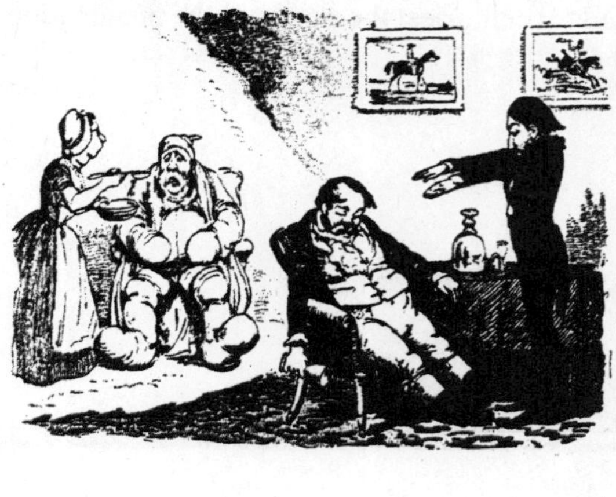

HYPNOSIS

An altered state of consciousness that can be induced by the self or by another person and during which conscious control is relaxed making the contents of the unconscious more accessible. In all measurable physiological respects, it does not differ from the waking state.

There are normally five basic steps to attain hypnosis, although actual methods vary. The most effective way of inducing hypnosis, even without step-by-step instruction, is to listen through earphones to magnified breathing sounds from the lower throat. This is done by a special recording device, but anyone with a soft voice can usually learn how to induce hypnosis.

1 The subject sits or lies comfortably; this limits physical tension and anxiety. This is the first stage of withdrawal from normal consciousness.

2 The subject is told to concentrate on the hypnotist's voice and actions to the exclusion of everything else. This reduces the number of environmental distractions.

3 The subject is told to listen passively and simply accept what is said. This limits the complex internal mental processes of evaluation and decision-making.

4 The subject may be asked to stare at a single object. This produces retinal fatigue, precisely what is required in hypnosis, so that the eyes are ready to close.

5 A sleep-like condition is suggested, and the hypnotist makes some trial suggestions to confirm that the subject has slipped into a hypnotic trance.

What can hypnosis do?
Several researchers have shown that hypnotherapy can relieve pain in terminal illness, be effective inducing healing in 50% of people over the long term and even make stubborn warts disappear when normal high-technology methods have failed.

Since commands to sit or stand will be followed under hypnosis, there seems to be no reason why we should not use hypnotic suggestion for healing.

Problems of hypnotherapy
An unconscious drive clashing with a suggestion made by a hypnotist, say about a dependent habit, may bring on a dangerous stress reaction if the habit provides an important crutch.

The other danger area is in the use of hypnosis for regression to uncover painful events that have been deeply repressed for self-protection. Thus, during hypnotic regression, recall is not always accurate.

AUTOGENIC THERAPY

A German psychiatrist and neurologist, Dr Johannes Schultz, was working in Berlin in the 1930s, when he began to develop hypnosis as a practical self-help activity for his patients. His autogenic training program consisted of exercises to attain passive relaxation in all parts of the body in six stages.
1 Feeling heaviness in all the limbs.
2 Feeling warmth in the extremities.
3 Calming the heartbeat.
4 Calming and regularizing the breathing.
5 Warming the solar plexus.
6 Cooling the forehead.
Neither the trainer nor the trainee/patient would direct these exercises toward an illness. The aim was to attain passive relaxation. This alone, claimed Schultz, was a healing state.

A pinch of optimism

Optimism is a very powerful force. It alters perceptions and moods, transforming misery and disinterest into joy and anticipation. Achievers are said to be eternal optimists, and small children are almost always optimistic. They believe that wishing hard enough for something will make it happen.

Believing you will get well from an illness is to be optimistic about yourself and the treatment. If the treatment is an apparently unrelated prescription, such as a rhyme to be repeated or a minor ritual to be performed, the result can be truly magical.

Ancient peoples often had little else to rely upon other than optimism. The act of doing something, such as reciting a magic formula or drawing a magic circle, gave shape to the hope for a cure. To the mind of the ancient savage, these rituals had a very realistic use.

The Abracadabra prescription
In use since the time of the Roman Emperor Caracalla, the Abracadabra formula would be written by the patient in full on the first day of treatment. On each succeeding day a letter is lost, relaxing the grip of the sickness, until it completely disappears as the last line is reached. The Abracadabra was also worn as a protective jewelry talisman round the neck.

The magic formula

A B R A C A D A B R A
A B R A C A D A B R
A B R A C A D A B
A B R A C A D A
A B R A C A D
A B R A C A
A B R A C
A B R A
A B R
A B
A

Using a magic ritual to force an illness to leave is not as crazy at it may seem. The optimism of children was perhaps why they cured each other's warts during an experiment described in 1953 by Professor H.J.Eysenck in his book *The Uses and Abuses of Psychology.*

The Eysenck wart experiment
One group of children was given normal medical treatment for their warts and the other group used magic.

The magic method began as each child made a large drawing of its own hand with the wart marked on it surrounded by a large circle. Every day a smaller concentric circle was drawn around the wart as magic exhortations were made until the wart was metaphorically squeezed out. To everyone's surprise, the magic method was far more effective than the medical treatment.

The drawing ritual
a First circle
b Last circle
c Wart

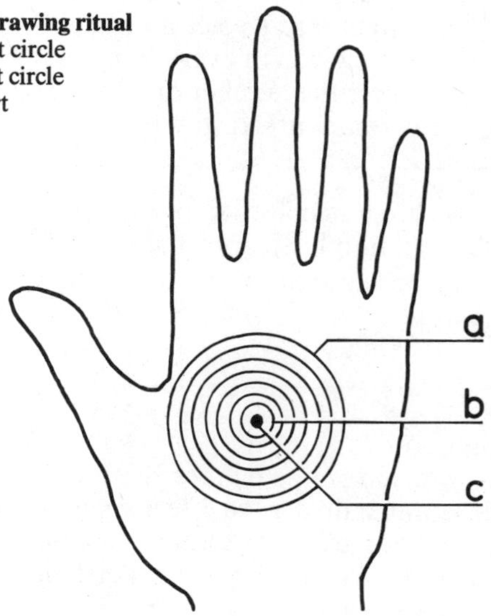

THE COMMON WART
By its very nature the wart is magical. It appears without obvious cause and generally disappears in its own time, seemingly regardless of treatment.

A wart, or verruca, is a small benign tumor on the skin caused by direct contact with a virus. Hence warts appear by contagion most often on the feet and hands. Warts and verrucas were traditionally regarded as blemishes. The common saying: "Will you love me, warts and all?" means "Will you love me, including all my failings?"

Some folklore methods to remove warts

Stringing
Take the stem of an onion and slice it length-wise until several fine, string-like pieces are produced. Then wrap the strings around the base of the wart, tying them as tightly as possible. In time the wart is expected to drop off.

Using herbs
Cover the skin surrounding the wart and apply the juice from several stems of the celadine flower. Slices of garlic may be applied instead. Repeat until the wart disappears.

Wart charms
- Charm it away with a kiss from your beloved (not a good idea, since warts are contagious).

THE MAGIC CIRCLE

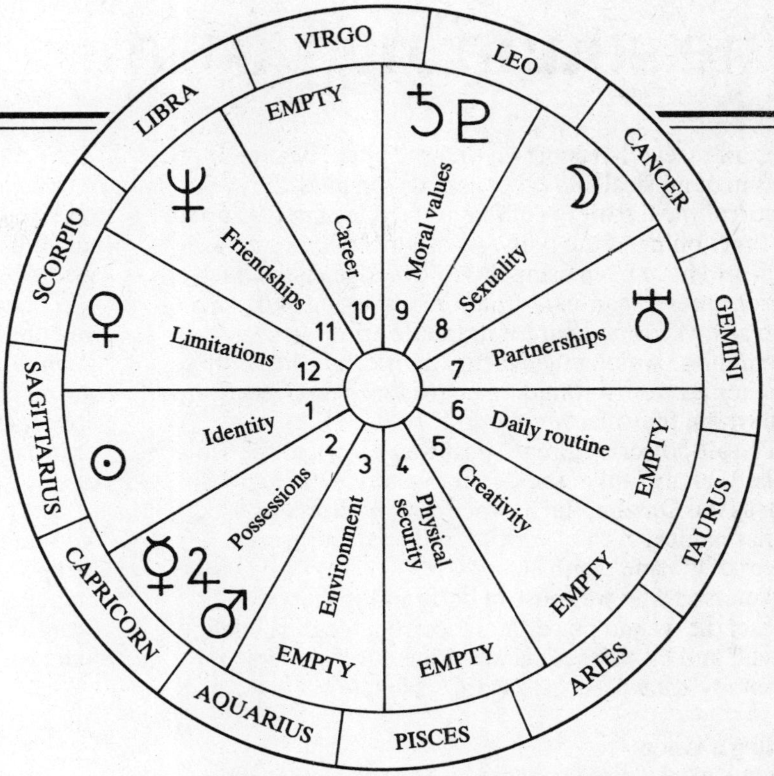

Key to the planets

☉	Sun	♃	Jupiter
☽	Moon	♄	Saturn
☿	Mercury	♅	Uranus
♀	Venus	♆	Neptune
♂	Mars	♇	Pluto

Throughout history, the circle has been a symbol for wholeness and harmony. The use of the circle in magic healing is to bring completeness by removing the evil that has caused disruption.

The incomplete circle is a feature of astrology. In a birth chart, it is said that the houses empty of planets are the areas of life that are lacking and should be filled to build a whole, satisfying life.

An astrological birth chart
The chart shows the positions of the planets at birth in houses numbered 1–12. The zodiac signs are around the edge and indicate the type of personality.

The chart is that of a woman who, after several false starts and mistakes, has finally "filled" the empty houses of her life by starting to build a career with a responsible job (**10**). This has enabled her to fill her needs for physical security (**4**), possessions (**2**), a daily routine (**6**) and an opportunity to develop creatively (**5**).

She has completed the magic circle and can now begin to develop all parts of her life to the full. The first step, as she explained, was the hardest for her: getting into the right frame of mind. Determined optimism enabled her to build bridges into her new life. Determination is the characteristic of her Capricorn sun sign. Optmism was the magic formula that helped to fill the gaps in her life.

- Wrap it in a cheesecloth soaked in sour milk.
- Run counterclockwise seven times around a church at midnight.
- Every night before retiring, expose the wart to the moon and say loudly: "Go wart, on this night, never more to be my blight."
- In the area of England around the old Roman city of Chester, the method was to rub the warts with a piece of bacon and push the bacon under the bark of an ash tree. The wart will disappear from the hand but remain as a knob on the bark of the tree.

Orthodox methods
Orthodox treatments include the application of a mixture of salicylic acid and podophyllum resin or of salicylic acid, lactic acid and flexible collodion.

Tying onion strings around a wart

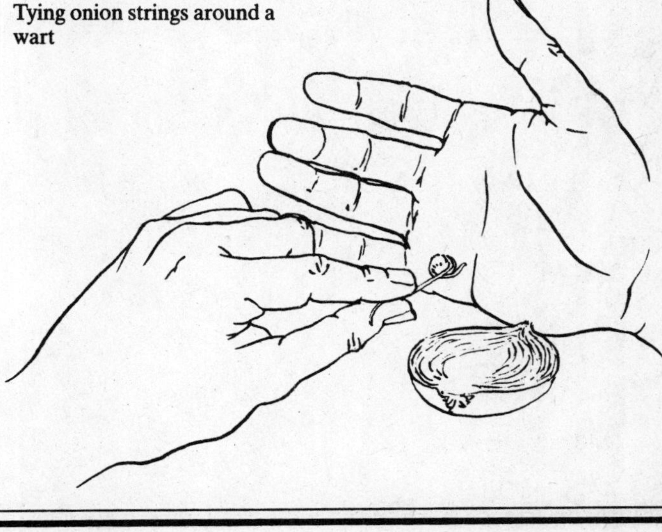

The sounding board

Modern research has shown that the pitch, beat and rhythm of musical and other sounds can alter the electrical wave patterns of the brain, which in turn affect the functioning of the body. Aboriginal peoples all over the world have been using this knowledge instinctively for centuries. Chanting, drumming, shaking and dancing have always formed part of dramatic primitive ceremonies. Among the North American Indians, these ceremonies were a sounding board for their Great Spirit, with whom they placed their faith.

The all-powerful Great Spirit was known to the Sioux as the Wakan Tanka: the Great Mystery. Other tribes, such as the Omaha, the Pawnee and the Iroquois used similar names; each of which signified the universal power of life and death.

A person who was pure in body and spirit could contact the wakan power and receive it for the benefit of himself and his tribe. This was done during a personal ceremony known as "calling the vision."

Calling a vision

Anyone who aspired to serve his tribe as a medicine man, a wise man or a great warrior must gain the power of the wakan before he could hope to succeed. A boy on the verge of manhood would go into a remote place to fast, meditate and lose himself in the forces of nature. Often he would stand and call into the solitude for a vision to appear. Eventually he would dream a vision of an animal that would help him to use the superhuman power that was flowing into him as he meditated. The animal might be an eagle, a bear, an owl or a crow. Throughout life, he could call upon the spirit of this animal to help him use his power wisely.

A young brave calling the vision of a buffalo

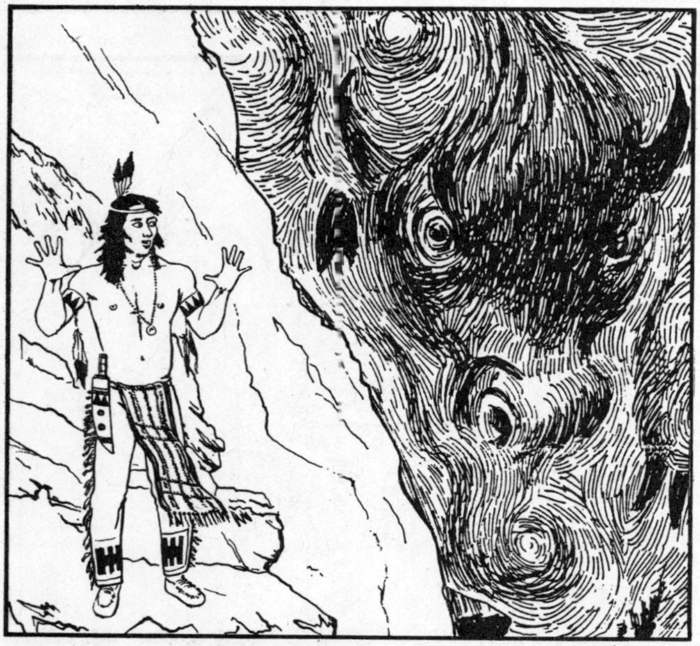

The American Indian medicine men

All the members of a tribe revered a man who had received in a vision the wakan power to heal. There might be several medicine men in one tribe, and they would live in seclusion, helped only by a wife.

The medicine men took part in all public ceremonies and undertook private healing ceremonies with sick members of the tribe. To conduct a healing ceremony, the medicine man would sit by the patient, chanting the appropriate medicine song, accompanied by sacred objects that also contained the wakan power: a rattle, a drum, the tail or horn of their visionary animal.

The patient had complete faith in the medicine man who himself had unshakable faith in the healing powers he had been given during his vision. The animal spirit helped to chase away the spirit that causes sickness and bring about healing. The rattle is often used to disturb and rouse the sick spirit.

A Papago medicine man from Arizona using the rattle and a deer tail

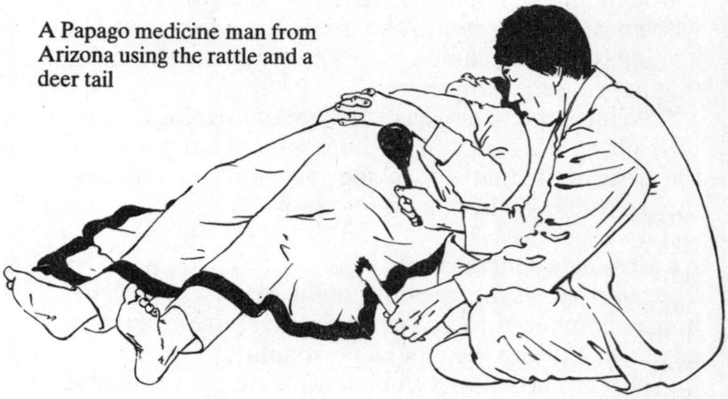

A Chippewa medicine man kneeling over his patient during a healing ceremony

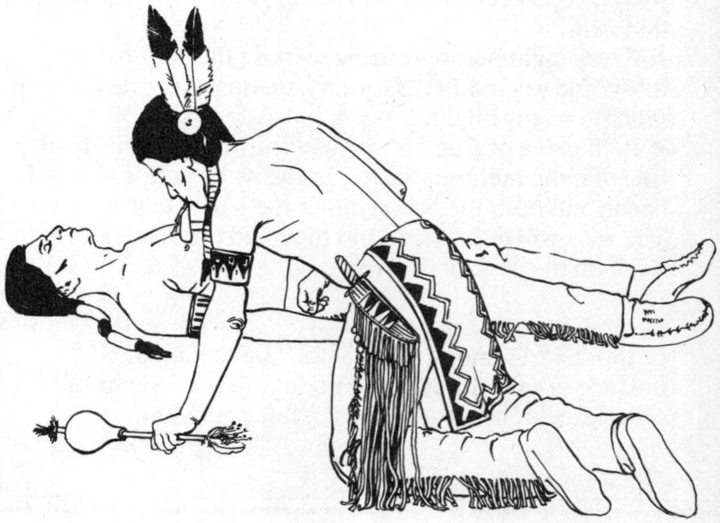

The religion of the Chippewa Indians
The Chippewa tribe of Minnesota believe that goodness ensures a long and healthy life and that evil will eventually destroy itself. The role of the medicine men is not only to heal the sick but also to undertake public ceremonies to prevent sickness and promote good health. These ceremonies are conducted by members of the Grand Medicine Society or Mide-wiwin.

Mide-wiwin men have undergone four initiations by calling the vision, and use medical songs and formulas received in visions by themselves and other members of the Society. The symbol of the Mide-wiwin is a small shell, similar to a cowrie, which itself has medicinal properties.

A translation of one of the Mide-wiwin songs is roughly as follows:

We dance around you, my life, a single tree,
I hear the spirit's voice around the sky,
I walk on half the sky,
I am in the crow, his skin covers my body.

This pictograph of medical songs (*below*) from the records of the Chippewa Grand Medicine Society uses mnemonics to remind the members of the Mide-wiwin of their sacred, healing songs.

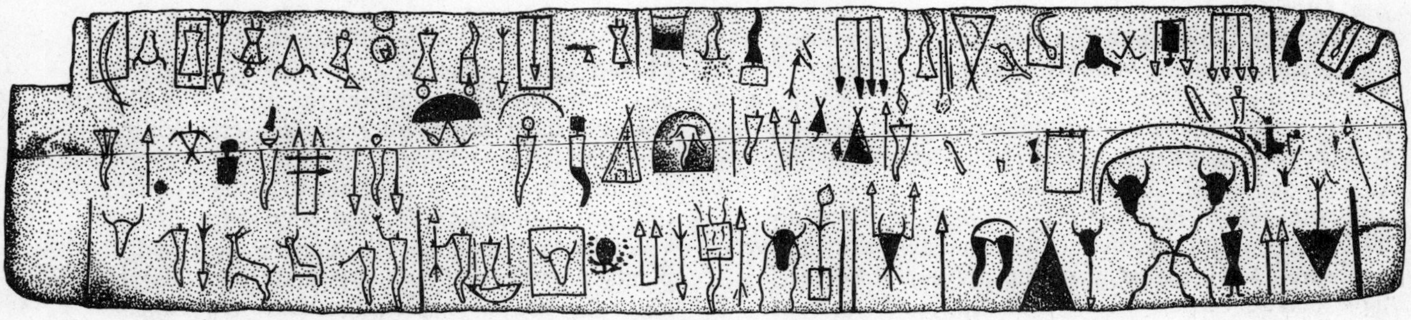

Indian herb medicine
Like all the tribes, the Navaho Indians believed that there is a spirit in everything that can be invoked by making the correct sound. When herbs are gathered for medicines special herb-gathering songs are sung to awaken the spirit of the herb, for it is this spirit that fights the spirit of the disease.

For a description of the ceremonies carried out by the Navaho medical "tremblers" refer to **Section Three: Magical rituals** (pp.60-61.)

The sounding board of healing
Other cultures use the repetitive sound of chanting, drumming or rattling to bring about healing; for example, Kido, a practice used by Korean Zen Buddhists, induces an ecstatic state of consciousness. Attained by chanting with percussion instruments for as long as 12 hours a day, the chanter is said to become one with the Bodhisattva of Compassion who will bring about healing.

In modern times, faith is still placed in the power of sound to heal. Music therapy is used both professionally and by amateurs to heal the disturbed mind and body. Many children who have felt alienated or unhappy in other ways have grown to love the music that gave them hope and taught them how to join in the pleasures of music-making with others.

For almost everyone, music of one kind or another is pleasurable and can take us into a dreamland, where we can throw off the stresses of the day and relax, becoming refreshed and rejuvenated. Whatever style of music is your sounding board, it has healing properties that can help to keep you well and "in tune" with life.

Malabar medicine man performs the Ottam Thullal dance at Trivandrum, South India

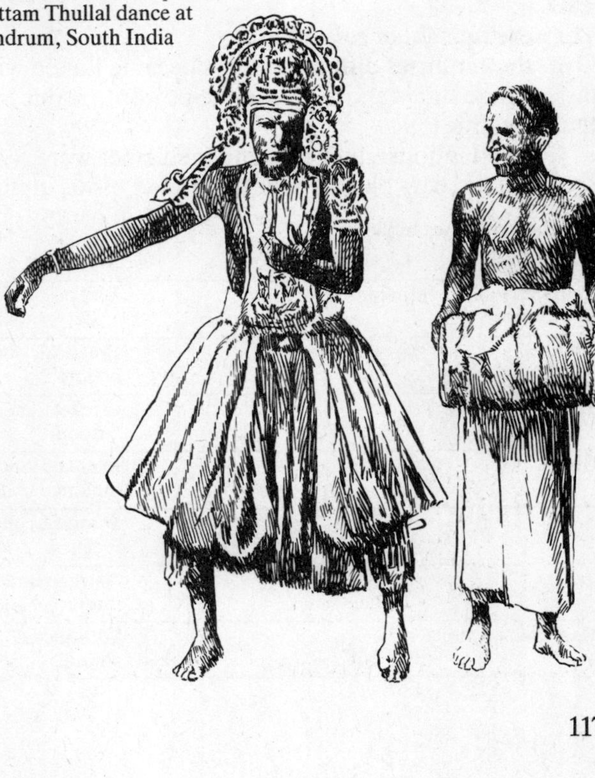

Rainbow health

It has been shown that a lack of light during winter gives some people a temporary depression. This seasonal depression is acknowledged by many medical authorities, and sufferers are urged to spend more time in daylight whenever they can and to use bright lights indoors.

The healing power of natural light has been applied for centuries. The sun-cult of heliotherapy was practiced by the Incas in South America, and Ancient Greeks spent much time sunbathing and airbathing, while other cultures were sun-worshippers.

The light of life

Scientists have proved that intense light enters the deep organs of the body and passes through the skulls of sheep, dogs and rabbits to activate photo-electric cells in brain tissue.

In addition to luminous animals such as glow-worms, all animals, including humans, emit light and radio waves of their own. In 1983 Dr G. Rein, a biologist at St Bartholomew's Hospital in London, England, reported that the electro-magnetic energy of healers affects enzyme activity and neurotransmission.

Sexual activity is also affected by light. In Piccadilly Circus in central London, the birds, mostly starlings, live exposed to the constant glare and colors of street lights and advertisements. It has been found that these birds remain sexually potent even during the normal period of impotency experienced by starlings living in a country habitat.

Even mammals that are color blind are influenced by colored light. Commercial breeders of chinchilla use blue light to encourage the conception of more females, which have thicker furs than males. In normal light chinchillas produce 50% males and 50% females; in pink light they produce 70% males and 30% females, but in blue light the percentages are reversed.

The development of color therapy

Over the centuries different colors became linked with different qualities and assigned the power to induce those qualities.

Colored lotions, unguents and medicines were recommended by philosopher Aurelius Celsius in the 1st century, and by the 10th century the magical properties of color were common knowledge, although not everyone agreed about those properties. Avicenna, an 11th century Arab physician, also related color to human temperament.

Probably the most spectacular claims for color were made in 1878 by an Englishman, Edwin D. Babbitt. In his book *The Principles of Light and Color* he linked colors with elements, minerals and functions of the body, claiming many instances of healing by filtering sunlight through stained glass.

Babbitt invented and sold aids to color healing, such as Chromo-discs, a Thermolune cabinet and a stained-glass window that could be used for healing minor ailments. A person sat inside the cabinet while sunlight was filtered through colored glass, bathing him in red, blue or green light.

Modern color therapy

Diagnosis involves examining the aura to establish the color shortage, using either a Kilner screen or the therapist's clairvoyance.

Filtered sunlight is then used to bathe the patient in the pure color required. Food, such as fruit and vegetables of the same color, may be suggested, and plants, flowers, artificial lamps and clothes should also repeat the color. While being treated, a person is encouraged to visualize the color during daily relaxation exercises.

In some instances a glass of water, wrapped in color filters, is left in the sunshine for several hours to absorb the required color directly from the sun's rays. The water is then drunk by the patient. In India, where color therapy is part of the Ayurvedic system of medicine, colored gemstones may also be used to focus the mind.

The Hygeia Clinic

Situated in Gloucester, England, the clinic is run by Theo Gimble, who is probably the foremost authority on color therapy today.

His father, Max Gimble-Seiling, worked for ten years with Rudolph Steiner (1861–1925). Together they devised a system of stage lighting to suggest various moods and went on to investigate the effect of colors on

The color rays used in therapy

Color	Attributes	Uses
Red: every shade from pink to maroon	Will power, life and vitality; courage	Blood and circulation; debility and depression
Orange	Practical, disciplined energy; intelligent action	Spleen, kidneys, digestion and chest conditions
Yellow	Intellect, mental activity, creativity and wisdom	Nervous system, the skin and some mental problems
Green	Sympathy, adaptability, harmony, diplomacy, stamina	Heart, nervous headaches and emotional disorders
Blue	Serenity, consciousness, self-reliance, idealism	Fevers, bleeding, irritations, nervous rage, anger
Indigo	Astringency, purity, spirituality and intuition	Eyes, ears and nose and all conditions of toxicity
Magenta and violet	Spiritual and mental equilibrium; psychic abilities	Sleeplessness, neuralgia, rheumatism and epilepsy

mood. The Anthroposophical Society, founded by Steiner, has done much research into the effect of colors and their significance in artistic expression.

Theo Gimble was influenced by all this work and has since developed color therapy comprehensively. He uses 16 filters to produce different colors in his color therapy room. While his books give exact instructions for color visualization for those who wish to apply self-help methods, he also runs training courses for therapists.

The Kilner screen
Dr J. Kilner, then a medical electrician in a London hospital, invented the Kilner screen for viewing a person's aura using a double plate of glass containing a cyanine dye.

He describes the human aura as extending about 18 inches in an ovoid shape around the body. It changes color and becomes duller and difficult to see during illness. He also found that some women were able to change the color of their aura at will.

Cobalt tinted glasses are also used. Many healers claim that only clairvoyants can see the aura.

THE ELECTRO-MAGNETIC SPECTRUM

Energy comes in the form of waves of varying length and frequency. At one end are gamma rays and x-rays (high frequency and short wavelength), at the other, radio waves and heat waves.

The primary light colors
Visible light is a narrow, fairly central band in the spectrum. It can be split into its component colors by refraction (bending) through a prism or crystal. Sunlight refracted through raindrops produces a rainbow.

Complementaries are made with two primaries. Indigo, for example, is cyan with more blue than green and a slightly lower intensity of light, resulting in the dark, greenish-blue of indigo.

Five bands of waves with similar properties
1 RADIO WAVES including laser beams; microwaves; wavelengths used for broadcasting radio and TV
2 INFRA-RED WAVES including radiant heat
3 VISIBLE LIGHT includes white light which contains a spectrum of colored light: violet, indigo; blue; green; yellow; orange; red
4 ULTRA-VIOLET RAYS cause sunburn
5 X-RAYS including gamma rays
a Heat waves
b Cosmic waves

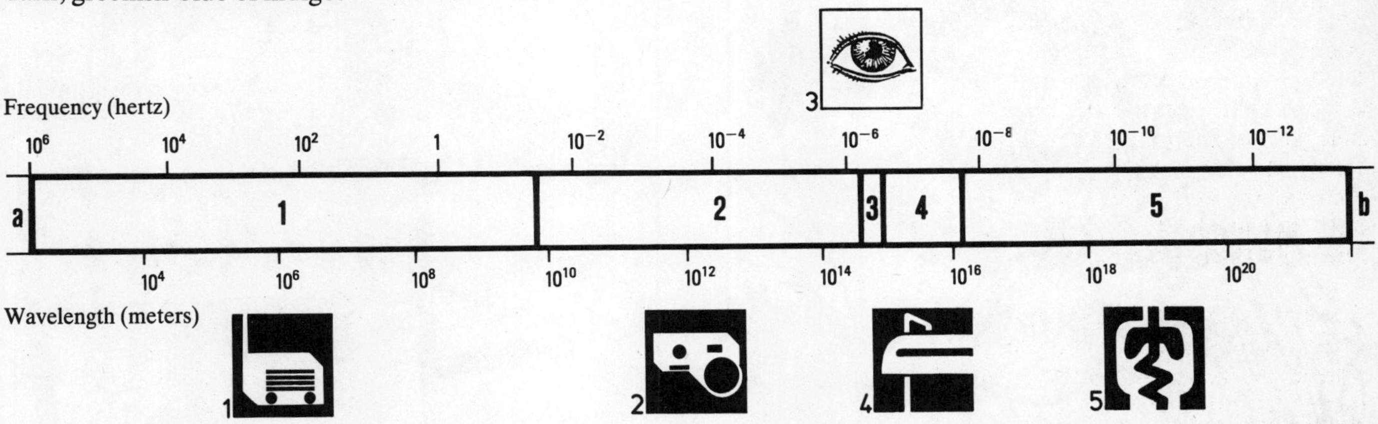

Chakra therapy
Some color therapists work via the chakras, the seven centers of intense energy down the spine. Each chakra is said to respond to a different color, which corresponds to the body function served by the chakra. It is unwise to try color therapy without a trained therapist, as exposure to the wrong colors can have negative results.

Correspondences claimed by chakra therapists

	Chakras	Location	Attribute	Color	Effect
1	Crown	Top of head	Spirituality	Violet	Clears the mind
2	Third eye	Bridge of nose	Clairvoyance	Blue	Stimulates
3	Throat	Thyroid	Intelligence	Cyan	Sensitizes
4	Heart	Centre sternum	Compassion	Green	Centers
5	Solar plexus	Just below navel	Feeling	Yellow	Impassions
6	Sacral	Base of spine	Sensation	Orange	Nourishes
7	Root	Just anterior to anus	Sexuality	Red	Reassures

Section six

ADAPTIVE POTIONS

Drinking, eating or applying a remedy are the first actions taken against all ailments in every culture. An ordinary family dwelling 3000 years ago would have a selection of tried and tested medicines, just as any modern home may have its shelf of pills for a headache, medicine for a cough or ointment for a wounded knee. Only when the remedy failed to cure the ailment would a doctor be visited.

In most instances the remedy worked. The menstrual pain would be relieved, the parasite removed, the bowels cleared or the spasm calmed. Herbs and other plant extracts were in use that are still appropriate today, such as castor oil, aloe and gentian.

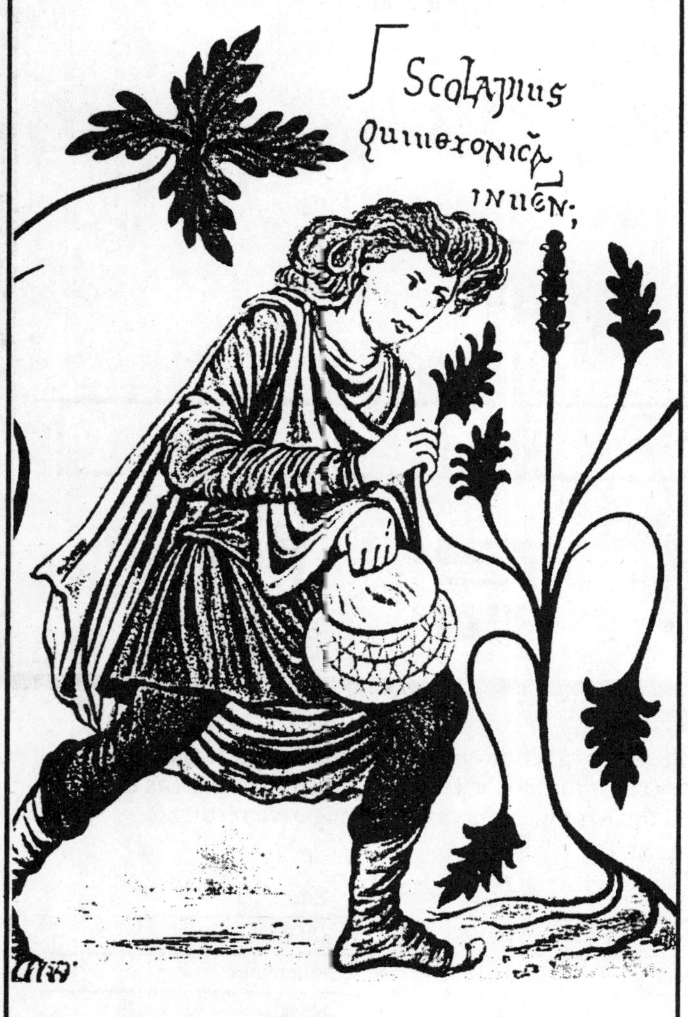

Herbs: Botanical enquiries lead to discovery of the healing properties of plants. Aesculapius discovers betony, from a 9th century MS.

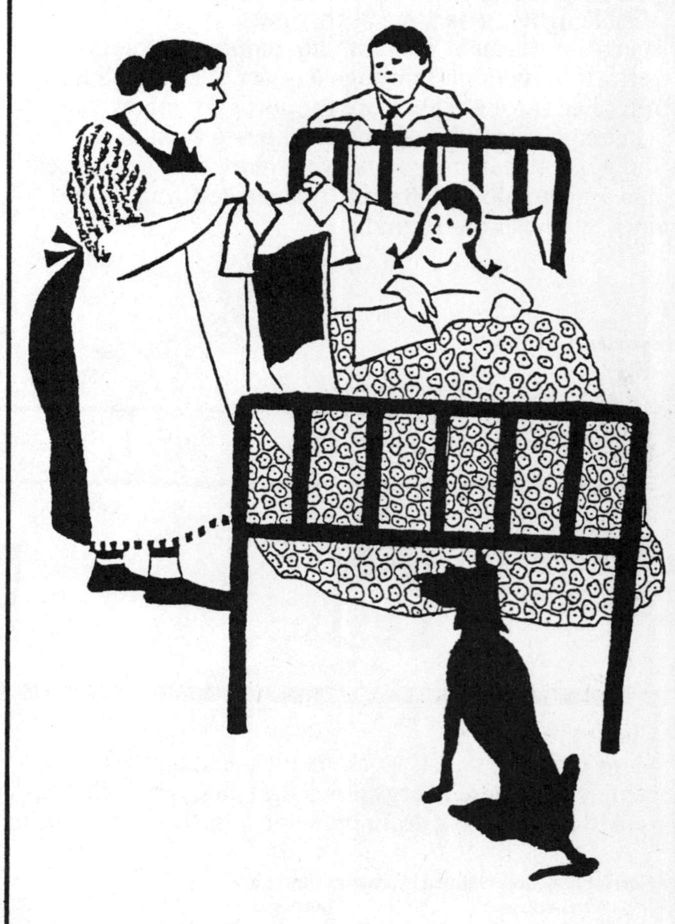

Old wives' tales: To cure a child's cough, greased brown paper was sewn under the patient's garment and worn until it fell off.

There were drugs and medicines for all occasions, some of which have a therapeutic effect, such as myrrh, which is an anti-microbial, and others that seem not only odd to us now but clearly dangerous, such as the feces of a horsefly used to calm a baby's tantrums.

Stories of remedies and their preparation were passed down through families, and many modern herbalists have gained much from this oral knowledge.

Special remedies, such as those prepared for homeopathic use, and special categories, such as mineral salts and flower remedies, are given careful attention in this section. It is easy to dismiss the old pharmacies as primitive, but that would be a great mistake, for of all the alternative medicines available today, many are direct descendants from an ancient medical folklore that made life easier for our ancestors, when they suffered from common ailments similar to our own.

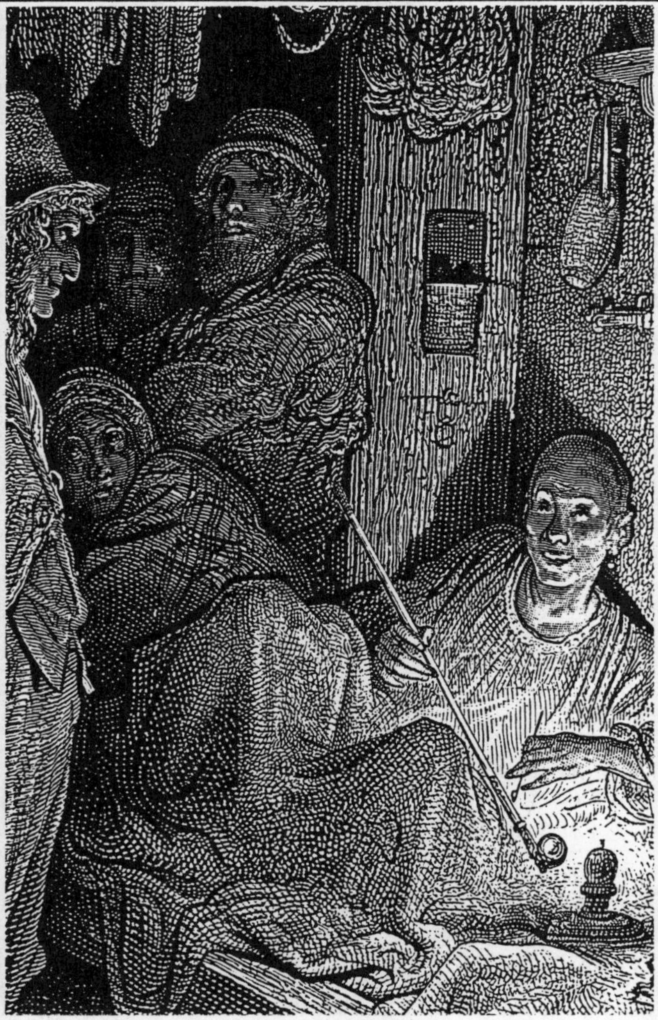

Drugs: Asian plants such as poppy-extracted opium began as medication and ended as widespread social addiction. Gustave Doré engraving of a Victorian East End of London opium den.

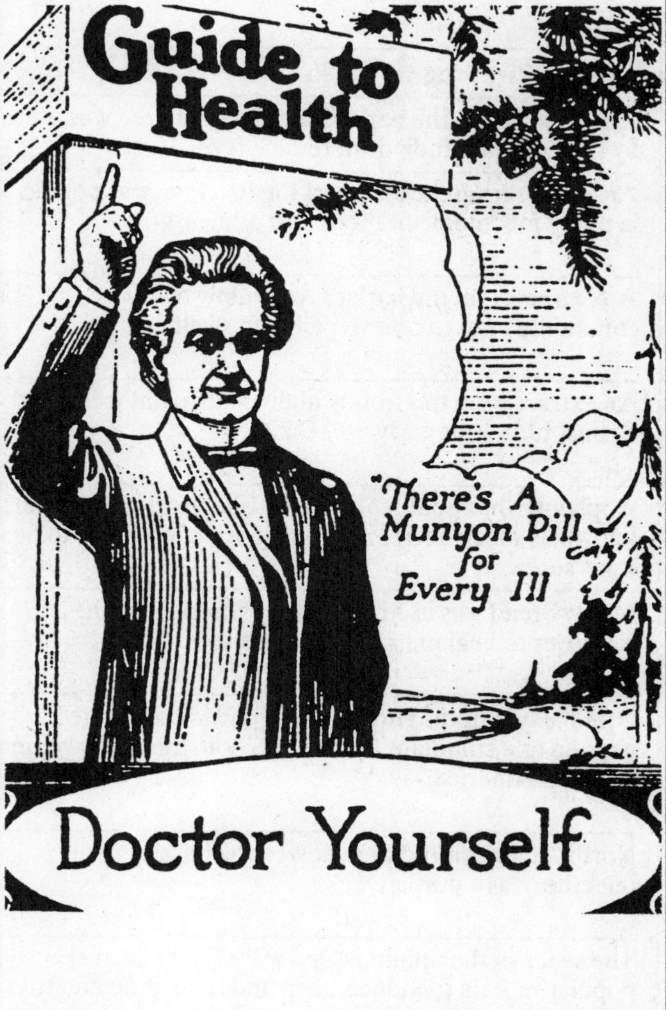

Placebos: Although the US Government had shown with tests that James M Munyon's pills were largely sugar, patients of the early 1900s continued to buy them in millions.

The primitive pharmacopoeia

Modern pharmacists are familiar with a range of drugs, medicines, salves, antiseptics, anesthetics, vaccines, cosmetics, contraceptives and many other concoctions whose use is spreading rapidily throughout the world.

There have been some disasters, such as the sedative thalidomide that in 1961 was found to cause limb deformities in the embryo. Some drugs also have alarming long-term effects; for example, in 1989 most health authorities recommended a 10-year limit on the use of oral contraceptives after a link was found with the occurrence of breast cancer. However, on balance, modern drugs and potions are life-saving or life-enhancing, yet many are not so new as we might imagine. Some of our most common drugs had their origins in the primitive pharmacopoeia

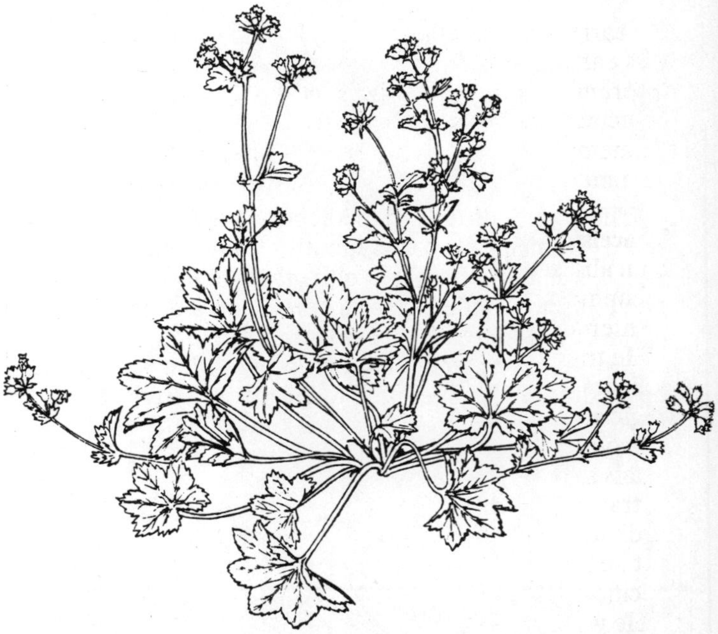

Lady's mantle or *Alchemilla vulgaris*, a small perennial plant, historically used to check bleeding and today as a herbal medicine to counteract excessive menstruation.

The primitive drug	The same drug in modern use
An extract from the bark of the cinchona tree was used by the Peruvian Indians to reduce fever.	Quinine, used by Europeans from the 17th century, treats malaria and other fevers.
An extract from the leaves of the foxglove was popular in many folk medicines for heart ailments.	Digitalis was for many years the only treatment for heart diseases until the discovery of beta-blockers and other new drugs in the 1970s.
An extract from the bark of the willow tree was commonly used to relieve pain and swellings.	Acetylsalicylic acid (aspirin) is still the basis of several hundred modern anti-inflammatory and pain-killing proprietory drugs.
An extract from the woody nightshade plant was used against tumors as early as AD 200.	The extract of woody nightshade was used with success in 1966 by researchers at the University of Wisconsin to treat a cancer in mice.
Applying a hot poultice of the crushed and boiled plant known as sheep-sorrel in rural America was used to heal open sores.	Oxalic acid (present in sheep-and wood-sorrel) is a very sour, poisonous acid with some antiseptic properties.
Moldy bread was used by soldiers throughout the centuries to heal their festering wounds.	Penicillin (*Penicillium notatum*) was the first antibiotic, discovered in 1928 by Alexander Fleming in bread mold.
Dried leaves of the shrub *Erythroxylon coca* were chewed as a stimulant by Indians, both men and women in South America.	Cocaine, derived from the coca plant, is still used medically as a mild anesthetic, although its illegal use as a stimulant is probably better known. It was an ingredient of Coca-Cola drinks until banned.
North American Indians chewed the bark of the buckthorn as a purgative.	Cascara powder, prepared from the dried leaves of the North American buckthorn, is infused or made into pills to treat constipation.
The seeds of the opium poppy were (and still are) popular in Asia to induce sleep and relaxation and to relieve pain.	Morphine, the alkaloid narcotic obtained from opium, is widely used in modern medicine for the control of extreme or terminal pain. Until the 20th century it was freely available on the open market as laudanum.
The evergreen leaves of the trailing shrub *ephedra* were used to relieve bronchial problems at least as early as Roman times.	Ephedrine is an alkaloid drug obtained from some ephedras, used for hayfever and asthma.

The early pharmacists
If an early pharmacist can be defined as a person who experiments with mixes of chemical substances to make medicines and other useful concoctions, then Paracelsus, Hahnemann and Ehrlich were probably the three most outstanding of the European pharmacists.

Paracelsus
Born about 1493 in a Swiss mining town, Aureolus Theophrastus Bombastus von Hohenheim grew up with an interest in medicine and metallurgy.

He traveled, took the name Paracelsus from his ancient Greek medical hero and dabbled in astrology, magic and alchemy. He went to extremes in all he did and soon became totally immersed in the chemistry of metals and the distillation of poisons he obtained during his travels. He believed that "the concealed finger of God" was in the chemicals with which he worked and that he only had to extract the correct substance to heal a specific disease.

He worked with many poisonous substances. He refined them to release their arcanum, or secret, special properties. He used arsenic, sulfur, strychnine, lead, copper, mercury, iron, silver and antimony, but all in tiny quantities. Accused of giving his patients poisons, he declared "all things are poisons; it is the dosage that makes them non-poisons."

Paracelsus was the first to treat specific diseases with specific medicines, ignoring popular ideas about evil spirits and sinful patients. After his death, the use of his medicines was enthusiastically adopted but in large doses, thus killing and maiming many people.

Hahnemann
Dr Samuel Hahnemann was born in Meissen, Germany, in 1755 and was disillusioned with the way medicine was being practiced. He traveled, taught Greek, Hebrew and Arabic and became familiar with the work of Paracelsus.

An Englishman returning from Peru introduced him to the bark of the cinchona tree, which had cured his malaria. Hahnemann chewed some of the bark himself and promptly got an attack of malaria, which soon passed. From this experience, he developed the idea that what cures a sick person will also produce the same symptoms in a healthy person. On this principle he refined some 4000 homeopathic medicines.

Ehrlich
The German Paul Ehrlich was born in Silesia in 1854. His work was similar in principle to that of Paracelsus and Hahnemann. Fascinated by dyes and how they would color certain tissues and not others, he set out to find a way in which a chemical could be aimed at an exact place in the body without damaging the surrounding tissues.

Moving to Frankfurt he set up a research team to find a cure for syphilis. His contemporaries thought he was mad to hope that a poison would seek out and kill a disease and leave the rest of the body unharmed.

After seven years, tests at a Berlin hospital cleared a syphilitic lesion in the throat of a male patient who was then able to speak again. The drug he refined was dihydroxyarsenobenzene dihydrochloride, renamed salvarsan. Although later changes have been made, Ehrlich had given the first successful chemotherapy treatment . . . or was it the first? Paracelsus had already successfully treated some advanced tumors with mercury chloride, some 400 years earlier. At least Ehrlich had the pharmacological work of Paracelsus and Hahnemann to thank for leading the way.

REFERENCE: For more information about Hahnemann and his remedies, refer to **Section Six: Homeopathic remedies** (pp.134–135)

THE COSMETIC PHARMACY
Painting the body for ritual purposes was usually done to ward off evil spirits, enhance potency or frighten adversaries during battle.

Woad was used by Ancient Britons as a body paint in battle. Woad is the blue dye from *Isatis tinctoria*, a biennial plant with arrow-shaped leaves and clusters of yellow flowers.

The use of cosmetics to cover blemishes was quickly developed as plagues spread across whole nations. While powdery yellow sulfur would heal small spots and sore throats, pox marks needed cosmetics.

In 16th century Europe, white lead, a mixture of lead carbonate and hydrated lead oxide, was the most popular base pigment for the face and shoulders. Rouge and blue veins could be added, and after the natural eyebrows had been burnt out, pieces of mouse skin would be stuck on above them. The whole face would then be given a polished sheen by painting it with egg-white. Pictures might also be painted on the forehead to hide pox marks. The saying: "Don't laugh, your face might crack" probably originates from these times; cracked dried egg-white would look messy and smell worse. Teeth were cleaned with pumice stone, salt or hydrochloric acid. Deaths from lead poisoning, which ate into the skin, were frequent.

By the time that Victoria was on the throne in Great Britain (1837), the fashion for makeup was in decline, and the young Queen preferred home-made skin care with simple recipes, such as rosewater washes.

Folklore remedies

Many recipes for herbal and other remedies have been passed down from generation to generation. Some remain localized, because a particular herb is only available in that locality. Other folk remedies have crossed national borders and found their way into homes all over the world, probably because they are effective.

Some popular folklore remedies in use today
For colds
Elderberry syrup is a sovereign remedy.
Rheumatism
Feverfew gathered from the garden and sprinkled on buttered bread is a simple but very effective remedy.
Varicose veins and sprains
Use a lotion of lead and opium. It will relieve all the pain.
For a bad chest or aching joints
Rub with goose grease.
For indigestion
Chew a sprig of parsley; it works wonders.
For sprains, bruises, aches and pains
Use comfrey (knitbone). The plant should be dried. Pour boiling water on the dry leaves and leave them to soak. Then bathe the sprain or bruise with the mixture.

A poultice can also be made by packing the mashed leaves around the area and then covering with a bandage. Comfrey soothes pain and helps healing.
An embrocation for all painful areas
½ fl.oz methylated spirits
½ fl.oz turpentine
½ fl.oz white wine vinegar
3 squares of camphor
Leave until camphor dissolves and dab on painful area.
For eczema
Pick some dock leaves and wash them.
Melt 1lb of pure lard in a dish. Add the dock leaves and cook in an oven at 150°C (302°F) for 1 hour. Leave to set for two days. Then spread the salve onto lint and apply to the spots. Make fresh salve every two days.
For constipation
The bulbs of squill, a seashore plant, should be dried and chewed as a diuretic and purgative. They can be crushed, infused with hot water and drunk instead.

Podophyllin, the yellow resin obtained from the roots of the may-apple tree, is useful as a purgative. Chop the roots and boil. Strain the liquid and drink some daily.

A traditional cure for warts was to place a live snail on them

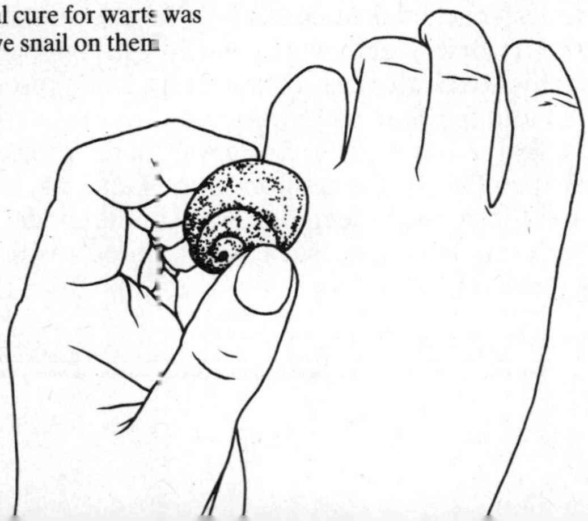

HERBALISM

Many home remedies were based on the use of plants, since most people used to live in rural environments. This branch of folk medicine has been developing as herbal medicine for over 5000 years. Manuscripts giving lists of herbs and their uses have been found in Ancient Egypt and China. Herbal knowledge was built up by a long process of trial and error.

During the medieval period superstition and sorcery became a necessary part of ritual healing ceremonies. For example, to ensure a herbal infusion would work properly, the patient might be required to walk seven times around a gravestone while reciting a Latin incantation.

During the 19th century herbal folklore spread widely; for example, when European emigrants arrived in America, they brought with them their native herbal folklore. This, together with the ancient knowledge of the American Indians, forms the basis of much modern herbalism in the USA. In the UK and Europe herbalism has a long history and is enjoying a revival.

How is herbalism therapeutic?
The herbalist aims to detect and restore normal functioning rather than attack a pathological condition. Only if the pathology is well entrenched may orthodox methods be recommended. Herbal remedies restore normal functioning by one or more of five basic approaches. It is thought that the combination of substances in herbal tinctures is more important than any single constituent. Tinctures themselves may also contain more than one herb.

Modern herbalists
The World Health Organization officially encourages local herbalism as a tool in the fight against poor medical services, and several large drug companies have begun to recognize the value of natural herbal remedies, since those concocted in the laboratory can never contain the variety of minerals and other substances that occur naturally.

Types of herbal practitioners
- Retail herbalists who sell remedies and give advice on their use.
- Professional medical herbalists who are trained and recognized by a professional institute. Many of these are orthodox doctors or recognized paramedics.
- Aromatherapists who use herbs distilled into essential oils and apply them externally during massage.
- Specialist herbalists in cultural medical systems, such as Chinese acupuncturists who use herbalism as an adjunct and the Hakims of Islam who practice Indian medical systems.
- Alternative medical practitioners, such as osteopaths, radionic technicians, dowsers, naturopaths and others, who may include herbalism as part of their practice.

Five ways in which herbalism aims to heal

1 By eliminating waste products

For example, senna contains anthraquinone glycosides, which irritate the bowels and cause elimination. Other herbs useful for constipation are alder, blackthorn, fennel, licorice, molasses, prunes and slippery elm.

2 By adjusting and balancing body processes

For example, the foxglove and, to a lesser extent, the lily of the valley for normalizing heart rate; also dandelion root for the liver, coltsfoot for the lungs and couch grass root for the kidneys. Fruit of the chasteberry tree is thought to balance the production of progesterone and estrogen by its action on the pituitary gland. Mistletoe, rose hips and lady's mantle help to normalize the menstrual flow.

3 By stimulating natural body responses

For example, chili, ginger and mustard contain acrid glycosides, which stimulate the blood vessels and improve circulation. Gentian and other bitter herbs stimulate the digestive processes. Comfrey has many herbal uses and is particularly helpful in clearing lung congestion and stimulating the lungs to work more efficiently. Oil of basil stimulates a brighter outlook.

4 By protecting against undesirables

For example, marshmallow root soothes and gives a mucilaginous protection against irritation. Witch hazel, tannin and other astringents form antiseptic coatings over tissue surfaces. Garlic fights both bacterial and fungal infections, and wormwood works against internal worms: onions are also useful.

5 By sedating body processes

For example, oats for nervous exhaustion and valerian for sedation. Hawthorn slows the heart rate yet increases blood flow, and licorice is excellent for calming stomach ulcers. Some herbs are useful against pain, such as oil of cloves for toothache and oil of peppermint for cramps and other pains.

A 16th century herb gatherer and a herbalist preparing his mixture with pestle and mortar

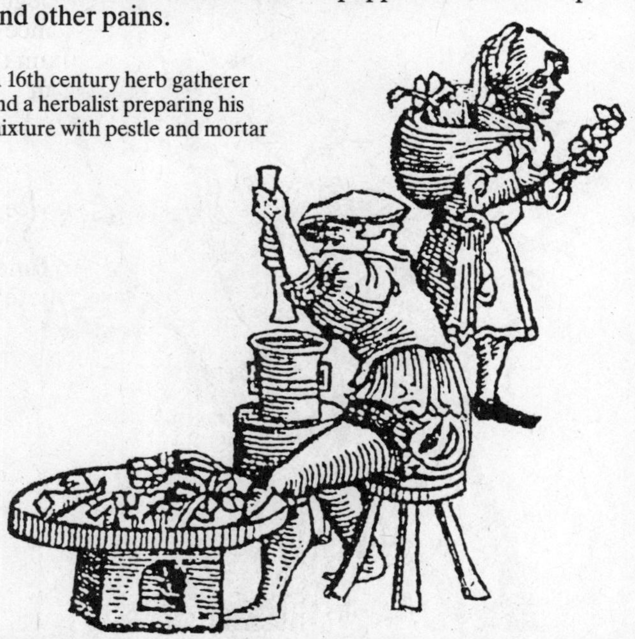

Early pathology finds a remedy

Desperate situations sometimes inspired remarkable solutions, which then entered the folklore tradition. Such was the case of the plant *Allium cepa*, the common, pungent onion.

Some of the history of East Indian medicine is recorded in Buddhist texts. One story tells of a piece of desperate pathological research undertaken by Queen Tisharakshita in the 6th century to find a remedy for her husband's condition.

King Ashoka was seriously ill. His feces were being forced back up his intestines and coming out of his mouth. His whole body smelled putrid, and he was close to death. He wanted to send for his son, Kunala, but the Queen knew that when her husband died she too would be expected to join him on his funeral pyre. Under this threat of death, Queen Tisharakshita rose to the occasion. She persuaded the King to trust her to heal him of his dreadful sickness, so he agreed to let her try, and he postponed sending for his son.

The Queen instructed the court physicians to find another man suffering with exactly the same condition as her husband, which they did. She then had the man killed and cut open. She personally examined his insides and discovered a large worm attached to the inner wall of his intestines that was blocking the passageway.

She took the worm out of the body and experimented with ways to kill it, using such things as peppers and salt, but the worm survived. Finally, she tried crushed onion and at last the worm curled up in a spasm and died.

The Queen then had to persuade the King that onions would cure his sickness. At first he resisted, because he was forbidden to eat onions by his religious sect. However, as his condition worsened, he gave in and drank nothing but the strong juice of crushed onions and was soon well again.

Throughout history strong-tasting onions and their near relative, garlic, have been recommended to keep illness and colds at bay. Some people still bite into a raw onion every day or take a garlic capsule to maintain good health. Garlic is said to have even greater potency than the onion.

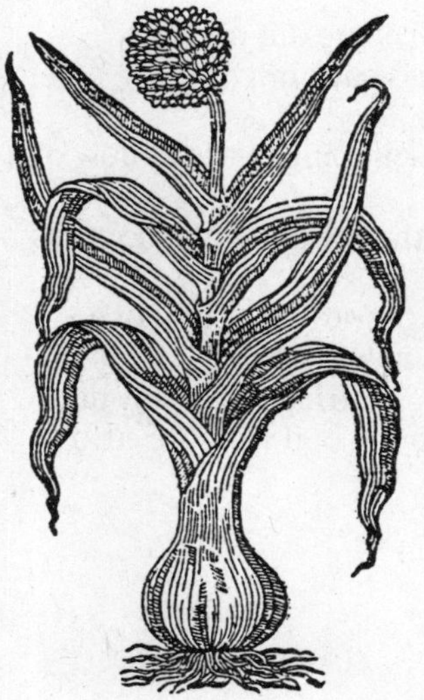

Garlic, from John Gerarde's *The Herball, or General Historie of Plants* (London 1597)

Old wives' tales

Ancient folklore stories about methods used to heal a plethora of human aches and pains are both comic and alarming. Many of them seemed to work, perhaps because of the power of suggestion. It was the older members of a community who carried in their heads all the medical experience of the tribe; in Europe it was usually the old women who were called upon to administer healing, and some believed they had the power of witchcraft ascribed to them by fearful gossips.

"Old wives' tales" is a phrase used in modern life to cast contempt upon these old methods ... yet some of them have been supported by scientific evidence. Because these methods were passed down through families by word of mouth, you may have some old family remedies of your own to add to this list. Do not count on the effectiveness of any of these to cure your ailment, however.

If you are fortunate enough to have an elderly person in your family, you will have a rich source of information about remedies used by their parents and grandparents, perhaps even a hundred years ago.

Small cuts
Wrap a cobweb around to stop the bleeding.

To cure a sore throat
Take a wool sock, which must have been worn for at least one week. Tie around the neck, with the foot under the chin. Keep on overnight. In the morning your sore throat will be gone (and so might your spouse!). This remedy is sometimes quoted as a cure for snoring.

Alopecia
Otherwise known as baldness, this condition has been a problem to men throughout history. A wife with a ready remedy was worth her weight in gold. One simple remedy was to rub a bald head with paraffin for several weeks; if you were lucky, the hair would grow back luxuriously. Baldness due to ringworm or infections was often treated with some success. Natural loss of hair was harder to reverse, and wigs have enjoyed popularity from time to time.

Hair-raising or another remedy for baldness!
Cover bald head with salt.
Incline head toward water.
The hair, becoming thirsty, will come out to drink.
Tie hairs in knots before they go back in!

Kentucky folklore

- Cure a cold by placing a nail-clipping in the hollow of a tree.
- Cure toothache by carrying the jawbone of a horse as far as possible, in secrecy.
- Relieve backache by having the seventh child of a seventh child walk up and down your back.
- Cure a boil by rubbing a greasy string on a rusty nail. Throw away the nail and touch the boil with the string several times a day.

PREVENTION IS BETTER THAN CURE
In primitive communities many superstitions were developed to ward off the evil spirits that caused sickness and other disasters. Divestment rituals and the carrying of lucky charms, mascots or amulets are two of the preventive superstitions that are still in common practice among people today.

In medieval England, protection against cramps, for example, would be sought by carrying a rolled-up eelskin or a hare's foot.

Divestment
Have you ever tossed spilled salt over your left shoulder?

If so, you are practicing a very old divestment ritual. Divestment was one of the many ways in which diseases were eradicated; it was also a method used to prevent evil forces from getting a hold on a person or a household.

Divestment is done by tossing something over the head or shoulder, or by throwing something over a gate, a tree, or even the roof of a house. In early Roman times, a stone or spear was thrown over the house during childbirth to protect the child. The stone or spear had to be one that had killed a human, a boar and a bear and thus was able to kill off any evil forces that might be around waiting for the newborn.

In this etching by Goya, a woman is seen taking the teeth of a dead man, an essential ingredient in protective potions. The blood of a hanged man was also said to cure leprosy.

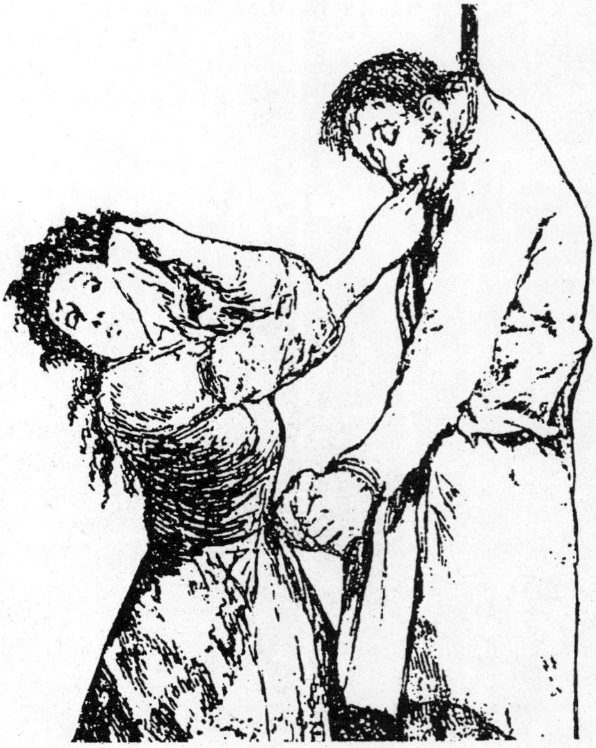

In Illinois two preventive actions were common in old folklore custom. The first extracted tooth used to be tossed over the shoulder to prevent any further tooth decay. When moving house, a person unrelated to the family carried the broom to the new house and threw it over the fence to ensure no evil had arrived with the furniture. Presumably, the person who carried the broom would carry any evil away with him.

In German folklore, the last egg of the laying season was associated with witches and was disposed of directly by the farmer, who stood with his back to the house and threw the egg over his own head and over the roof of the house. If, by mischance, the egg hit the house, it was a sign the building would be struck by lightning or attract other misfortunes.

In Anglo-Saxon times in Britain, a notched stick was the medium which could be used to carry actual or potential disease away from the homestead. To dispose of the evil, the stick must be thrown over the shoulder from a bridge into running water.

Emblems of good luck: Painted eyes on a Greek drinking cup to ward off evil; The horse shoe (*right*); and the four-leaf clover are positive bringers of good luck.

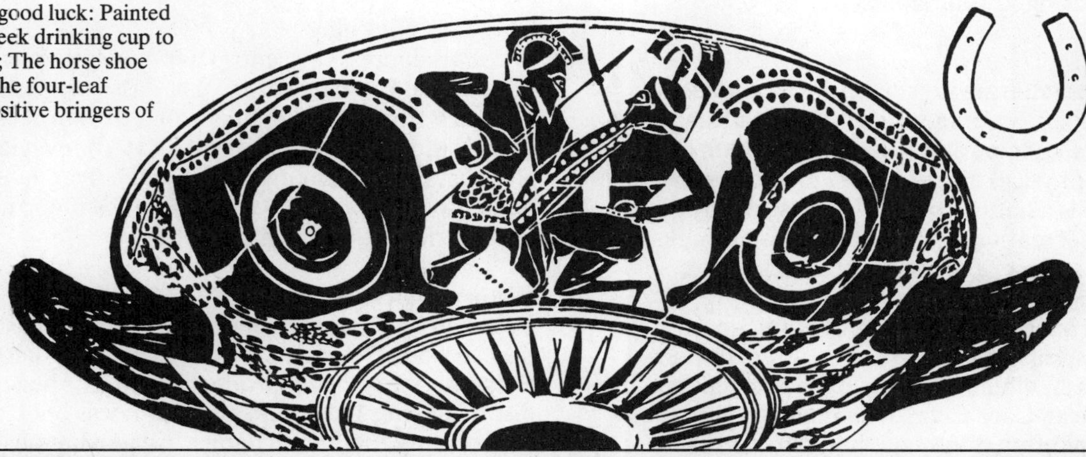

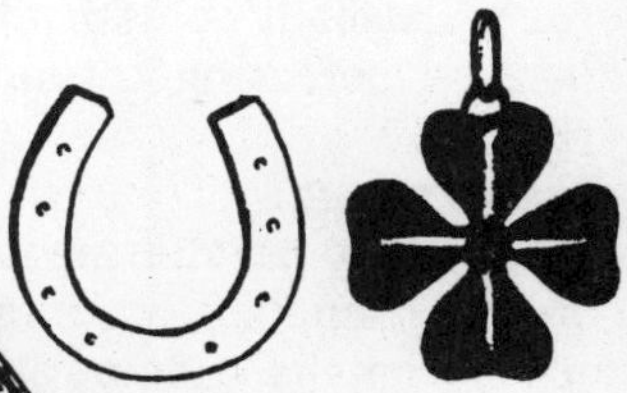

18th century quackery?

Joanna Stephens in the 1730s claimed she had invented a potion to cure gallstones, the recipe for which she would disclose for £5000 ($25,000). Although her claims were attractive, nobody raised enough money. Eventually, her suggestive persuasiveness resulted in the British Parliament setting up a commission of well-known doctors to investigate her claim, using the potion she had invented.

Most members of the commission said it worked and were convinced of its "utility and efficiency." Consequently the £5000 was paid to Joanna Stephens and she revealed her prescription . . . a potion which included crushed egg shells, squashed snails, hips and haws, roasted black soap and honey.

The old and the young

It was taboo in many communities to allow young children near sick or very elderly people. It was believed that the sick or weak person would draw strength away from the young, who would be helpless to resist. Adults, it was thought, were better able to look after themselves. However, in communities where children were regarded as chattels, an infant would be sent to live with a sick person in order to help him or her get well.

Sacred water

In the folklore of Finland, healing could be aided by washing with water drawn from a sacred spring by the community Tietäjä or wizard. He had to be paid in silver which had been taken from a corpse. The washing had nothing to do with hygiene, although it obviously must have made a difference. The sacred spring water was used to wash away the evil spirits who were causing the sickness.

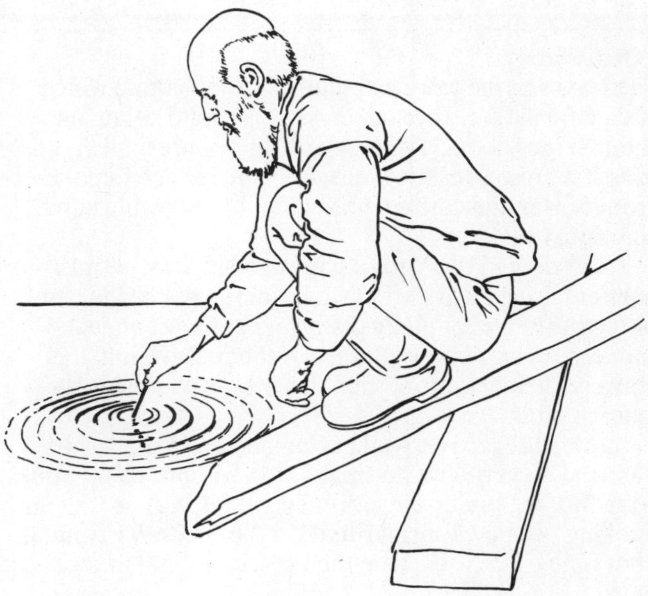

Drugs for all occasions

Throughout recorded history, and probably long before that, drugs have had a powerful appeal to the human race for their psychotropic effects. Often quite wonderful mental and physical experiences they provided, both in a social context and when used as a potion against pain, depression and stress.

However, the drug that is prescribed at a clinic or bought illegally on the street in the 1990s is often of a very different quality from the same drug used in its plant forms by primitive societies. The prescribed drug may be a synthetic version of the original drug; the street drug will usually contain additives to increase the quantity, increasing its profitability.

What is a drug?
A drug is a mind-altering substance, for example cocaine, cannabis, morphine and codeine. Substances such as digitalis, quinine and cascara, that are taken for their effect on physical functions, are medicines, although there is a natural overlap. The same drug can be medicinal, recreational or addictive, for example, alcohol can be a tonic, a pleasant social drink or a life-threatening addiction.

Many drugs have become a part of ethnic social activity, for example in Turkish coffee, French wines, West Indian hash, Chinese opium, Japanese teas and the original American Coca Cola. A summary is given here of some mind-altering drugs and their derivatives.

ALCOHOL
Three kinds of alcohols are drunk for their intoxicating effects: ethyl alcohol in wines, beers, spirits, liqueurs; methyl alcohol in solvents, anti-freeze, etc; iso-propyl alcohol in toilet waters, after-shave etc.
Alcoholic liquors are made by fermenting apples, grapes, grains, which may be malted or roasted, and other sugary things. Beers may have hops added for flavor. Some drinks are matured such as malt whiskies that are kept in casks for 10 years and some cognacs are only at their best after 50 years. Liqueurs originated from herbal medicines made in the Middle Ages and are spirits flavoured with secret herbal recipes. Absinthe, a favorite of artists and writers during the 1800s in Paris, was a drink containing 60–80% spirits and flavoured with wormwood, which attacks the nervous system; it is now widely banned.

Fortified wines such as sherry, port and vermouth are a combination of wines with brandy or one of the neutral spirits and flavorings.

The effect of alcohol
Alcohols depress the central nervous system and release inhibitions. Excessive alcohol releases urges that are normally kept well under control. Alcohol causes dehydration, malnutrition and loss of body heat. Regular, heavy drinking damages the liver, lungs and heart. A concentration of 0.15% in the blood causes mild intoxication, 0.6% endangers life.

History of alcohol
Beer and berry wines were being drunk at least as far back as 6500 BC and an Egyptian papyrus dated 3500 BC, describes alcohol production. Spirits began to be distilled about 1000 years ago, but it was only in the late 19th century that brand names became famous.

CANNABIS
Cannabis has been used for centuries in all the countries where it grows naturally, such as India, North Africa and the West Indies.

The tough fibres of the male *Cannabis sativa* plant are used to make hemp ropes. The flowers of the female plant produce the sticky resin which is cannabis, although the most common form is a mixture of leaves,

TOBACCO
The leaves of the tobacco plant contain nicotine which has a dual nature. In small doses it is a mild stimulant and in larger doses, a depressant. In its purest form, it is the most poisonous substance known. Tobacco smoke produces tar and carbon monoxide, both of which are poisonous.

According to the Vedic scriptures in India, people were enjoying intoxication while smoking, chewing and eating the leaves of many plants, including cannabis. Tobacco was probably another of them. Certainly the Maya civilization, at AD 500 in Mexico, was using the tobacco plant.

In 1565 tobacco arrived in England and for 20 years was used by herbalists to treat lung and sinus complaints. Then in 1586, under the patronage of Sir Walter Raleigh, smoking became a social ritual. In the 1600s, Virginia, in what is now USA, became the tobacco capital of the world.

Some countries prohibited its use and imposed dreadful punishments: smokers were pilloried in Switzerland, decapitated in China, suffocated by smoke in Persia and exiled from Russia with a split nose.

Tobacco became big business when the Bonsak automatic rolling machine was patented in 1841. It could do the work of 40 employees who had previously rolled cigarettes by hand. Snuff, which is ground, flavored tobacco, became popular in the 1700s.

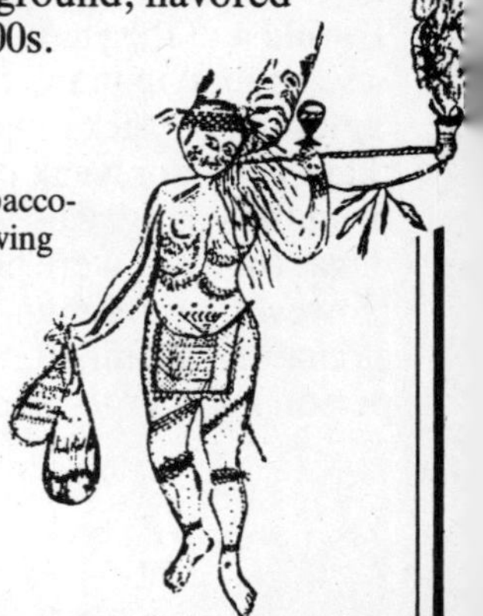

American Indian pipe tobacco-smoker, 16th century drawing

flowers, stalks and seeds ground together.

The caked resin from North Africa, known as hashish, is often put into a local, spicy confection called majoon. There are dozens of variables and a similar number of names, including dope, grass and marijuana.

The most concentrated form is hash oil which is made by grinding it down, mixing with alcohol and straining out the cellulose solids. The solvent evaporates leaving a sticky, green oil which can be further refined to the colorless and tasteless THC i.e. tetrahydrocannabinol, which is the psychotropic content of cannabis. THC was eventually synthesized in 1966 and has yielded probably up to 80 derivatives, some of which are used for drug withdrawal, anxiety, depression and convulsions. In the mid 1800s, cannabis was the standard treatment for migraine in London.

COCAINE

Cocaine is contained in the pulped leaf of the South American coca plant. The Indians who live in the thin air of the high Andes, consume on average two ounces a day, which contains virtually all the vitamins necessary for good nutrition. It is a mild physical stimulant, tones the digestive muscles, aids breathing, acts as an aphrodisiac and keeps the muscles of the larynx in good order. Coca wines have been in great demand from singers and orators alike.

Like the opium poppy, the coca plant grows in profusion. Both plants have many advantages to offer and both are easily abused when the active ingredients are extracted from the plants. Cocaine has a powerful and short-lasting effect on the central nervous system. It can be a stimulant and an anesthetic, depending on the form and quantity taken.

Recreational coke is obtained in the main from the *Erythroxylum coca* plant that grows on the slopes of the Andes in Peru, Bolivia and Equador.

Four ways of using the coca leaf.

1 The leaf can be mixed with lime and chewed.
2 The leaf can be made into a paste for smoking.
3 The pasta can be converted into the crystalline powder, cocaine hydrochoride, known as snow, toot or snort, and be sniffed.

Sniffing, or snorting, is said to induce confidence, suspend fatigue and hunger and enhance concentration, stamina and imagination. The effect wears off after about an hour.

4 The most potent form of cocaine will not dissolve in water and cannot be injected or sniffed so it is smoked with a water pipe to cool it. This is called freebasing and has an effect like a massive orgasm, without relief: the body is left screaming for more. Frequent or high doses lead to the very opposite and a toxic psychosis can result.

The Brompton Cocktail

Known as a speedball on the street, the Brompton Cocktail is a mixture of heroin and cocaine given to terminally ill patients, sometimes with the addition of a little brandy. The effect is a euphoria greater than either drug taken alone. For the terminally ill it has been a blessing and a wonderful relief from the unbearable pain of some diseases.

THE NARCOTIC ANALGESICS

This family of drugs, known as the opiates, all derive from the opium poppy, *Papaver somniferum*. Opium seeps out of the slit seed-pods as a milky juice which dries into hard blocks which have to be boiled and seived several times to remove impurities before the final paste is dried and smoked. Many other drugs are extracted from opium, including morphine, heroin and codeine.

The joy plant

In Sumerian texts thought to be about 6000 years old, the opium poppy is referred to as the joy plant. Most peoples in the Middle East used poppy juice for body and spirit. In the 3rd century BC, the Greek philosopher Theophrastus discussed the medical use of opium in his records and the Chinese used opium as a medicine from the 7th or 8th century AD when the Arabs took it to China.

It was not until the 17th century that the Chinese took to smoking opium and in 1729 the Chinese Emperor made it illegal, which drove the practice underground. The habit was encouraged by the British who exported opium grown in Bengal to China, despite the opium wars with the Chinese authorities, who tried to control the situation.

Opium in Europe

Paracelsus, the Swiss physician who lived from 1493 to 1541, is often regarded as the first pharmacist. He began using opium as a medicine, mixing it with alcohol and calling it laudanum. Successive physicians added sherry and spices and by the 17th century it was the standard treatment for pain and was used by most people to block out the pains of daily life.

In 1821 Thomas de Quincey published his book *Confessions of an English Opium Eater* in which he described the horrors of his own addiction to opium, gained from using laudanum to cure severe neuralgia while studying at Oxford University.

Opium smoking and the drinking of laudanum was commonplace among all social groups, from rural outbacks to the opium dens of London's docklands. Similar practices were to be found throughout America and Europe. Opium was a universal addiction long before its derivative, heroin, became a problem of modern drug-abuse and international economics.

The hallucinogens

Information about these drugs is on the next page.

Mystical excursions

Drugs which alter sensory perceptions are collectively known as hallucinogens. Most people who take hallucinogens are doing so to go on a 'trip' or a mystical excursion during which there are extreme, unusual and often wonderful visual and auditory experiences, such as swirling colors, moving surfaces, sounds from inanimate objects and sensations ranging from tickling to a religious encounter. There is also a loss of the sense of time, a visual perspective that is elastic and doubts about the self and others.

Depending on unconscious factors and his general state of health, a person may have a good trip and feel positively enlightened or have a bad trip full of horrific experiences.

Since the loss of ego is part of the hallucinogenic excursion, there is the risk of an ensuing psychosis. This happens when a person continues to be out of touch with his or her ego-identity after the trip is over. This is only likely if a psychotic state was already impending.

What is reality?
There is a valid point of view that suggests we only perceive a partial reality anyway, so how can we judge the accuracy of enhanced perceptions? Some people, such as artists, composers, poets, nuclear physicists, inventors and others with eccentric perceptions present us with many strange views of reality. So it may be that some hallucinogenic perceptions are just another aspect of a reality that is far more complex than we imagine. For example, under powerful microscopic enlargement, the human skin is a jungle of hairs, cracked skin, sticky oils, dirt, heaving humps and hollows and an assortment of living, crawling bacteria. Due to even more powerful enlargement techniques, nuclear physicists are discovering patterns in the random movements of micro-particles, called fractals, which reveal beautiful curved, repeating patterns very similar to those drawn by some people under the influence of LSD.

The 19th century Dutch artist Vincent van Gogh painted exciting but diverse views of reality, for example in his picture of sunflowers.

THE HALLUCINOGENS
These are the psychotropic drugs found in traditional magical plants, such as certain mushrooms, toadstools, belladonna, henbane, the mandrake root and many plants of the *Solanaceae* family, which have been used for 2000 years as medicines, aphrodisiacs and to bring more excitement into sexual and social activities.

European sorcerers and witches used them in the Middle Ages for healing, for inducing mystical experiences and for dispatching enemies. The difference between a therapeutic and a lethal dose of most of these plant extracts is quite small. Physical dependence does not occur and the mental effects are so powerful that psychological dependence is rare.

The drugs in hallucinogens are from the chemical family known as the indolealkylamines, which interfere with messages being passed through the brain because they are similar to one of the neurotransmitters in the brain, known as 5-hydroxytryptamine.

The best known of the hallucinogens is probably LSD (d-lysergic acid diethylamide) which is derived from a fungus called ergot, which grows on rye and other grasses. A similar substance, LSA (d-lysergic acid amide) is found in the seeds of the morning glory plant and psylocybin is found in certain mushrooms. Many drugs similar to those found in plants are now being chemically synthesized in laboratories and are usually named by their initials, such as MDA, PMA, DMT, and PCP which is called angel dust or the peace pill. North America has the greatest variety of plant life containing hallucinogens and many of the synthetic varieties are made in the USA.

Drawing inspired by LSD trip

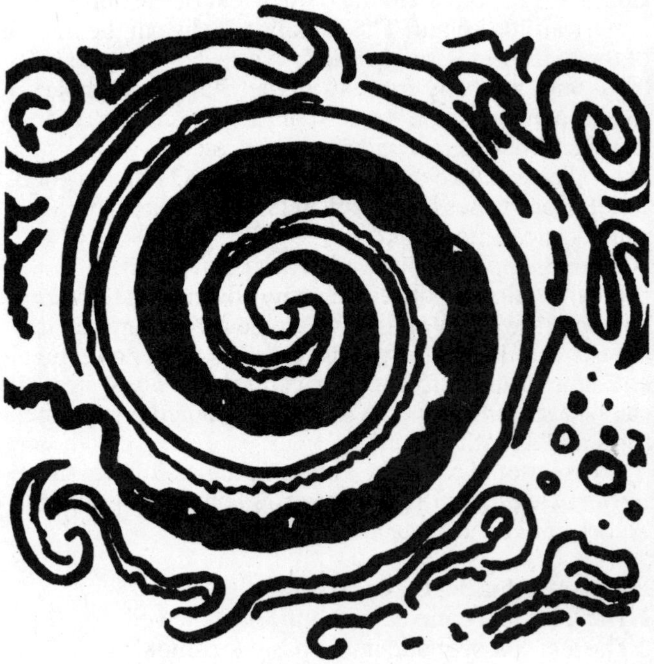

St Anthony's Fire
In medieval times, many village people in Europe suffered from an affliction called St Anthony's Fire, during which they had severe convulsions, hallucinations and limbs that appeared blackened by fire, but which were actually gangrenous.

No cure seemed to work except a pilgrimage to one of the shrines dedicated to St Anthony. Strangely, people who visited the shrines often were cured, except for the loss of limbs due to gangrene, so the cure was attributed to St Anthony. The actual reason for a cure was that during their pilgrimage people fasted and did not eat rye bread, which was infected with the fungus, ergot, which contained LSD. Large doses of LSD constrict the blood vessels, as well as affecting the transmission of information in the brain.

Synthetic LSD
From 1918 onwards, Swiss-based chemists Dr Arthur Stoll and his younger associate Dr Albert Hoffmann began making the ergot alkaloid in its pure chemical form. And several similar synthetic compounds were tried out for pain-relief from migraines, childbirth and geriatric complaints. It was not until 1943 that Hoffmann discovered the powerful effect of taking the pure synthesized LSD, describing himself as "transported into other worlds" while riding home on his bicycle. As with all LSD trips, the effects lasted about 12 hours after which time he slept well.

The trip must have been alarming, as these chemists had no knowledge of hallucinogens at that time. After further experiments, it was decided that what they had discovered was a very powerful psychomimetic, i.e. a drug that could produce temporary psychoses and could perhaps be used to explore and understand mental illnesses such as schizophrenia.

The clinical use of LSD
After World War II psychiatric departments in many hospitals were using this synthesized LSD on their patients. It was thought to be especially useful for loosening neurotic repressions more quickly, thus shortening the time normally required for Freudian analysis. Alas, the effect was catastrophic for many patients: the released material was too much and too powerful, leaving people more confused and frightened than before and in some cases making the illness worse.

Psychiatric patients were subjected to doses far too high and even given injections which would create an immediate hallucination and panic in a healthy person.

Because LSD seemed to bang the brain into spewing forth an incoherent stream of sensations and changed the perceptions of people, army and intelligence officers thought it might be useful to incapacitate the enemy or even to reverse the effects of brain-washing.

Cures for all manner of things were claimed, from drug addiction to arthritis, hysterical deafness and skin rashes. Eventually, as a result of research in the US in 1960 and elsewhere later, the clinical use of LSD was restricted and eventually ended when authorities in most countries became alarmed by reports of problems increasing due to widespread recreational use.

Mescaline for the Mescaleros
In the 19th century, parties of Mescalero Apache Indians collected supplies of the peyote cactus when they raided areas of Mexico, and took them back to their homelands.

The peyote is a spineless cactus, *Lophophora williamsii*, native of Mexico and Southwest US, and the hallucinogen, mescaline 143, is found in the knobbly buttons on the head of the cactus. When extracted, it is a white, crystalline powder, which the Apaches used for healing and for religious rituals.

The effects of mescaline are similar to those of all hallucinogens and have been described in detail by Aldous Huxley, the British writer (1894–1963) in his book *The Doors of Perception*, which he wrote in 1954.

The domestic and recreational use of hallucinogens became widely popular in the 1960s during the hippie culture. Interest in mescaline was stimulated by the Mexican writer, Carlos Castenada in his several books, such as *Tales of Power*, published in 1974. In his books, Castenada describes the experiences of a young novice at the hands of a wily old Indian shaman, Don Juan, who fed him peyote mescaline. The dose was small enough for the novice (Carlos) to be capable of describing the knowledge he gained during his experiences. Knowing, for example, the exactly right place to sit in a room, was one of the early wisdoms he gained and guided by Don Juan, no harm befell him on his journey of discovery.

MAGIC MUSHROOMS
While there are only about a dozen species of mushroom in Europe that contain hallucinogens, there are over 100 in the US. A guide to mushrooms and toadstools is essential for anyone wishing to identify edible or hallucinogenic varieties, such as the Liberty Cap mushroom, *Psilocybe semilanceata*. While it is estimated that 8lb of the Liberty Cap would be lethal, considerably less can do damage, so the recommended amount is only two or three of these mushrooms. Even then, the amount of the drug in each mushroom varies. The Liberty Cap is a small, elegant mushroom about 2½ inches tall on slender stems. They grow in lines and have yellow-brown sharply conical caps.

The Fly Agaric
This mushroom, the *Amanita muscaria*, is another of the hallucinogenic mushrooms that can be very easily, and fatally, mixed up with other members of its genus. *Amanita phalloides*, the Death Cap and *Amanita virosa*, the Destroying Angel.

Reports about the Fly Agaric reached Western Europe from Siberia in the 18th century. Many Siberian tribes were familiar with its intoxicating effects and they had also noticed that its active contents were quickly expelled from the body via the urine, unmetabolized. Thus the habit of drinking urine during intoxication extended the period of the 'high' or trip. Although the tribespeople would drink each other's urine, they didn't indulge in their reindeer's urine, although the animals were fond of eating this particular fungus. This leads one to wonder if the reindeer lived on a permanent hallucinogenic high?

Which potions?

In medieval England, manuscripts, written by hand in Old English, recorded recipes and methods for use in the arts of leechdom, wortcunning, and starcraft.
Leechdom: the art of physical healing.
Wortcunning: the knowledge of herbs.
Starcraft: using wisdom from the stars.

Some potions contained items that we might find obnoxious and were often prepared by ritual processes to add to their potency. The ingredients were intended to cure, either because they did have some healing properties or because it was believed certain things had a contagious or a sympathetic magical influence.

Most of the examples of potions are given here in modern English, but an extract and some literal translations from one medieval manuscript are shown because the language itself is delightfully archaic and has a flavor of magic about it.

Yellow jaundice: a literal translation
"From gall disease, that is from the yellow, comes great evil; it is most powerful of all diseases; when there wax [grows] within unmeasured humors, the tokens [symptoms] are these: the body becomes bitter and yellow as good silk; under the tongue be swart [swollen] veins and his urine is yellow."

The treatment for yellow jaundice was:
"Let him blood from the lung vein, give often a stirring drink; give a stone bath. After make him a drink of sorrel in wine and water. Then every morning in the bath, give him mulled ale, it will amend the bitterness of the gall."

This treatment, like so many, involves blood-letting from "the lung vein," the intention being to remove bad blood tainted by the evil disease.

Original Old English version

[4]Oꝼ ᵹeal adle ſio biþ oꝼ þæꞃe ᵹeolƿan · cymeþ ᵹꞃeaꞇ yꝼel ſio biþ ealꞃa adla ꞃicuſꞇ · þonne ᵹeƿeaxeð on innan unᵹemeꞇ ƿæꞇan þiꞅ ſinꞇ ꞇacn · ꝥ him ſe lichoma eall abiꞇeꞃað ⁊ aᵹeolƿað ſƿa ᵹod ſeoluc · ⁊ him beoð undeꞃ ꞇunᵹan ꞇulᵹe ſƿeaꞃꞇe ædꞃa ⁊ yꝼele ⁊ hím bið micᵹe ᵹeolu · læꞇ hím oꝼ lunᵹen ædꞃe blod ꞅele him óꝼꞇ ſꞇyꞃᵹendne dꞃenc ſꞇanbaðu ᵹelome. [6]Ƿyꞃc him ðonne ſꞇilne dꞃenc óꝼ omƿꞃan on ƿine ⁊ on ƿæꞇꞃe ⁊ ón þam baðe ᵹehƿilce moꞃᵹene dꞃince mylſce dꞃincan ſio ᵹebeꞇ þa biꞇeꞃneꞅꞅe þæꞅ ᵹeallan.

ARE MODERN AND MEDIEVAL SICKNESSES SIMILAR?

One of the medieval leech manuscripts contains remedies for a long list of illnesses including:

- headache;
- old headache;
- ache of half the head, known as megrim (migraine);
- swollen eyes;
- white speck in the eyes;
- worms in the eyes (presumably maggots);
- obscured vision and bleared eyes;
- pain or worms in the ear;
- toothache and hollow teeth;
- mouth broken inside;
- neck pain;
- cancer;
- cough and lung disease;
- throwing up blood or bile;
- the yellow disease;
- pain in the stomach, loins, spleen;
- womb or belly pain;
- stones waxing in the bladder;
- obstruction of fecal discharge;
- diarrhea and worms (tape worms);
- joint pains;
- warts;
- leprosy or elephantiasis;
- constant thirst;
- gripe and ache of all guts;
- burning with fire, liquid and sun;
- dry disease;
- shooting pains;
- broken bone and dislocation;
- tear from a hound;
- bite from the gangwayweaving spider;
- man not being able to kindle a child;
- woman having a dead bairn inside;
- woman bleeding too much;
- having worms bore holes in skin;
- lunatic man;
- lice;
- poison;
- prick by a thorn or reed;
- palsy (fits);
- fig disease;
- sore knees or feet;
- too much bleeding from a blood-letting incision;
- soured milk (blamed on bad temper);
- skull that is bound up;
- meat that will not digest;
- prating (talking) women;
- temptations of fiends;
- a wen (corn);
- elfins and night goblins;
- temptations of the devil;
- wild heart;
- carbuncles;
- cheek blotch.

SOME LEECHDOMS AND WORTCUNNING

In medieval England several remedies were often given for each disease; either so they could be used together, or if one didn't work another could be tried.

In case a man ache in the head (from a blow)
1 Place the crushed root of crosswort on a red fillet and bind the raw meat to the head.
2 Crush the seeds of mustard and rue and mix with oil. Put into hot water and bathe the head with it often.

For the pock disease (smallpox)
A surprisingly large number of people survived attacks of smallpox, though they were left badly scarred. Some of the salves mentioned were designed to remove the sores leaving no scars.
1 Crush onion, houseleek and fieldmore (carrot); add clear ale and leave for three nights. Drink a cup each morning.
2 Boil water in a pot, add honey and skim foam away until it stops foaming. Sip often as hot as you can. Smear the pock (the sores) with honey where it may be breaking out.
3 Boil butter, yarrow, githrife, the flower of red nettle and drink.
4 Another remedy is bishopwort, attorlothe, springwort and burdock mixed in ale.
5 Against the pocks freely employ bloodletting and drink a bowl full of melted butter.
6 If pocks break out, delve away at each one with a thorn and then drip alder wine into the raw holes. Glovewort boiled in butter will soothe the pocks.

Some ways to treat poisoning
1 Crush betony, marche, wormwood, fennel and radish into ale and drink it.
2 Stand betony and the small attorlothe in holy water. Drink the water and eat the worts (herbs).
3 For a snake bite, wash a black snail in holy water and drink it. Also put as much betony as weighs three pennies in three bowls of wine and drink it all.

How to treat the "dangerous disorder in which a man, they say, unnaturally speweth his feces through the mouth. They say he belcheth often and all the body stinketh foully."
1 Let the man drink dill mixed in oil and take a loaf of hot bread soaked in oil. The blood of a reremouse or a bat, cut up, is smeared on the man.
2 For inner sores and wounds of the gut, take sweet oil mixed with harts marrow, wild mint and hot water.
3 Fennel and coriander in wine hot with a red iron. Let him have as much as he can drink for three days, and it will cure him.
4 Mark his name on a hazel twig and score three notches. Then rub in some blood from his sores and throw the stick over your shoulder into the stream. Or better, throw it backwards between the legs while running away from the stream.

For late digestion (night-time indigestion)
Rue, vinegar, beet and red nettle were among 54 remedies given by medieval physicians for this troublesome condition. Fasting was advised, and mallow was recommended to be eaten with sprouts every third day. Warnings were given that if the condition is not treated the result will be dropsy, liver pain, swelling of the spleen, retention of urine, bloating, bladder stones and sand in the guts! Finally, the night fiends would take over with terrifying results, such as permanent cramps and misfortunes.

Salves for abscesses, tumors and infected wounds
1 Mix sorrel, salt, ribwort, egg, soot, burnt loam, fine flour of wheat, oak rind, appletree bark and sloethorn. Use this to cleanse the wound.
2 Burn sulfur in a copper vessel and rub it to fine dust. Sieve through a cloth and mix with a little old soap. Soften with a little virgin honey and apply with a mallow leaf.
3 Turn milk into cream and then to butter without the water. Add oakrind taken from the north side of the tree and crush together. Apply to the wound.

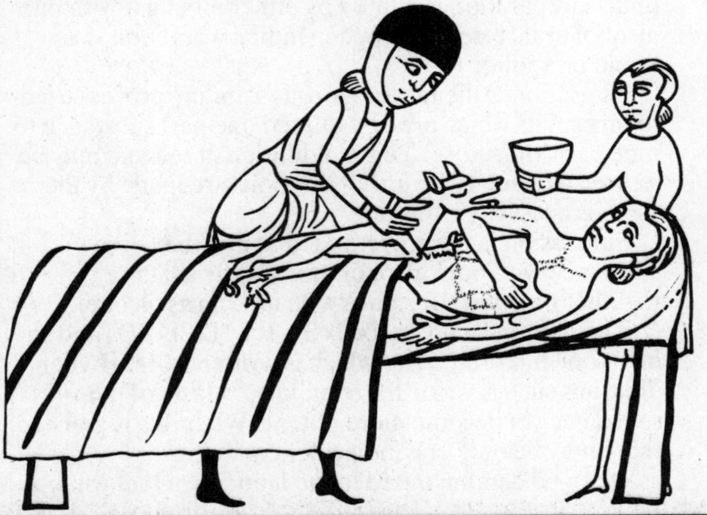

Treating a prolapsed intestine by laying the body of a dying animal on the patient. This poultice-type treatment was taught at the famous medieval medical school of Salerno, Italy, 11th century onward

Homeopathic remedies

Hippocrates, the Greek physician who lived in the fifth century BC, was the first to record in his medical books the homeopathic principle that like cures like. However, it was not until 1811 that Dr Samuel Hahnemann, from Leipzig, published a practical system of healing based on this principle. Homeopathy is now widely used in Europe to treat disease by prescribing minute doses of substances that would produce in a healthy person symptoms similar to those of the disease.

The birth of homeopathy

Hahnemann was interested in the effect of substances such as herbal preparations and root and bark extracts. He was experimenting on himself with an extract of quinine from the Peruvian cinchona bark which was the common treatment for malaria. He was surprised to observe that the substance produced in himself the same symptoms as it was used to cure.

Over several years he tested hundreds of substances on healthy volunteers, observing any deviations from the normal that were produced. These deviations he listed as symptoms, in some cases as few as five or six, in others as many as 3000 or more.

He then matched the symptoms of his patients with the symptoms produced by the tested substances. To do this accurately, he had to devise a thorough method of diagnosis, which involved recording the patient's answers to many detailed questions.

How much is the correct dose?

The new skills of homeopathy practised by Hahnemann were successful except in a few cases, when the doses given seemed to make the disease worse. Since his aim was to cure without adding to the harm already caused by a disease, he began to give smaller and smaller doses, diluting the substances in pure water.

Unfortunately, the more dilute the solution, the less effective it was therapeutically. At least this was the case until Hahnemann made a startling discovery. He was testing different ways of preparing the homeopathic solutions when he found that by shaking the dilutions violently, they retained their medical potency despite repeated dilution. A substance might be diluted 100 times, yet be more effective than a stronger solution, providing it has been shaken very thoroughly during its preparation. This process was called potentization and the diluted remedies were known as potencies. A typical homeopathic practitioner would have in excess of 2000 potencies from which to choose one or more suitable for a particular patient.

A theory of disease

Hahnemann always treated the patient not the disease. He found that different combinations of potencies were required by different people who at first glance appeared to be suffering from the same disease. He also found that while acute conditions were easily cured, only temporary relief was gained in many chronic situations. He concluded there were inherited and acquired disease tendencies that he called miasmas.

His opinion that some people had a lower natural vitality, and therefore greater vulnerability, led him to state that there could be no such thing as disease without the ground in which it could grow. Disease only occurs when the vital principle of a person's body cannot cope with changes occurring in the body.

FUNDAMENTAL CHARACTERISTICS OF LIVING THINGS

Ways in which all living things behave automatically, regardless of human will power, are fundamental to understanding how homeopathy works.

- An organism is constantly renewing and repairing itself, for example by replacing blood and skin cells. Consequently a living organism has the capacity to overcome the cause of a disease.
- Only the organism itself can achieve a cure. All homeopathy can provide is the extra stimulus.
- An organism is sensitive to substances that will stimulate a cure; in other words, to that which is homeopathic to the patient's condition. The word homeopathic means of similar pathology, i.e. similar symptoms of disease.
- When an organism is curing itself homeopathically, the symptoms will first briefly intensify and then will move from the internal organs to the less important organs and will disappear in the reverse order in which they appeared.

IS HOMEOPATHY MAGICAL?

People new to the concept of homeopathy often find it incredible that such large dilutions can have any effect at all. The early practitioners were convinced by their results and claimed that the substances left their mark in the water with which they were diluted.

This was known as imprinting and now has scientific evidence to support the claim that greater dilutions are more potent.

The preparation of homeopathic remedies

After its extraction, usually from a plant, the substance under preparation is diluted by either mixing it with pure alcohol or lactose powder, depending whether it is a liquid or a solid.

Tituration is the fairly vigorous grinding process used to mix solids which are first diluted one part substance to nine parts of lactose. This is a dilution of ten and may be written as 1x or 1D. Further dilutions are made by the same process of tituration.

Succussion is the process used to mix the liquid substance with pure alcohol by violently shaking together one part substance with nine parts alcohol.

The dilutions may be 1x 2x 3x, (or 1D 2D 3D) and so on to one hundred times which is written as 1c. Higher dilutions such as 5c or 10c contain very little of the substance yet become more potent. When 12c is reached there may be only one molecule remaining.

It can be demonstrated in the laboratory that while a

THE BALANCE OF HEALTH

The healthy see–saw illustrates how the extra homeopathic stimulus alarms the body and makes it spring into action more quickly and effectively against disease.

The unhealthy see-saw shows how homeopathy may only stimulate temporary relief, when the health of the organism is chronically off-balance, perhaps due to inherited factors or to an inappropriate lifestyle. It is thought that environmental factors contribute to many chronic diseases and homeopathic doctors recognize that some people are simply luckier than others and are born with a potentially better basic health balance. Some doctors claim there are no incurable diseases, but that there are some incurable people.

It should be noted that homeopathy is not used exclusively. It would be useless to try and cure an emergency that must be treated surgically, such as a burst appendix.

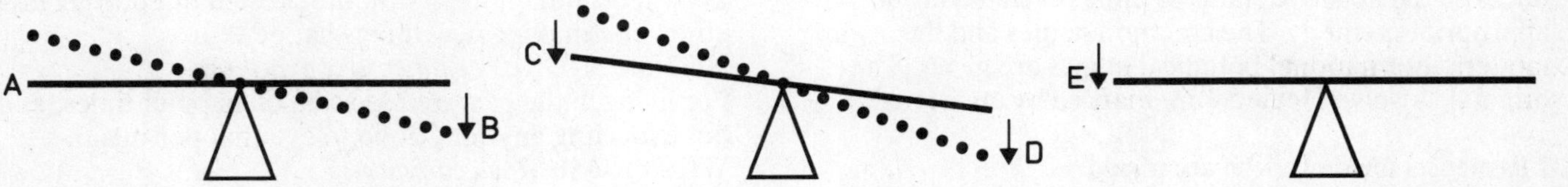

The healthy see-saw

A A natural healthy balance
B Disease upsets balance
C Body makes a natural response to disease
D Homeopathic stimulus pushes body further off-balance
E Body makes response to disease and the extra stimulus

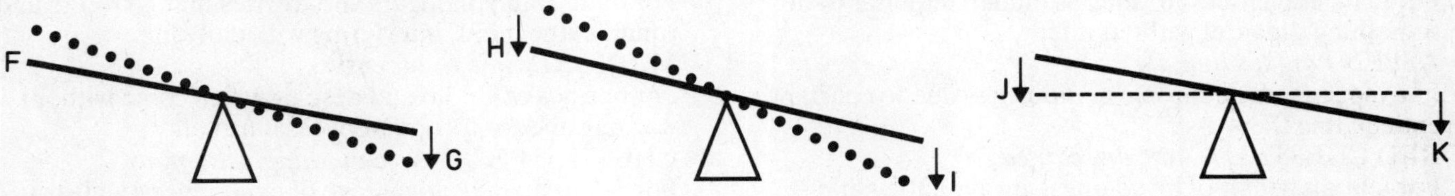

The unhealthy see-saw

F Health is chronically off-balance. Body constantly trying to re-adjust, has depleted energy
G Disease upsets balance further
H Body makes extra effort to respond to disease
I Homeopathic stimulus pushes body further off-balance
J Body responds to extra stimulus bringing temporary relief
K Body returns to "normal" chronic situation because fundamental situation is the same

large dose of a poison kills, a minute dose of the same poison can stimulate the cellular function vital to produce a natural antidote.

How can it be that a solution that may no longer contain any molecules of a substance can still be therapeutically potent? Some people thought it was all a matter of suggestion and placebos, but that answer is no longer the only one available. Modern nuclear physics is now producing evidence that the early homeopaths were right. A molecule can leave its mark in a dilutant. Modern biochemists and nuclear physicists have shown that substances can leave an imprint of themselves upon a dilutant, providing there is enough energy available for them to do so.

The grinding and shaking of substances increases the energy potential of their molecules, so while remedies may be given to patients in low concentration, they contain high energy states, patterned in the same way as the original molecules. It has also been suggested by physicists that imprinted patterns can replicate themselves. If this is so, it would explain the increased potency of a remedy even beyond the 12c dilution.

What seemed like magic in Hahnemann's day would appear to be scientifically acceptable today. For more information about the homeopathic approach used by Dr Edward Bach, refer to the following pages entitled **Flower remedies**.

Flower remedies

In the 1920s, a system of treatment was developed by Englishman Edward Bach based on homoeopathic principles but using the 38 Bach Flower Remedies. This was not in itself very revolutionary; it was his method of diagnosis that initially made him an object of ridicule by his contemporaries, both in the orthodox medical profession and among respected homoeopathic practitioners.

Bach ignored any physical indications of illness and diagnosed a condition by observing the patient's mental attitude. He then treated the mental state with a small selection from his 38 remedies.

Edward Bach's career

Trained in orthodox medicine, Dr Bach was a bacteriologist at the University College Hospital in

THE BACH FLOWER REMEDIES

Bach identified 38 mental attitudes, which he grouped under seven negative states of mind, each having an appropriate remedy. The common names and the modern international botanical names are given. The original "Twelve Healers" are marked by an asterisk.

1 Remedies for those who are afraid

ROCK ROSE* *Helianthemum nummularium*
An emergency remedy for fear due to an accident or a sudden shock. Also helpful for anxious onlookers.
MIMULUS* *Mimulus guttatus*
For secret fears about everyday things that could happen, such as loss, illness, the dark or loneliness.
CHERRY PLUM *Prunus cerasifera*
For fears about oneself, such as hidden impulses to do something dreadful without intent.
ASPEN *Populus tremula*
For vague fears or chronic nervousness due to constantly anticipating the worst.
RED CHESTNUT *Aesculus carnea*
For fear on behalf of loved ones, always anticipating dreadful things that might happen to them.

2 Remedies for those who are uncertain

CERATO* *Ceratostigma willmottiana*
For lack of self-confidence when making decisions and always seeking advice and reassurance.
SCLERANTHUS* *Scleranthus anuus*
For indecisiveness when choosing between two options because both points of view seem to make sense.
GENTIAN* *Gentiana amarella*
For being easily disheartened by small setbacks or loss of confidence when faced with a minor challenge.
GORSE *Ulex europoeus*
For hopelessness due to lack of faith in any kind of treatment for an illness, although many may be tried.
HORNBEAM *Carpinus betulus*
For doubting one's own strength to continue carrying the burden daily life has become.
WILD OAT *Bromus ramosus*
For frustration due to having energy, ambitions and experience but not knowing which way to go next.

3 Remedies for disinterest in the present

CLEMATIS* *Clematis vitalba*
For vague unhappiness with the present but putting little effort into making new things happen.
HONEYSUCKLE *Lonicera caprifolium*
For living in the past, reminiscing on happier times, and not expecting anything good to ever happen again.
WILD ROSE *Rosa canina*
For resigning to life's troubles without reason and without effort to improve the situation.
OLIVE *Olea europoea*
For extreme exhaustion due to mental or physical suffering, when daily life has no pleasure in it.
WHITE CHESTNUT FLOWER *Aesculus hippocastanum*
For undesirable thoughts and worries that go round and round in the mind, interfering with daily life.
MUSTARD *Sinapis arvensis*
For periods of gloom and despair which come without warning and for no apparent reason at all.
CHESTNUT BUD *Aesculus hippocastanum*
For failure to take advantage of experience and learn from mistakes or good advice.

4 Remedies for loneliness

WATER VIOLET* *Hottonia palustris*
For isolation due to talent, introversion, self-reliance or independence.
IMPATIENS* *Impatiens glandulifera*
For isolation due to quickness of mind, impatience or desire to proceed without delay at own speed.
HEATHER *Calluna vulgaris*
For people who cannot be alone and seek companions regardless of their suitability.

5 Remedies for over-sensitivity to influences

AGRIMONY* *Agrimonia eupatoria*
For chronic joviality, cheerfulness or good humour which hides anxieties. Such people may drink a lot.
CENTAURY* *Centaurium umbellatum*
For good-natured, willing helpers who do more than their share of work, neglecting their own needs.
WALNUT *Juglans regia*
For occasional distraction from own ambitions and ideals by others with strong convictions.
HOLLY *Ilex aquifolium*
For dissatisfaction with oneself, suspicious thoughts, or jealousies that are without foundation.

London when he first came across the practice of homoeopathy. Subsequently he worked at the London Homoeopathic Hospital and eventually ran a private practice combining orthodox medicine and homoeopathy.

Convinced that simple remedies were God-given, he gave up his practice and retired to Wales to study flowering herbs and trees, selecting those that had a curative effect on the seven main mental attitudes that he observed to be synchronous with illnesses. In common with homeopathic doctors, he treated the person not the disease.

Bach published details of the first flower remedies in 1933, calling them the Twelve Healers. Before he died in 1936 he had made a collection of 38 remedies which he used with remarkable accuracy.

6 Remedies for despair

LARCH *Larix decidua*
For a sense of inferiority and failure, and no attempt to make enough effort to succeed.

PINE *Pinus sylvestris*
For discontent with one's own performance, despite hard work and even in success. For blaming oneself.

ELM *Ulmus procera*
For occasional doubts while carrying out a purpose in life for the benefit of humanity.

SWEET CHESTNUT *Castanea sativa*
For extreme anguish when a situation can no longer be endured and only death or destruction seem to remain.

STAR OF BETHLEHEM *Ornithogalum umbethlatum*
For refusal to be consoled, comforted or to progress when unhappy, in distress or grieving for a loss.

WILLOW *Salix vitellina*
For bitterness or resentment, finding it impossible to bring anything positive out of an unjust adversity.

OAK *Quercus robur*
For extreme bravery in a hopeless situation because the self is not allowed to fail.

CRAB APPLE *Malus pumila*
For those who feel unclean and want to change themselves but often ignore the real problem.

7 Remedies for over-concern for others

CHICORY* *Cichorium intybus*
For over-protectiveness and always putting things right for children, relatives and friends.

VERVAIN* *Verbena officinalis*
For always struggling on according to strong, wilful, fixed beliefs and trying to convert others.

VINE *Vitis vinifera*
For domineering people who try to persuade others always to accept their ideas.

BEECH *Fagus sylvatica*
For intolerance of imperfections and a desire to help everyone to become perfect.

ROCK WATER See note
For people who are tough, strict and self-denying and want to appeal to others by example.

Note: rock water is literally the water from any natural rock spring known to have healing properties.

The condition of the mind affects the body

From his observations of people, Bach concluded that mental attitudes, such as fear, anxiety, mistrust or possessiveness provided excellent environments for the invasion of illness. When the patient's outlook became more positive, through the use of the flower remedies, the illness would leave, because it could no longer survive.

Even Bach recognized that damage already done by an illness might not be reversible but he was sure that much sickness could be avoided by changing mental attitudes. Thus his remedies were also used to prevent disease and to reduce the effects of unavoidable conditions.

How to prepare and administer the remedies

Warm, morning dew is collected from the flowers or fruit of the appropriate plant. Alternatively the flowers may be placed in a bowl of pure spring water and stood in the sun for several hours. The water or dew is then bottled with a few drops of brandy to preserve it. This is then labelled as a basic stock bottle.

When illness strikes, the patient's dominant attitudes to life are sought from among those listed. Usually more than one applies, so two or three remedies may be chosen. Normally not more than six stock remedies are used. Ten drops are then taken from the stock bottle and added to pure water in a one ounce bottle and shaken. Four drops of this dilution would then be taken four times a day for as long as necessary. There are no side-effects or dangers in taking these flower remedies.

How does the Bach method work?

Nobody is sure how these remedies work. There is little traceable chemical evidence in the diluted stocks and it is thought that the flowers leave a unique pattern in the water which then affects the body.

REFERENCE: For further information see **Section Six: Homeopathic remedies** (pp.134–135) and **Section Five: Hidden patterns** (pp.102–103).

Natural remedies

A natural remedy is one that has been successfully tried and tested over a long period of time by successive generations in a local environment. It may be a particular diet or potion made from plants and animals that thrive in the local habitat. A collection of such remedies form the basic folk medicine peculiar to that area.

Are natural remedies universal?
When looking for successful remedies to adopt, it may be more appropriate to take into account the whole way of life, rather than try to isolate only one aspect. This has been found to be true by researchers seeking to find the ideal diet to promote a long and healthy life.

In the 1960s, American researcher Dr Alexander Leaf tried to understand the secret of longevity by studying the eating habits of people who live long, active lives. For his study he visited three such communities, all of them in remote mountain regions.

Dr Leaf made detailed recordings of the eating habits of village people in Vilcabamba, Ecuador, in a Hunza settlement of Kashmir and in Abkhazia, Georgia in the southern Soviet Union. In all of these communities the number of people living healthy active lives over the age of 100 was approximately 300 times greater than in the US.

He and his team were delighted to find that the dietary habits of the first two communities closely matched the low animal-fat, low calorie diet recommended by modern Western medical opinion.

Unfortunately, in Abkhazia his findings were quite the reverse. The healthy, happy, long-living Georgians ate more food high in animal fat and calories than average Westerners, to which they added substantial quantities of wine, bread and pastries.

So how did these people retain such good health and usually only reach the peak of their working lives between 70 and 80 years? Nobody has yet answered that question satisfactorily.

While a natural remedy may be a successful part of local folk medicine, it may not work for others unless account is taken of the whole way of life; inherited factors, upbringing, daily habits and environment will also play their part.

HONEY AND APPLE CIDER VINEGAR
One of the best investigations into the universal use of a natural remedy was undertaken by Dr D.C. Jarvis, whose medical practice was in his native Vermont, in the US. Over a period of twenty years, he and his colleagues in 32 states studied the remarkable effects of the folk medicine of Vermont, in particular the use of honey and apple cider vinegar as a preventative and a cure. Dr Jarvis published his findings in 1958.

The honey and cider vinegar way of life in old Vermont
At the time of Jarvis' investigations, most people in Vermont worked on the land well into their seventies and eighties. Dr Jarvis was curious to discover how so many people in the community achieved such good health and longevity.

Clearly the daily exercise of work was enjoyed by these rural people and seemed beneficial to everyone. He noted that each person, man or woman, worked at their own steady pace and their movements were strong and graceful. Sudden jerks, painful tensions and exhaustion were avoided.

One of the most popular tonics used by the rural Vermonters was apple cider vinegar, of which there was a plentiful supply locally. It was commonplace in the diet of both humans and animals and was used to ward off colds, increase the stamina of new-born animals and relieve aches and pains.

Dr Jarvis and his study group observed the effects of this remedy on their patients, both people and animals, and were surprised at the beneficial results obtained when just two teaspoons of the local, dark honey, mixed with two teaspoons of apple cider vinegar, were sipped on rising in a morning, as a general tonic. The honey was not essential to the results, but it did make the sour cider vinegar palatable.

Why was this simple, natural substance so popular and evidently so effective? Dr Jarvis concluded that it helped to maintain a healthy acid/alkaline balance in the body. It should be noted that different acids have different effects on the body. Apple cider vinegar has a positive effect but other acidic foods, such as oranges and grapefruit had a negative effect.

Dr Jarvis also recommended that oats, corn or rye be used instead of wheat and honey instead of cane, maple or beet sugar.

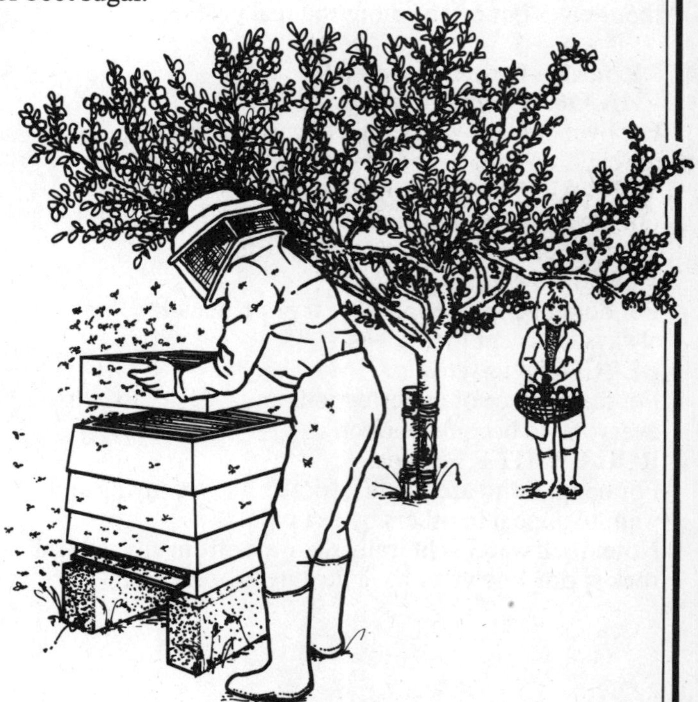

ACIDS AND ALKALIS

Acids

These are sharp, sour substances that have a strong smell and neutralize alkalis. The chemical formula for hydrochloric acid is HCl. By adding it to an alkali such as dilute sodium hydroxide, NaOH, common table salt and water will be left. The reaction is written chemically:

$HCl + NaOH = NaCl + H_2O$

acid + alkali = salt + water

Alkalis (or bases)

These are opposite substances to acids, they taste bitter and have a soapy feel. If too much is eaten a lot of digestive acid is released into the stomach resulting in indigestion. A mild alkali in the form of indigestion tablets will quickly neutralize the excess acid.

Measuring strength

Chemists measure the strength of acids and alkalis by numbers called pH numbers. Strengths can be measured with universal indicator papers which change colour.

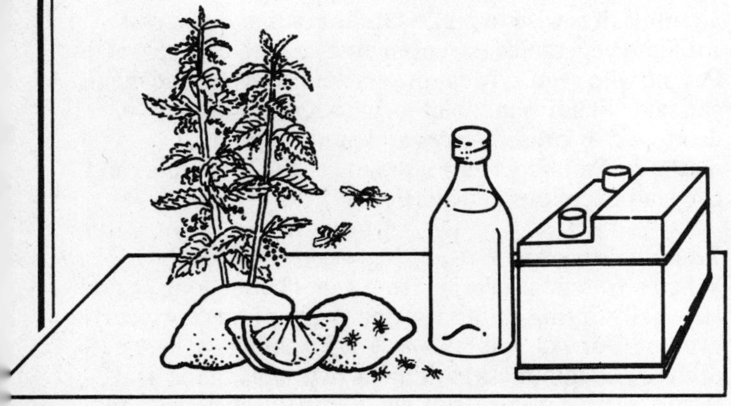

All these things contain acids. Some acids are very weak and others are strong enough to dissolve metals: Vinegar, lemons, car batteries, nettles, ants, bee stings.

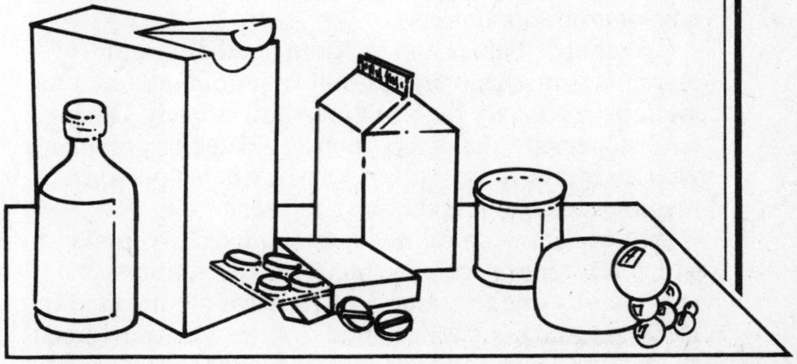

All these things contain alkalis, some of which are very mild and others are caustic and will burn: Washing soda, baking soda, cows milk, ammonia, indigestion tablets, soap.

MAKING NATURAL REMEDIES WORK FOR YOU

According to Dr Jarvis and other researchers since, an acid reaction in the urine, tested before eating breakfast is the best indicator of good health.

Testing the urine

Neutral litmus papers or universal indicator papers can be bought from drug stores which can be dipped into a sample of urine taken on rising. If the urine is alkaline, the indicator will turn lilac-blue; if acid, it will turn pink-red.

It is normal for the urine to change from acid to alkaline and back again throughout the day as meals are eaten and as the body has periods of activity and rest. Under normal healthy conditions, the urine will show an acid reaction first thing in a morning before eating. The urine will turn alkaline for short periods during the day but if alkalinity persists, an adjustment should be made to diet and to the way of life, and cider vinegar taken three times daily.

Acidity of the urine

Dr Jarvis observed that urine turned acid, and stayed acid, under the following conditions:

- when the weather was settled, even though cold
- when the body was warmed, e.g. by baths, sun-bathing, physical activity, warm clothes, warm air
- when a person was relaxed or at peace
- when a person had no illness
- when the body was feeling pleasure
- when mental work was interspersed with short periods of day-dreaming, walks or chats
- after hard physical work that was relaxing
- after physically pleasurable recreation

Alkalinity of the urine

Dr Jarvis observed that the urine turned alkaline, and stayed alkaline, under the following conditions:

- two days before a drop in weather temperature
- when the body was cold, e.g. by thin clothing, cold air, immobility, lack of sun, cold drinks or food
- when a person was worried or under extra stress

just before the onset of illnesses such as chickenpox, sinusitis, hayfever or ashthma

- when the body was in pain
- after prolonged mental work
- after hard physical work that was exhausting
- after physically stressful recreation

REFERENCE: For more information about the acid/alkali balance, refer to **Section One: The balance of life** (pp.14–15).

An alphabet of vitamins

Vitamins are substances in food which are essential to the normal growth and nutrition of people and animals. Some orthodox Western doctors and many alternative practitioners recommend the use of vitamin supplements in certain circumstances, such as after surgery, while dieting, when under extra stress at work or to prevent winter colds.

Most people can obtain their normal vitamin needs from eating a sensible diet which includes some fresh foods without preservatives, raw vegetables and fruit.

A concentrated excess of vitamins A and D can be dangerous, so anyone with high blood pressure or heart problems should always consult a doctor before taking any vitamin supplements.

In general, babies and children need different amounts from the average adult requirement and some vitamin needs vary between men and women. During natural periods of change, such as old age or pregnancy, vitamin intake is naturally adjusted when a person responds to changing dietary preferences.

Most countries have a recommended daily intake, to which reference should be made, as the amounts can vary slightly due to cultural and environmental factors. However, the body is designed to cope with nutritional changes and fluctuations providing there is no overall nutritional deficiency. Unfortunately there are many instances of vitamin deficiency in the well-fed areas of the world, due to the refining of food which also removes the fiber content.

Protecting vitamins

As indicated in the table, several vitamins are susceptible to excessive heat or light, so the storage of food in a cool, dark place has always made good sense and the modern refrigerator serves the purpose.

Freezing food does not appear to affect most vitamins except Vitamin E which is destroyed by freezing. All vegetables, especially green ones, will lose their vitamin content if over-cooked or if bicarbonate of soda is added.

Since canning, roasting and frying destroy so many vitamins, it is wise to make sure that some fresh, raw fruit and vegetables are eaten every day to compensate. People who regularly eat pre-packed convenience meals can take vitamins in tablet form to replace those destroyed by preservatives and modern refining methods. Smoking destroys many of the B vitamins and can lead to serious deficiencies.

Vitamin deficiency

When a vitamin is missing from a diet over a long period, especially during childhood, many symptoms are clearly evident. For example, the lack of Vitamin A causes eye disease and blindness in millions of people in the Third World, scurvy is the result of vitamin C deficiency and rickets a symptom of insufficient vitamin D.

ORTHOMOLECULAR MEDICINE

This is the treatment of human disease by varying the concentration of substances normally present in the body, in particular large doses of vitamins.

The term orthomolecular was coined by the American Dr Linus Pauling, who was the 1945 Nobel Prize winner for chemistry. He was interested in the use of Vitamin C to prevent and cure the common cold. Later he became involved with others in orthomolecular psychiatry which treats depression and schizophrenia with large doses of the C and several of the B vitamins, both of which are essential to brain and nerve cells.

Orthomolecular psychiatry

In Britain, schizophrenia is largely regarded as a problem of family relationships, but some psychiatrists, particularly in the US, are now convinced that schizophrenia is a biochemical problem. The American pioneer of orthomolecular psychiatry, Dr Abram Hoffer, regards many mental diseases as due to vitamin dependency states.

Vitamin dependency is described as a condition in which the body is unable to absorb or metabolize certain vitamins from food normally containing those vitamins. To correct the situation, orthomolecular psychiatrists prescribe extremely large doses of specific vitamins so that at least some will be absorbed into the blood stream.

Evidence that absorption may be the problem points to the changes in the digestive tract suffered by those who have celiac disease. Celiacs are given large doses of vitamins because it has been shown that they have difficulty absorbing certain vitamins in the gut. Some long-term schizophrenias are accompanied by changes in the gut lining that are similar to those seen in celiac disease. Of course, there must be other factors at work, since people with celiac disease are not schizophrenic.

In the 1970s, Dr R.F. Smith, an alcoholism expert, claimed to have a 77% recovery rate over a two-year period with 507 alcoholics at the Brighton Hospital, Detroit, using massive doses of vitamin B complex. Many similar studies have been undertaken but there are no final conclusions. Claims have also been made of damage caused by megavitamin therapy, often prescribed by unqualified people. It is clear that orthomolecular medicine must pay attention to the whole, individual person. It may be just an old saying that what is one man's meat is another man's poison, but there is wisdom in it that we would do well to remember.

Vitamin therapies often form a part of the broader based nutrition therapies that are growing in popularity. For more information see **Section Four: What's in a diet?** (pp.82–83).

THE COMMON VITAMINS

† Fat soluble vitamins are stored until required.
* Water soluble vitamins are not stored in the body so need to be eaten daily.

Vitamin	Function	Some food sources
† **A**: retinol; needs vitamins C and E to be effective. Destroyed by canning, frying, food preservatives, some fertilizers and drugs.	Reduces susceptibility to infection or air pollution; helps digestion of protein and building of bones, blood and good night vision; keeps skin supple.	Fish oil, eggs, milk, cream, butter, margarine, green and leafy vegetables, broccoli, carrots and liver. 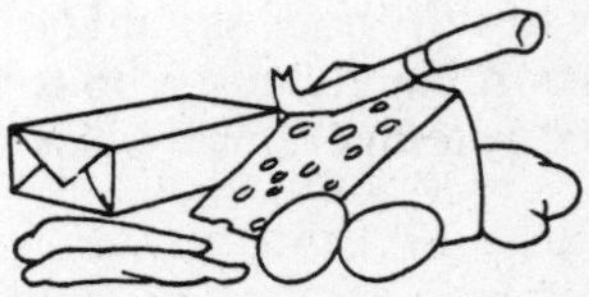
* **B** complex: 15 different compounds which must be taken together or they will lose their value. Destroyed by most antibiotics, sugar, alcohol, food refining methods and some drugs including the contraceptive pill. Individual B vitamins can be affected by deep freezing of meat and canning.	Essential to metabolism of carbohydrates and the function of nervous system; maintains muscle tone, and health of skin, hair, eyes, mouth and liver.	Brewer's yeast, torula yeast, fish, meat, seafoods, whole grain breads and cereals, green vegetables, peanuts, peas, eggs, molasses and wheatgerm. 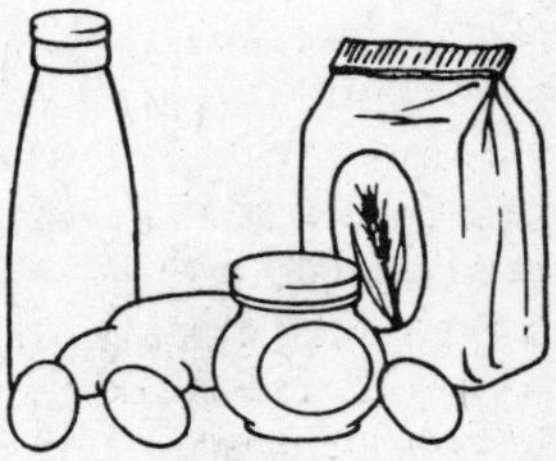
* **C**: ascorbic acid; best taken in small amounts every mealtime as it only stays in the body for 3–4 hours. Destroyed by oxygen, light, heat and many common drugs such as aspirin.	Prevents hemorrhage; fights bacterial infections; aids healing of wounds and scars; prevents colds and allergies.	Fresh fruits and vegetables, rose hips and green peppers, potatoes 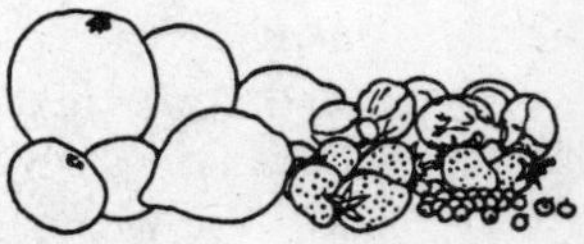
† **D**: a combination of substances including calciferol; best combined with Vitamin A. Destroyed by food preservatives, canning, frying and some fertilizers and drugs.	Essential for bone formation, heart function and normal blood-clotting; stabilizes nervous system.	Fish liver oil, eggs and dairy products; produced by skin on exposure to sunlight. 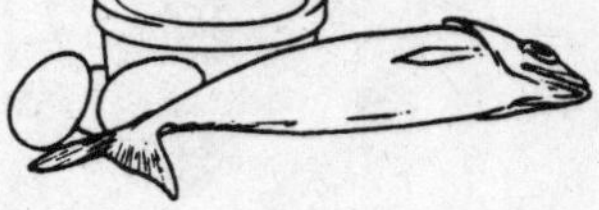
† **E**: tocopherol; only stored in body up to 3 days. Destroyed by light, air, frying, food freezing and some drugs.	Essential for stamina; facilitates work of other vitamins; protects against natural poisons; retards aging; increases fertility of both sexes helps to prevent miscarriages; heals burns and scars; aids focus of eyes in middle age.	Cold pressed vegetable oils; whole seeds, nuts, eggs, soybeans, wheatgerm oil and leafy vegetables. 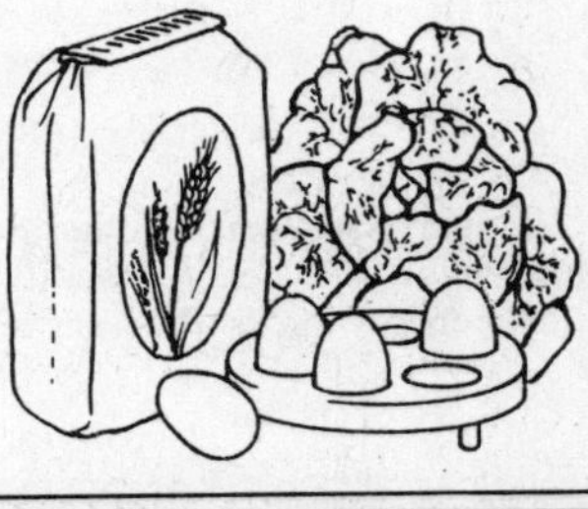

Section seven

HOW ARE YOU?

What is a healthy body? Is it one that functions effectively at any age, despite injuries, disabilities or inborn handicaps? Or is a healthy body one that is almost perfect . . . and if so, what is perfect health?

Is there a size, shape, color, weight or proportion that a healthy body should be? How strong, supple or coordinated must a body be to pass as healthy? Can the body temperature, pulse rate and blood pressure all be within normal limits and yet the person be unhealthy?

How important are inherited factors and family upbringing? How much effect can the local environment have on the health of the people who live in it? How important are lifestyle and the absence of stress?

This final section is devoted to both scientific and traditional methods of diagnosis and some of the signs that are said to indicate a healthy or an unhealthy body.

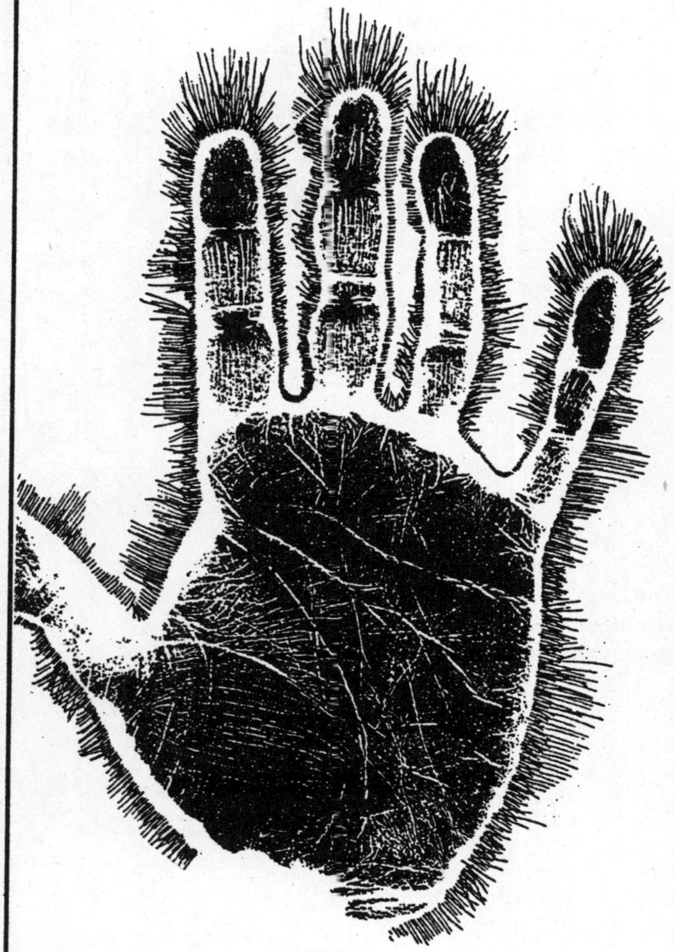

Life energy sources: Whether the "aura" of a hand is a true indication of its healthy condition or not. All living forms contain *inner* energy forces which sustain them.

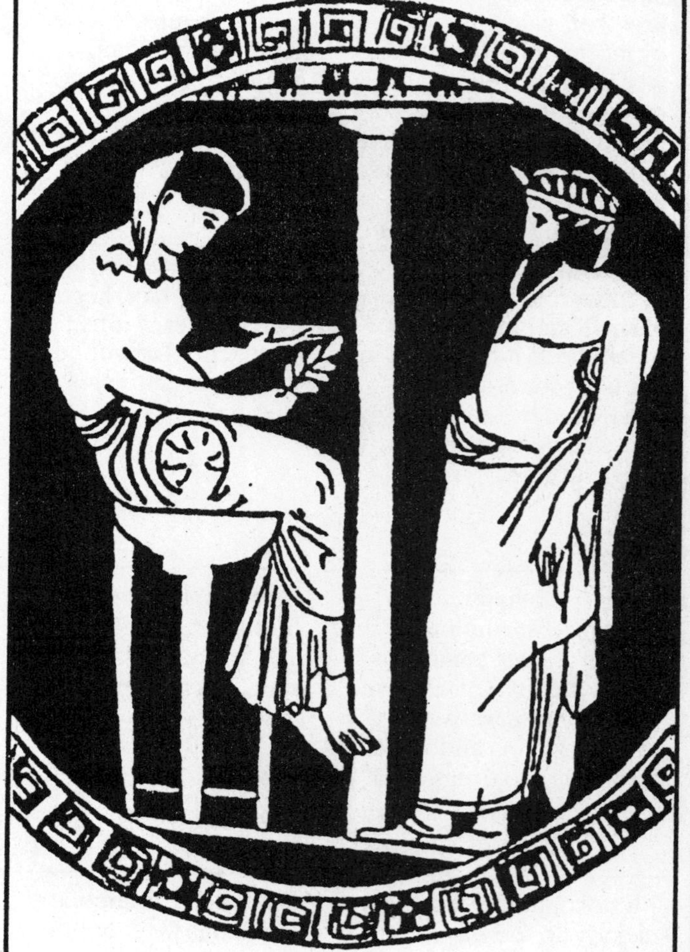

Faith: Health without faith is life without hope. Ancient Greek gods were consulted through the medium of an oracle (here, Apollo's priestess of Delphi) to diagnose health conditions.

The scientific methods used by practitioners of alternative methods are similar to those used by modern Western doctors. They are based on observations and measurements; however, their different viewpoints become clear as they are described.

What is a doctor looking for, a disease or a state of being? Is the diagnosis designed to pinpoint the cause of particular symptoms or understand the conditions that brought about the state of ill-health? Furthermore, does the diagnosis also indicate the treatment, or is that a quite separate decision made by the doctor?

In the modern world health checks, screening and medical examinations for jobs are common practice, so one of the many possible diagnoses made by the modern doctor is that of good health. Other approaches are more predictive of likely outcomes.

Finally, the possible effect of combining many different approaches is discussed. In the end everyone must make their own choice about which type of diagnosis and treatment to accept.

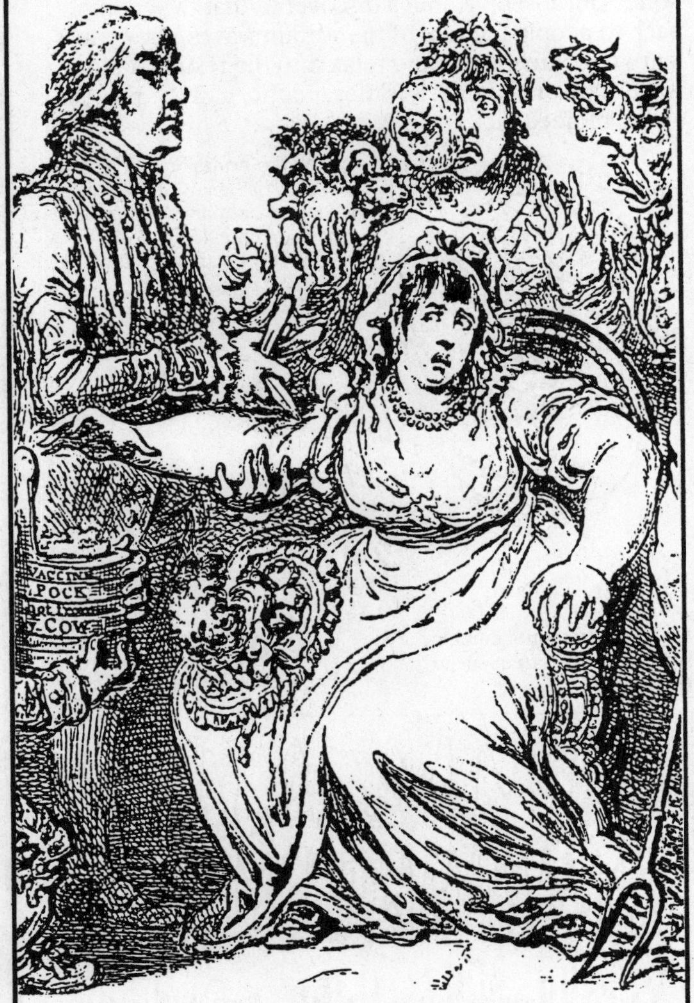

Orthodox and unorthodox: English satirist James Gillray "Cow-Pock" cartoon of 1802 for the Anti-Vaccine Society ridiculing Edward Jenner's new smallpox vaccination. What is unorthodox may become orthodox.

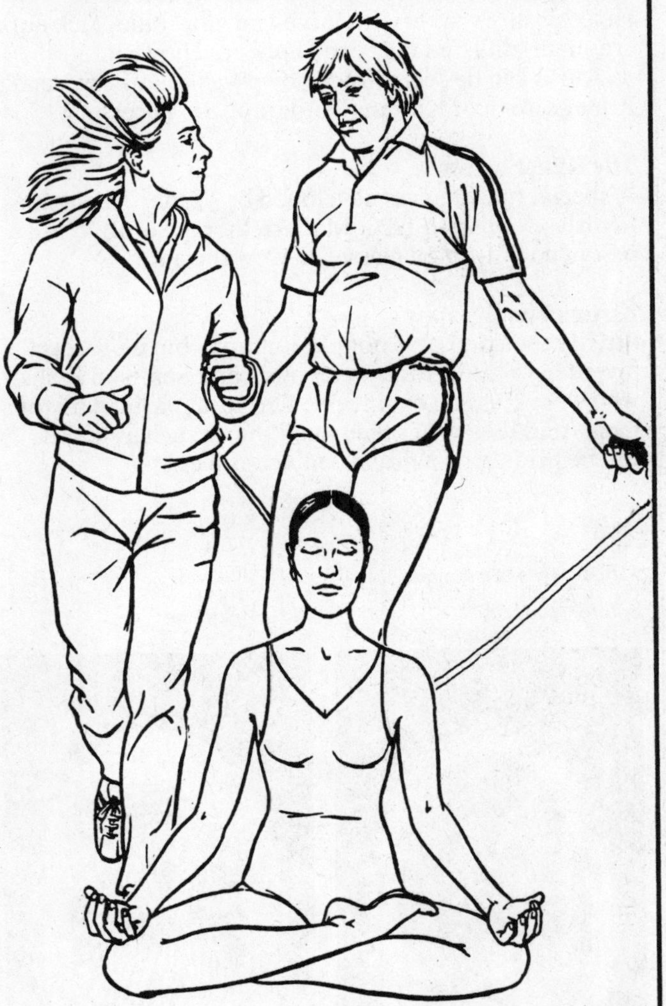

East and West: The ancient oriental arts of yoga and meditation combined with western physical exercise can produce well-being that has the best of both worlds.

Diagnostic alternatives 1

Traditional, Western allopathic diagnosis relies on asking the patient questions, making measurements and internal examinations.

Alternative medicines may also use some measurements but rely on diagnostic processes quite alien to the allopathic doctor. Because small changes can be detected taking place in the body, many of these methods can be used prophylactically, i.e. to prevent illness developing.

Further diagnostic alternatives can be found on the following pages.

Advantages of alternative diagnostic procedures
1 Preventive because they reveal a predisposition toward a particular physical weakness.
2 Realistic because they recognize that disorders affect the whole person so assessment is of the whole person.
3 Inexpensive because they require very little equipment.
4 Accurate because most diagnostic methods are used throughout treatment to assess progress and adjust treatment.

AURA DIAGNOSIS

The pulsing energy field surrounding all living things is called the aura. When a person is ill or in the process of sickening for something, a disturbance in the color, size and rate of pulsation of the aura can be detected. Healthy auras are bright, large and glow blue. Sick auras are small, dull and may even appear yellowish.

Auras can be seen directly by psychics; otherwise a Kilner screen or Kirlian photograph are necessary.

The Kilner screen
A special type of glass developed by Walter J. Kilner, a British scientist, in 1920. Modern therapists often use a pair of cobalt-tinted glasses to view the aura.

Kirlian photography
Strictly speaking, it is not photography but a process invented in the 1930s by Valentina and Semyion Kirlian, who were Russian engineers. The aura, particularly of hands and feet or of other small things such as leaves, can be printed by a direct contact process.

Kirlian prints of a thumb aura:

Before treatment

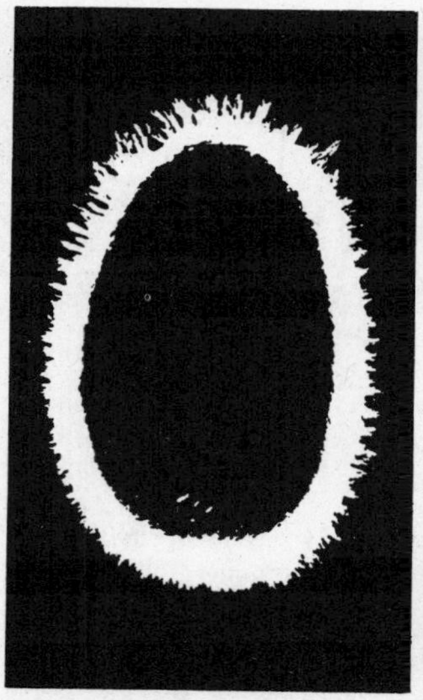

After treatment

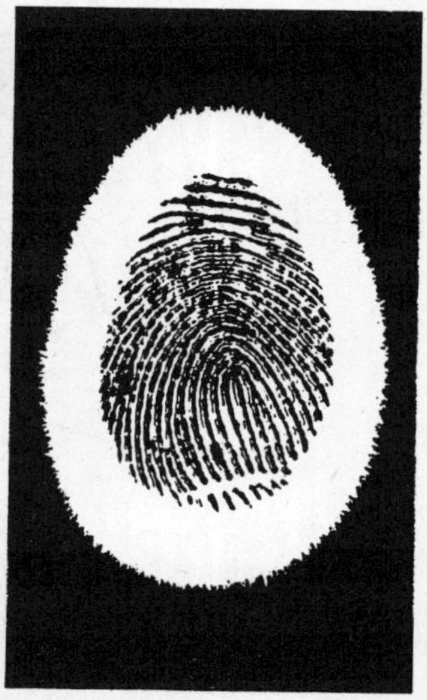

ELECTROENCEPHALOGRAPHY

EEG for short, this is a graph showing the electrical pattern of brain waves measured via electrodes attached to the scalp and is generally used in traditional medicine to detect brain damage and disease. In the 1950s the American Joseph Kamiya discovered that by feeding back to people the rate of their brain waves, they could learn to control them and relax into the resting alpha-wave state. This in itself is therapeutic, and the process is called biofeedback.

Detecting brain waves
1 Electric signals ripple across the brain as millions of brain cells fire repeatedly.
2 Electrodes at intervals along the head reveal a set of brainwave traces.

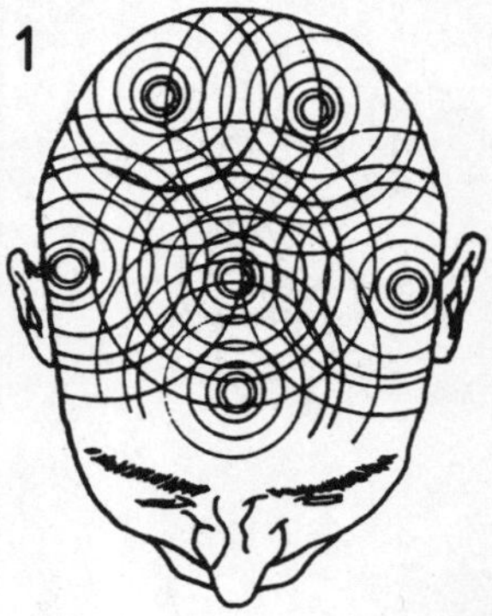

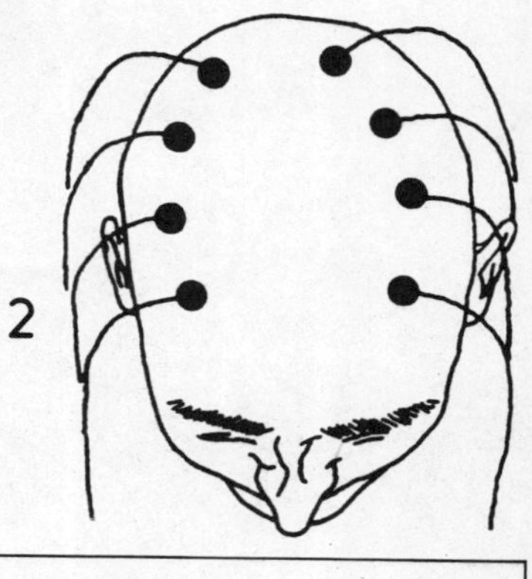

One wave trace may combine waves of several frequencies (here shown below it).

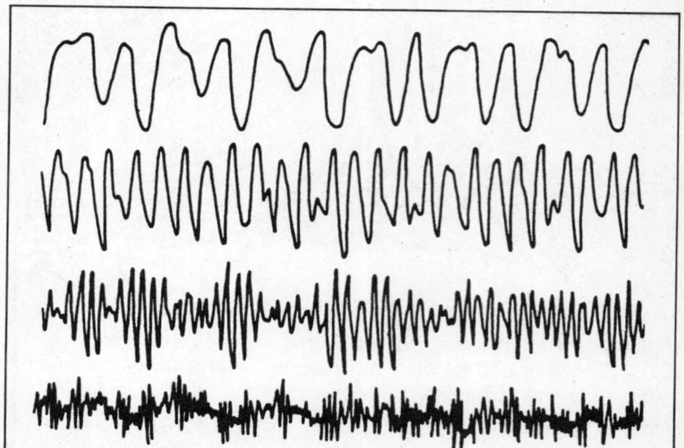

EYE DIAGNOSES

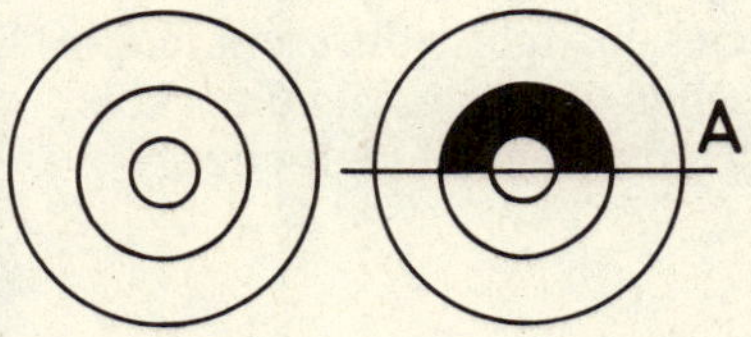

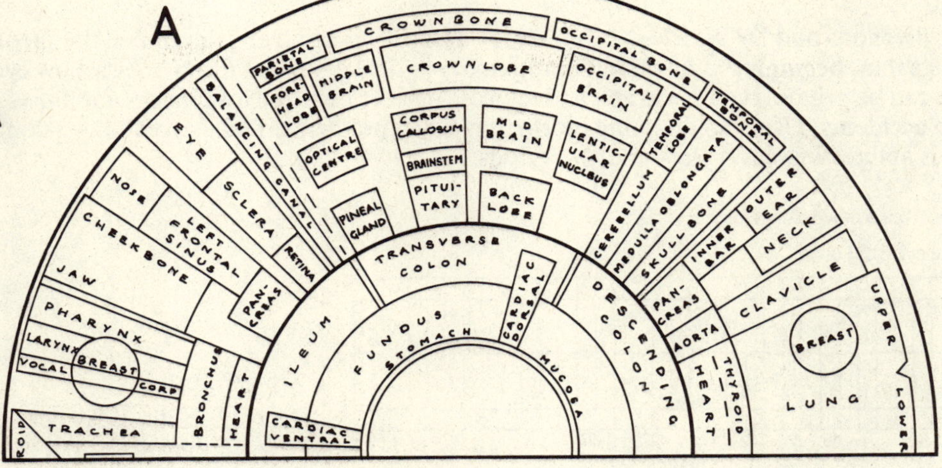

A shows half the iris of the left eye and the relevant Iridology chart

IRIDOLOGY

The iris of the eye is the colored, muscular region that controls how much light enters the eye through the pupil. The condition of the iris has been used for over 3000 years to diagnose conditions of the body. This method is called iridology and, in modern terms, is a study of the neuro-optic reflex.

The Chaldeans recorded readings of diseases from the eyes, and the process of iris diagnosis was known to the Ancient Chinese, Japanese and Indian cultures. There are also references to iridology in the medical writings of Hippocrates.

The most comprehensive study of iris diagnosis was undertaken by an Hungarian physicist, Dr Ignatz von Peczely, who lived from 1822 to 1911. He first drew the modern form of iridology charts. Many medical people have added their observations over the years, matching physical condition with marks on the iris of the eyes.

Iridology is done by an eye-to-eye examination that may take 30 minutes for each eye. A properly trained, experienced iridologist will be 75% correct. The percentage can then be increased by using high definition photographic enlargements of the irises of both eyes.

Disadvantages of Iridology

Because almost anyone can get hold of an Iridology chart and start comparing it with their own irises, problems arise from ignorance.

It should be noted that to attempt self-diagnosis is unwise. There are so many possible interpretations of a mark on the iris that only careful study of other features will determine which interpretation is correct. A particular mark on the iris can also indicate good health.

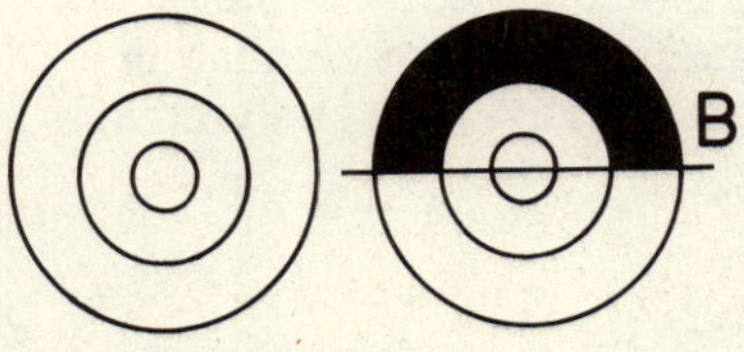

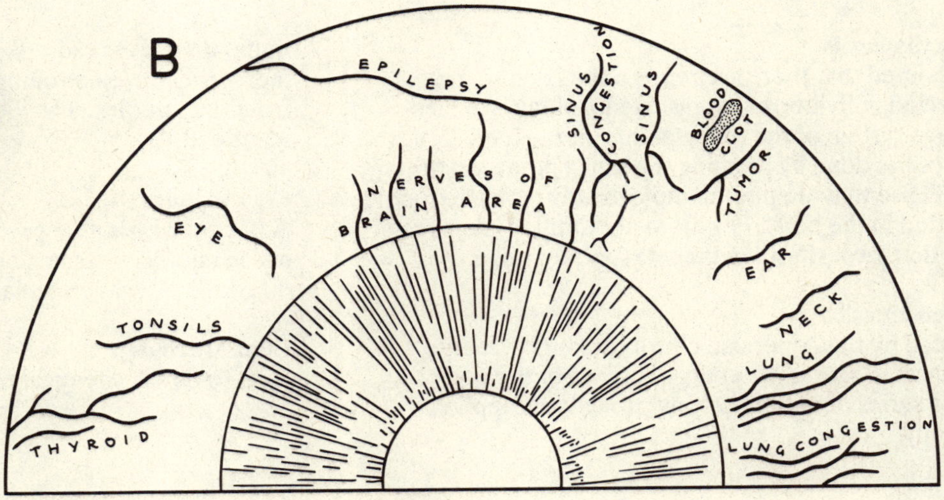

B shows half the sclera of the left eye and the accompanying sclera diagnosis chart

SCLEROLOGY

This is a method similar to Iridology but the sclera or white part of the eye is examined for changes. This is a less reliable method, as discolorations and marks tend to appear and disappear quite frequently on the sclera.

Diagnostic alternatives 2

BIORHYTHM DIAGNOSIS

Dr H. Swovoda and Dr W. Fliess in Vienna and Berlin respectively, developed the theory of biorhythms which suggests that, beginning at birth, our emotional, physical and mental activities follow cycles of slightly different length. These can be printed out on a graph and indicate days of high and low energy and times when we are most vulnerable, say, to accidents. Using an on-going biorhythm chart, problems can be avoided by taking advantage of high-energy periods and resting during low-energy periods.

Sections from a biorhythm chart

Physical cycle: 23 days

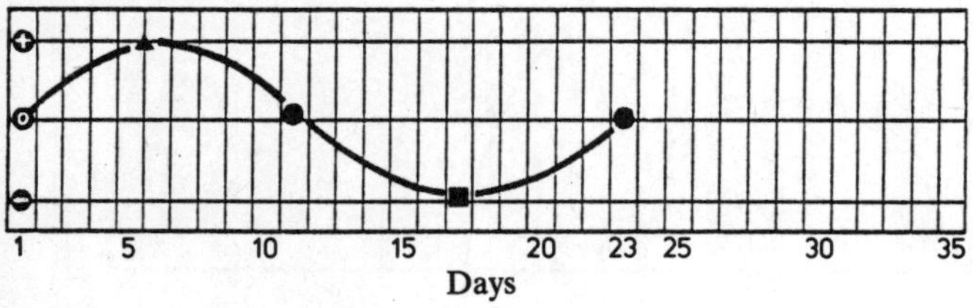

Emotional cycle: 28 days

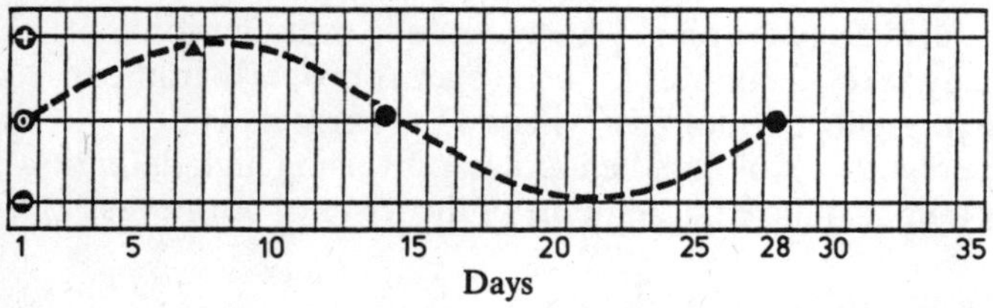

Intellectual cycle: 33 days

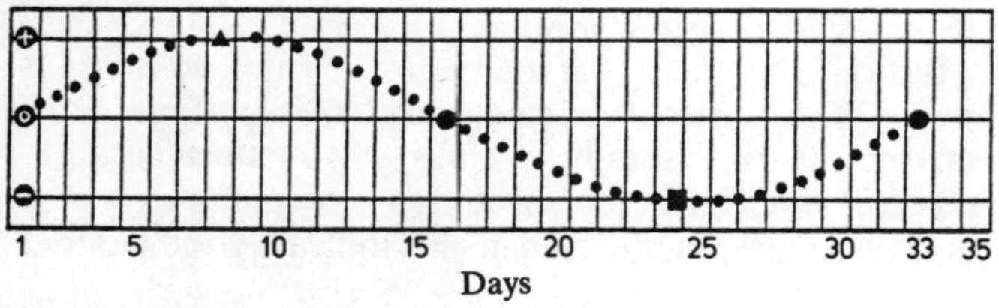

A triple critical day occurs when all three cycles cross, even if they are not in the same phase. On these days, which happen once a year, prudence is the best policy when planning demanding activities.

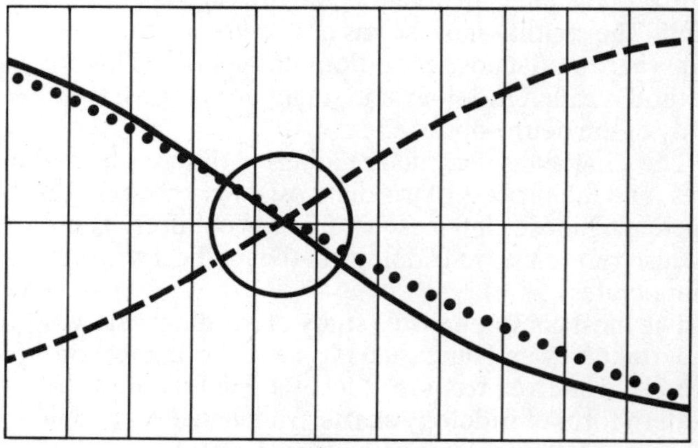

Reflex diagnosis
It is claimed that there are reflex points on the feet connected with internal areas. Reflexology is a deep massage system of the reflex points on the feet. Reflex diagnosis is done by pressing the reflex points on the feet. Those that are painful indicate areas where trouble is located in the body. For more about this system, refer to **Section Two: It's all in the sole** (pp.50–53).

Applied kinesiology
Invented by the American chiropractor Dr George Goodhart to assess the energy balance of the body by using a series of muscle-testing procedures applied manually.

Radionics
Radiesthesia is a method of diagnosing by a process of dowsing. The movements of a sensitive pendulum held over a sample of hair, blood or saliva are noted and a treatment is chosen by finding the same pendulum-swing when held over a number of remedies, usually homeopathic. In radionics, the diagnosis is done by measuring the electromagnetic vibrations emanating from the samples. The vibrations are then analyzed and identified.

Clairvoyance
A person who is able psychically to see disturbances inside another person's body is using clairvoyant diagnosis. This is a special talent.

Clinical ecology
Tests to detect chemical allergies.

CHINESE DIAGNOSIS

Used by acupuncturists and practitioners of related therapies. Four methods are used:
1 Observing physical appearance and smell.
2 Hearing the quality of breathing and tone of voice.
3 Asking questions and examination by palpitation (discovering if pain is felt on applying pressure in certain areas). This method is used in traditional medicine.
4 Making a pulse examination. This is by far the most complex as there are 12 pulses, one for each of the 12 meridians or pathways connected to regions where major organs are situated. The strength and quality of each pulse is noted.

An acupuncture doctor will take the pulses of a patient over a period of time, comparing the patient's normal rate with any changes. What is a normal pulse for one person may not be normal for another, since the pulses reflect not only physical make-up but emotional characteristics. The times at which pulses are taken is also noted, as some will be stronger at different times of the day.

Positions of the pulses, six on each hand

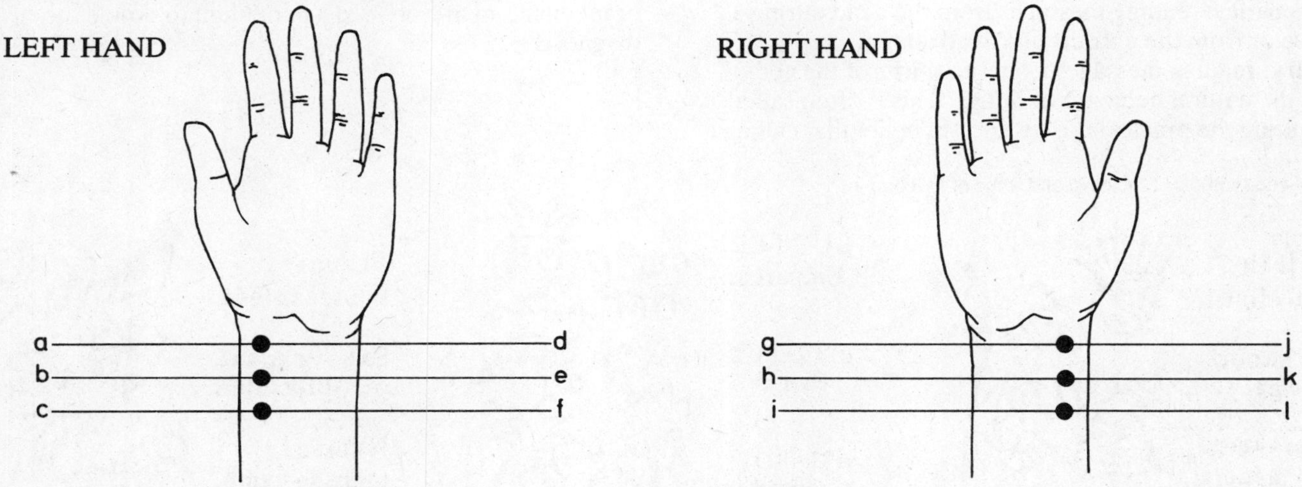

Superficial pulses
a Small intestine
b Gall bladder
c Bladder

Deep pulses
d Heart
e Liver
f Kidneys

Deep pulses
g Lungs
h Spleen
i Circulation/Sex

Superficial pulses
j Colon
k Stomach
l Pericardium

SPAGYRIK ANALYSIS

Spagyrik therapy is a sophisticated combination of diagnosis and treatment that was first developed in Germany. However, it is based on a very ancient practice of drinking one's own waste products.

A small amount of blood, urine or saliva is processed leaving a clear liquid which crystallizes on cooling. The crystal formation is said to be unique to each person and can be read by an experienced practitioner. The pattern reveals potential problems and specific existing disease, degeneration and the effect of external stresses.

Small amounts of the crystals are given to the patient in liquid form. This stimulates the body's immune system by being given back its own information. This process is homeopathic.

Herbs that match the crystal pattern may also be used. The Spagyrik process is used repeatedly to assess, progress and continue treatment, the body itself regulating what it needs to stimulate self-healing.

Spagyrik crystal patterns

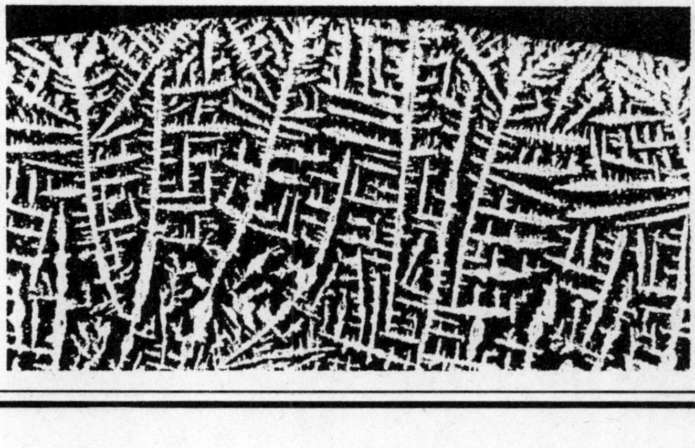

Divining the diagnosis

Divination is the art of using magic, fortune-telling and folklore beliefs to foretell outcomes. Divination has been used over the centuries to diagnose sickness and make a prognosis, the purpose of which was to discover which evil spirit was causing the disease and what had to be done to pacify or remove the evil one. Divination was also used to establish paternity and to ensure conception.

Diagnostic divination
Three sources of information have been used to find the cause of a sickness. Two examples of each are given.

1 Divination from the spirits
Necromancy: reading messages from the dead during a seance or from the entrails of a dead animal.
Augury: reading messages from the spirits of the gods from the natural behavior of things. This is often called consulting the oracles. It is an ancient belief that calling a person's name gives the power to summon them, so the gods were called upon by name. Similarly, the devil can be evoked by calling his name or the name of one of his number. Hence the old sayings: "speak of angels" and "speak of the devil."

2 Divination from the natural world
Astrology: consulting the positions of the planets.
Geomancy: reading patterns made by the earth, for example, as sand is thrown to the ground.

3 Divination through a human medium
Oneiromancy: interpreting the dreams of the patient.
Clairvoyant dowsing: consulting a shaman, witchdoctor or medicine man who uses a pendulum to dowse the diagnosis.

Names and symbols of the devil and some of his company

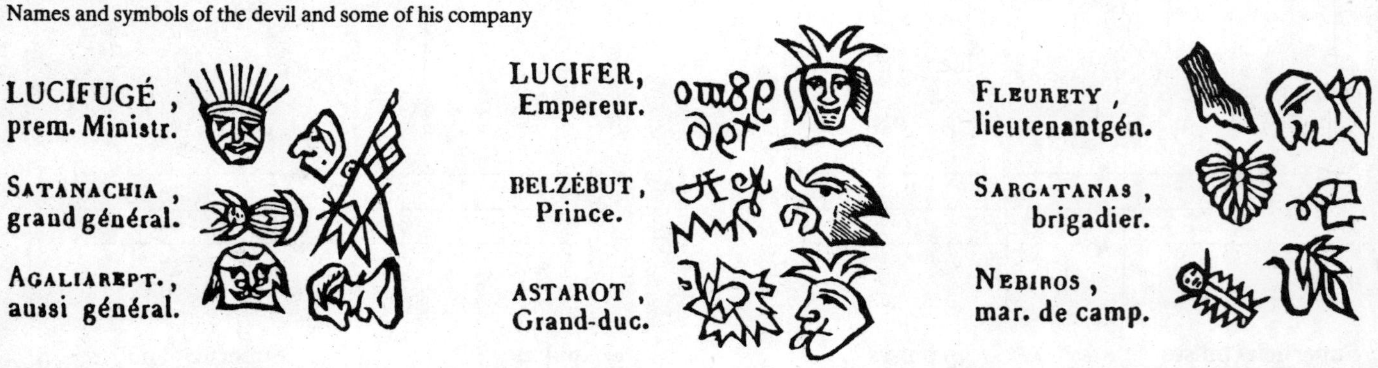

CONSULTING THE ORACLE
The Zande were a sophisticated community of people who lived in remote central Africa between the Rivers Nile and Congo. Their approach to diagnosis was both scientific and magical.

When a Zande fell ill, it would first be assumed that he had a disease that was due to natural causes. He would be questioned about his symptoms, in very much the way a modern doctor might question his patient. He would then be treated with local drugs, which were known to all the older people in the community. Only if these failed was it assumed that magic done by a witch was preventing a cure.

The relatives would possibly consult one or more oracles. Two questions would be asked of the oracle: where it would be safe for the sick person to live in order to recover and the name of the witch responsible for the disease. Anyone in the community could be a witch using good or bad magic.

When the witch was named, often to his or her surprise, the witch had to be persuaded by the witchdoctor to leave the sick person in peace, so his treatment by the drugs could be completed. There follow the oracles the Zande used:

The three-sticks oracle
Three pieces of wood were carved and stood in a quiet place overnight, one resting on top of the others. Only if they fell was the reply to the question negative.

The rubbing-board oracle
Everyone can carry a small rubbing board around in a little bark bag, to be consulted on many minor matters. Larger boards can be kept at home. Everyone makes his own board, which is an oval table shape (the female part) supported by two legs and a tail and a lid which fits the surface of the table (the male part).

The board is transformed into an oracle by being carved and having hot juices and oils rubbed into it. It will then be placed in a new barkcloth and buried under a pathway for two days. Those who walk along the path are said to take away all coldness from the board; it is most important that the board does not become cold. To use the rubbing-board oracle, juice of the Kaffir apple is rubbed onto its surface. The lid is replaced, and a question is asked of it. If the lid sticks when rubbed, the reply is negative; if it moves easily, the reply is positive.

How to use a dowsing pendulum
Any fine thread and a small crystal, a round button, pendant or a ring will make an excellent pendulum for dowsing answers to questions.

The pendulum is suspended from the left hand while questions are asked. A swing will indicate an answer. Questions must be phrased to give a yes/no answer. The pendulum is said to swing for a yes answer and remain still for a negative answer.

Sample questions that would evoke yes/no replies
- Will the sickness stay a long time?
- Will the disease leave before the new moon?
- Should he (the patient) remain in this village?
- Can the witch be named? (A series of questions could be asked, or an oracle could be consulted to ascertain the name.)

When questions are close to the truth, the pendulum will become more agitated.

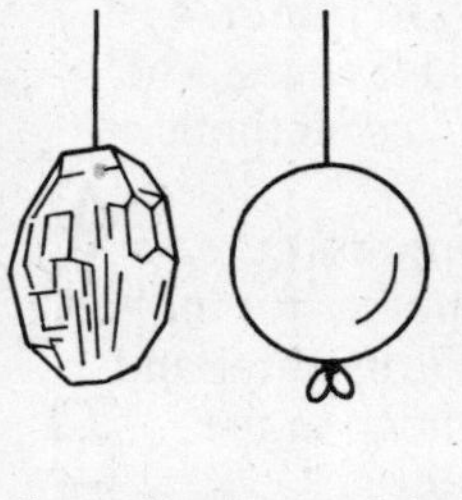

Some dowsing pendulums

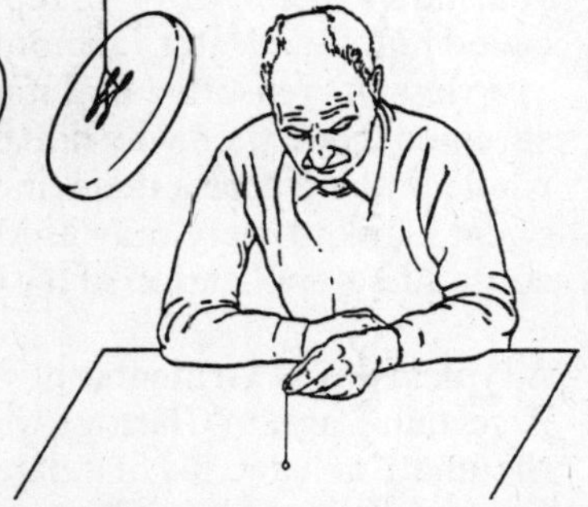

The termites oracle
The relatives have to find a termite nest and run. Two twigs (one yes, the other no) from different trees are stuck into the ground on the termite run. A question is asked, and the termites are requested to indicate the reply during the night. The next day the answer is divined from which of the twigs has been eaten by the termites.

The poison oracle
This was the most reliable of all the oracles and the most expensive, so minor questions were eliminated by using the other oracles, leaving only one important question for confirmation by the poison oracle.

A substance known to the Zande as *benge* was prepared from a forest creeper as a red powder, which was then mixed with water to form a paste. Liquid from this paste was then squeezed out into the beak of a small fowl, which would suffer terrible convulsions. The substance was chemically similar to strychnine. The death or survival of the fowl was taken as an answer to the question put to the poison oracle, and indeed the results were final according to ancient Zande laws.

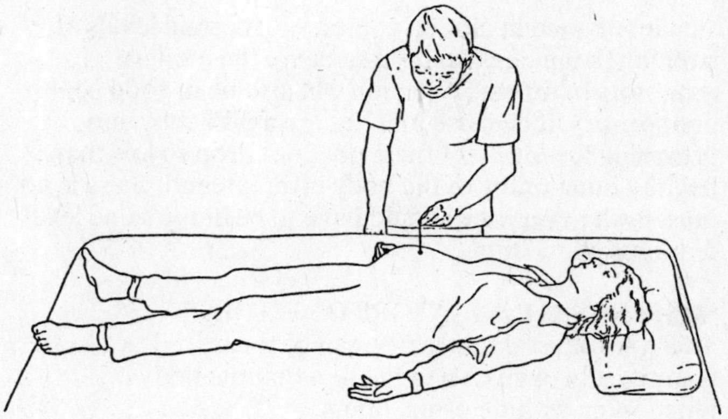

Using a wedding ring dowsing pendulum to detect the sex of an unborn child. With most operators, the pendulum will swing backward and forward (**A**) to indicate a boy, and around in a circle (**B**) to indicate a girl

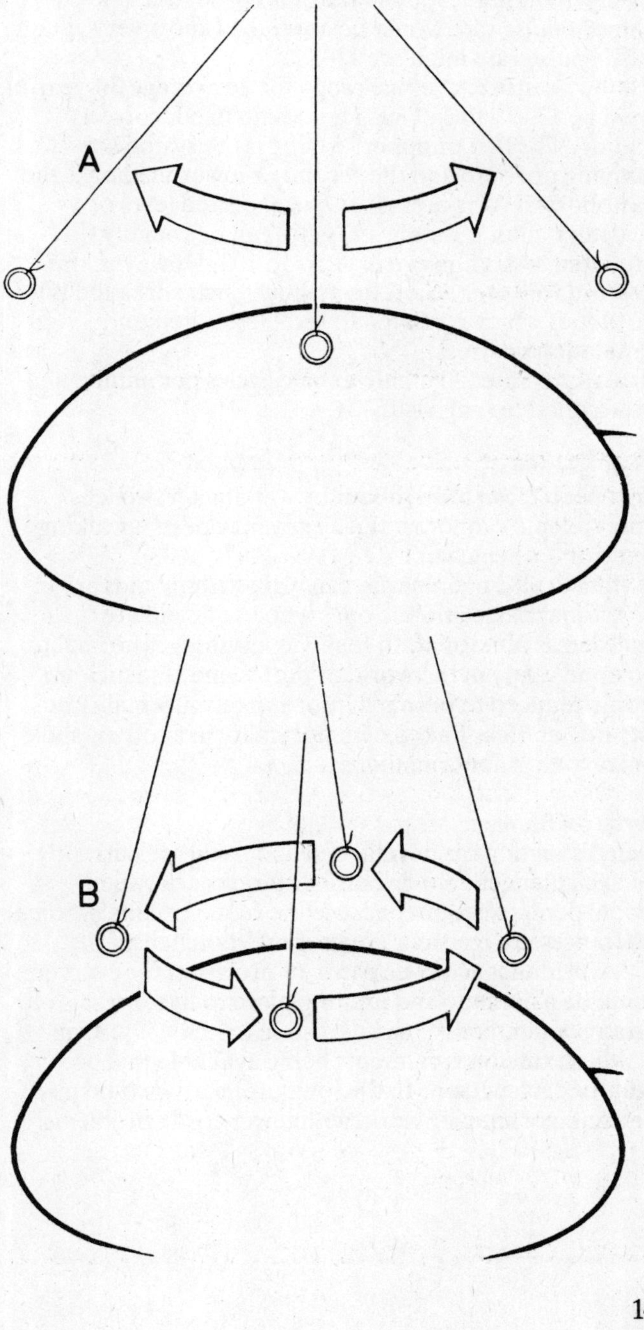

How fit are you?

A state of good health combined with certain levels of strength, suppleness and stamina are the modern indicators of fitness. A person can also be in good health but not very fit because muscles are a bit flabby, but providing the level of fitness does not drop so low that healthy functioning of the body is threatened, there is no reason why everyone should have to be at the same level of fitness all the time.

SOME BASIC INDICATORS OF FITNESS

There are several things that can be measured scientifically to give an indication that the body is functioning within normal limits.

- Body temperature: 98.4°F (36.8°C), the acceptable range being 98–98.6°F (36.7–37°C). Above 100°F (37.8°C) is regarded as a fever.
- Resting pulse rate: the average is 72 pulse beats per minute and the acceptable range is 60–80, but a fit athlete's pulse rate would be around 40 and a very young baby's pulse rate might be 120.
- Blood pressure: average range for an average 30-year-old could be 120/70 to 140/80. There is no fixed, correct reading. The first or upper reading is the systolic or pumping pressure and the second or lower reading is the diastolic or resting pressure. The expected level of a particular adult's systolic pressure can be roughly estimated by adding age in years to 100. However, this pressure will alter according to how much adrenalin is in the blood, which is related to level of excitement, stimulation or stress.
- Breathing rate: 20 inhale/exhale cycles per minute and the acceptable range is 16–24.

What is normal?

Most people can move about by walking on two legs. Other people cannot do this. They may need a walking frame or a wheelchair.

Statistically, people who can walk without aids are in the normal range and the ones who use an aid are regarded as abnormal. In reality everything is normal to someone. Only in the world of profits and statistics are people reduced to norms. Unfortunately, normality in one area of life is linked with normality in another, and similarly with abnormality.

Variety with parity

Such distinctions as normal and abnormal are currently being challenged, not because differences between people don't exist, but because the requirements of some differences are ignored, creating additional disparity.

A world that achieves parity of provision for everyone would be a humane and exciting place to live, for it is our differences that make us interesting to know. Parity in healthcare means treatments being available that are right for each person. In the long run, parity would pay for itself in a happier world with fewer costly problems.

THE HEROIC WATER CURE

Western medicine has tended to match the treatment to the illness regardless of the person. Since each person is unique, it would seem reasonable to assume that only certain treatments are suitable for certain types of people under certain circumstances.

Water treatments, for example are of two main kinds: hot or cold. Some doctors who ran the hydrotherapy programs at various spa centers, that developed in Europe in the 19th century, swore by heat treatments; others insisted that cold water was the only valid water treatment. One infamous cold water spa was the one at Gräfenberg, 2000 feet up in the mountains of Austrian Silesia (now known as Jesenik, in Czechoslovakia). It was run by Vincenz Priessnitz, a farmer's son, who became famous for his hydrotherapy cures-without-drugs, and rich in the process. He combined cold water treatments with lengthy exercise and mountain air.

Priessnitz claimed his cures made people fitter than they had ever been, although according to rumor, a person had to be fit to undertake his water cures. The *Journal of Health* of 1852, reporting on his methods, called him the 'Water Demon'.

Priessnitz reasoned that if a cold compress cured a sprained ankle then why not a cold compress for the whole body to cure a deep disorder? Warm water and sweat blankets were only used to add shock to the consequent application of icy cold water.

A typical day at Gräfenberg

A certain Captain Claridge who suffered from rheumatism listed his first day of treatments at Gräfenberg as follows:
4 a.m. dip in the cold spring;
an hour in the sweat blanket;
cold plunge for three minutes followed by a long walk;
breakfast, with cold, spring water to drink;
10 a.m. five minutes under the cold douche;
warm sitz bath and foot bath for 15 minutes each;
another cold douche – it's like gravel on my back;
a long walk until lunch at 1.p.m.;
wet-sheeting (skin massage with wet sheets);
an ascending cold douche for the genitals;
another long walk, a head-pack and cold sponge-down;
warm sitz-bath and foot bath for 15 minutes each;
9.30 p.m. in bed with feet and legs bound in cold, wet bandages. Up at 4 a.m. the next day. After three months, the Captain had walked 1000 miles and was cured of his rheumatism.

The cold douche

A modified version from Dr Grindrod's *Malvern: Past and Present*. The water would fall 10–14 feet for women and 19 feet for men. The head was protected or the patient bent forward to avoid being hit on the head by the water which fell with considerable force, massaging the back, and the legs and arms. The treatment lasted anything from 2 minutes to even an hour for the bravest. Are you fit enough to take a cold douche?

WE HAVE DIFFERENCES

There are at least two types of people in the world: male and female. The typical male body is broader across the shoulders than at the hips, while the typical female body is narrower across the shoulders than at the hips.

Then there are variations among both sexes, such as tall thin people, short fat people. Age alters the body which may also shrink in height. The diet, exercises or medical treatments needed at different ages to keep different types of people fit may be as many as there are types of people.

No one type of person is the epitome of fitness. There are many different types of people who are all fit and healthy. So when assessing your personal fitness, you should always take into account your body type.

Assessing your own weight

Folk medicine suggests that you are at your ideal weight if the measurement twice around the wrist equals once round the lower part of the neck, and twice around the neck equals once around the waist.

An American Dr Lulu Hunt Peters has the following rule for estimating your ideal weight:

1 Measure height in feet and inches without shoes.
2 Take the number of inches above or below five feet and multiply by 5½.
3 If taller than five feet, add result to 110.
If shorter than five feet, subtract result from 110.
4 The final number is your ideal weight in pounds.

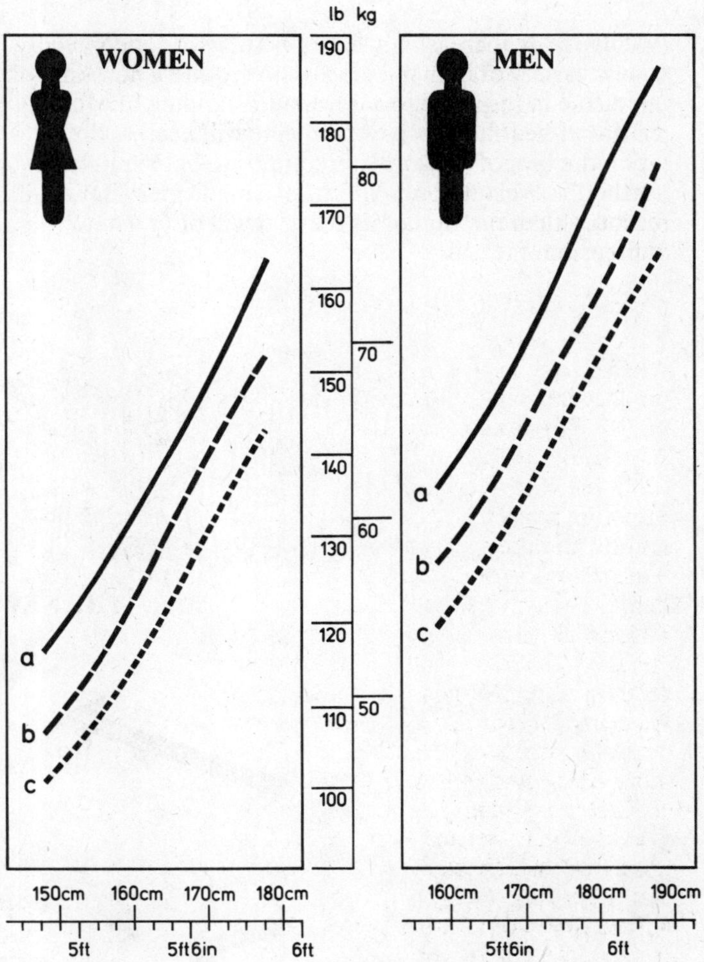

Graphs show desirable weights
a Large frame **b** Medium frame **c** Small frame

WHAT TEMPERAMENT ARE YOU?

Every primitive medical system was aware there were broadly different types of people. Knowing your own type would help you be aware of danger signals, by knowing how your own type reacts to excessive pressure and strain, which in the end often leads to illness.

The four temperaments

Hippocrates, the ancient Greek physician, identified the four main types of person as phlegmatic, melancholic, sanguine and choleric, each representing one of the main body fluids. When in good health, the four humors would be balanced. When off-balance, one of the body-fluids would fail to work properly, according to personal tendency.

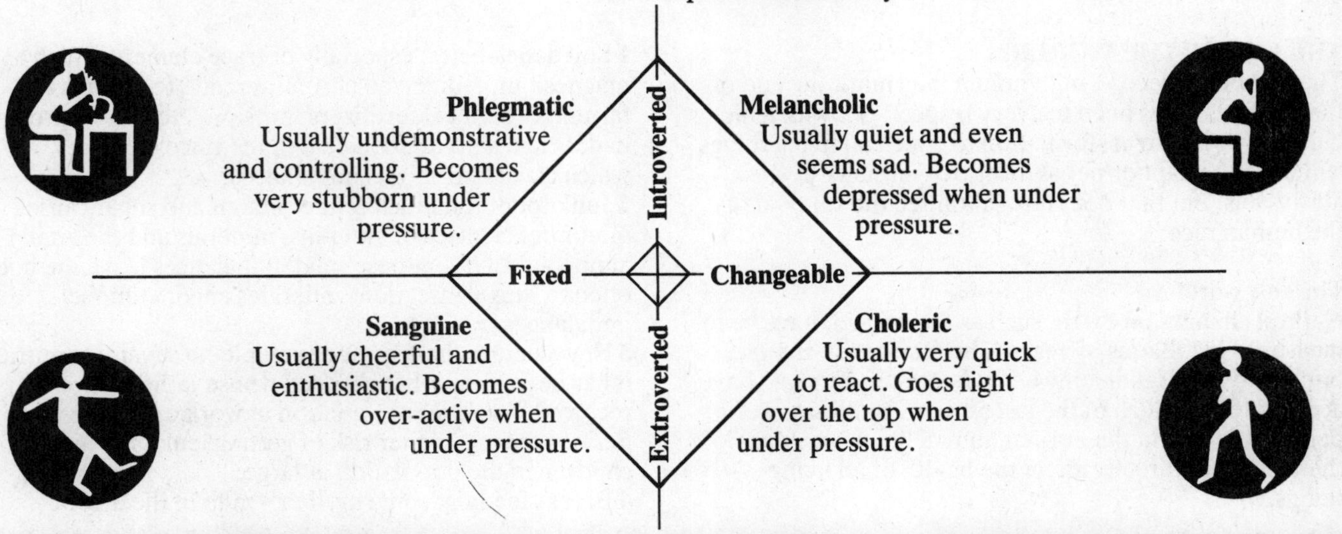

The best of both worlds

We live in an increasingly new kind of world, peopled by a new variety of human beings who require a new kind of medicine in response to a new understanding of what causes ill-health. This new medicine will need to draw upon the best of all worlds: a composite of Primitive, Orthodox Western and Alternative medicines. But it will be more than the sum of its parts; it will offer a new dimension.

The new medicine will be truly "magical" because it will often be impossible to know exactly why a treatment works, yet it will have an entirely scientific basis.

To use this new medicine the doctor must take a holistic view of the patient, which will inevitably involve the patient in a partnership with the doctor. Gone will be the doctor-patient heirarchy that has existed in both Western and Alternative medicines.

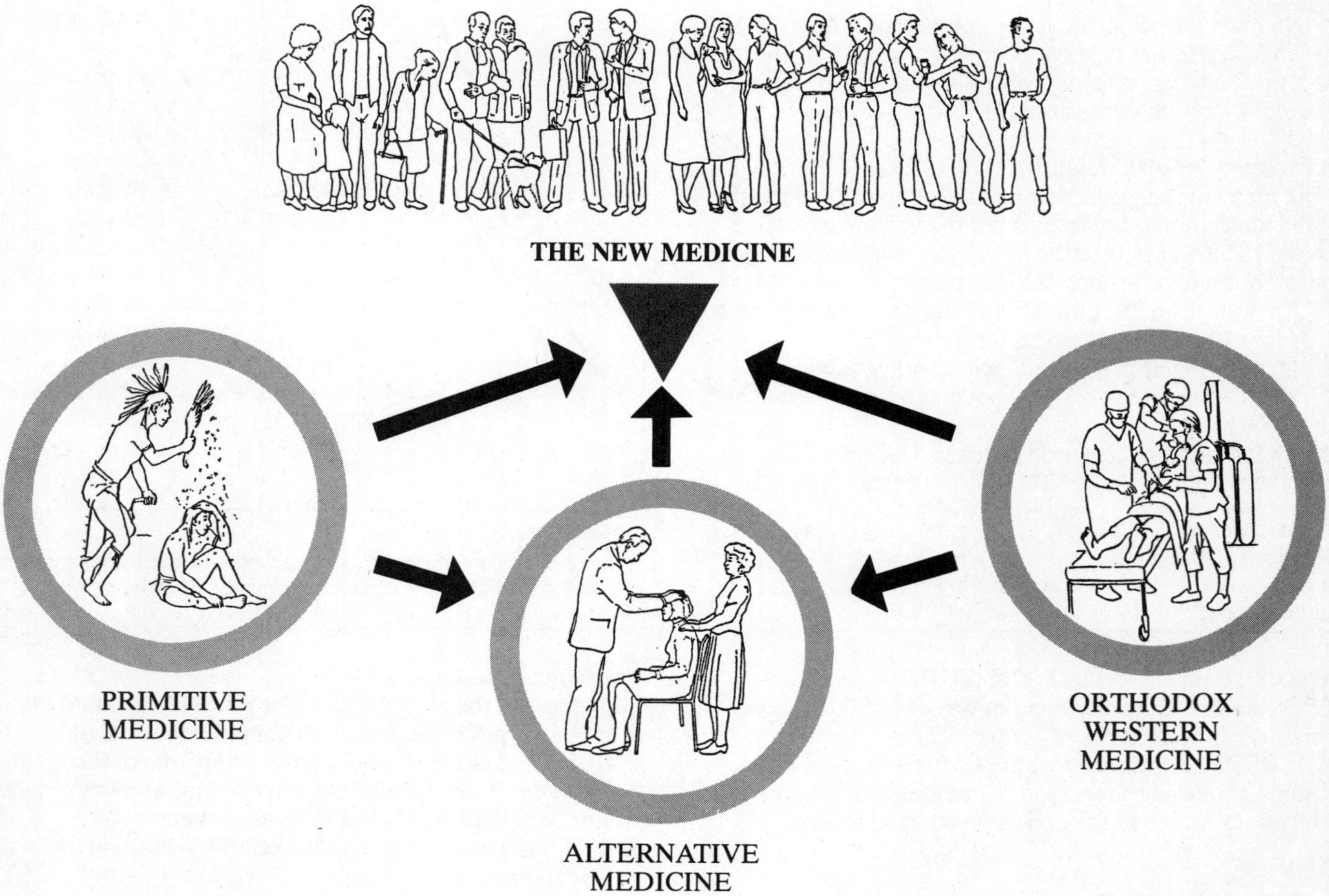

THE END OF THE WORLD?

The end of the second millennium may mark the end of the world as it has been in every respect, not with a big bang, but with a transformation to which all living things will have to adapt or perish. Nature will survive, she always has, but that does not guarantee the survival of the human race.

The new world

Natural changes on earth, such as the ice age, have been measured in millions of years. The man-made changes to our world have taken only a few hundred years and have accelerated so much in the last 50 years that they are perceptible within the normal human life-span. Many of these changes directly affect the health of all living things.

1 Soil deficiencies: especially of trace elements, such as magnesium, iodine and chromium, due to intensive farming, chemical fertilizers, erosion, etc. Foods grown in deficient soils are deficient in the trace elements, which causes hormonal imbalances.
2 Junk food: too much refined starch and sugar causes minor deficiencies of vitamins, minerals and the vital amino acids. Even these small imbalances leave the body open to fungal infections, allergies and metabolic imbalances.
3 New genetic changes: for example, in several countries it has been found that children whose fathers have received low doses of radiation at work over long periods, have a higher risk of getting leukemia than children in the population at large.
4 Breast-feeding: some mother's milk in the diet of

infants stabilizes the developing immune system and contributes many essential antibodies which will prevent later allergies and fungal infections. Cows' milk does not achieve this.

5 Environmental pollution: from agricultural, industrial and household chemicals, putting greater strain on the immune system. Immunity is also weakened by long exposure to electro-magnetic fields, to continuous vibration and to certain levels of noise.

6 Prolonged negative stresses: emotional, mental or physical, and despair itself, all weaken the immune system leaving it vulnerable to infections from fungi, such as yeasts, allergens such as pollen and dust, and an astounding variety of viruses.

7 Allopathic medicines: such as steroid hormones, antibiotics and the birth control pill are all thought to be involved in the enormous increase of allergies among younger generations, especially women. Immunization programs weaken natural immunity.

8 Animal feeds: hormones, antibiotics and offal from other animals given to farm animals to fatten them are also implicated in human immune-deficiency diseases and are known to support fungal diseases in humans.

The new person

Dr Allen Scott Levin, a clinical ecologist from San Francisco is of the opinion that the average citizen of the 1980s was genetically and biochemically different from the average citizen a generation earlier in the 1950s, due to the effects of the changes in the "new world", as listed above. The new person is more likely to have a weakened immune system, and therefore be more vunerable to infection, particularly from viruses.

The cause of ill-health

At the centre of all ill-health is the malfunctioning of the body systems due to the failure of the immune system to defend the body against its invaders, e.g. bacteria, viruses, allergens, etc.

THE VIRUSES

There is nothing new about viruses. They have always existed, invading living things and causing diseases. The apparent increase in virus diseases may not be due to an increase in viruses but to the number of people they inhabit who have a weakened immune system.

Different viruses cause varieties of influenza, the common cold, AIDS, chickenpox, hepatitis, herpes, shingles, measles, rubella, mumps, smallpox, typhus, yellow fever, Lassa fever, glandular fever, and some cancers, including 80% of cervical cancers.

Viruses are also thought to be important in a variety of very different diseases such as rheumatoid arthritis, multiple sclerosis, clinical depression, ulceration and schizophrenia. Viruses are implicated in a newly recognized twentieth century disease, known around the world by many different names, such as Myalgic Encephalomyelitis, Post-viral Fatigue Syndrome or Yuppie Flu.

How are viruses spread?

They can pass into the body by contact with other people or animals, or they can be picked up from the air we breathe and the water we drink. Viruses are unavoidable, but we need not allow them to take over.

What is a virus?

A virus is a parasitic, submicroscopic organism that consists of a central core of nucleic acids, i.e. RNA or DNA, enclosed in a shell-like protein. In this state it remains inert and can exist in animals, plants and the human body for years.

If a weakness enables one virus to invade a cell, then it will disrupt the cell's DNA, and use this genetic protein to reproduce itself because it cannot do this unaided.

A healthy body reacts with a sequence of immune responses, including producing an anti-viral protein known as interferon, which prevents the viral growth from spreading.

The attempt to synthesize effective anti-viral drugs has so far evaded the allopathic drug industry. Anything that destroys a virus will also destroy the cell tissue it inhabits. It may be that instead of trying to treat only part of the problem, i.e. the virus, a more holistic approach will have to be made. This is likely to be one of the major tasks of the new medicine.

The new medicine

Immune-related diseases, allergies and fungal infections are all on the increase. Learning how to build our natural immunity against these diseases will be a main task of the new medicine.

There are already indications that some conventional Western doctors are beginning to look for ways in which the whole body can be stimulated to protect itself more efficiently against an increasing variety of viruses. In particular a correct diet is being advocated, which is one of the bastions of holistic naturopathy.

Dowsing and magnetic therapy, for example, are being used by specialists who would previously have thought such methods madness. A dowsing device, such as a swinging pendulum, is thought to respond to the electro-magnetic field of the body. Dowsing is used by some nutrition specialists to decide if a particular food is suitable for a patient. Magnetic therapy is claimed to affect the ion balance in the body.

The new medicine will be involved with self-help and prevention as much as cure. As more and more is understood about the effects of the new world on our immune systems, more can be done to counter these effects by building strong, resilient immune systems.

The role of amino acids, lipids, vitamins and minerals is an area of growing research. All this knowledge will be essential to the new medicine.

It may rest with all of us to find ways to live in the world that do not produce irritants and other dangers that threaten the delicate balance of our vital immune systems.

Glossary

Names in parentheses, e.g. (medical), refer to the system from which the meaning of the word is derived.

ABREACTION
Powerful emotional discharge of previously repressed feelings, sometimes accompanied by insights.

ACID
A sour, sharp substance, such as vinegar or lemon juice, that can be neutralized by an alkali.

ACUPUNCTURE
Preventing and curing disease by stimulating selected points on the skin with fine acupuncture needles.

ALEXANDER TECHNIQUE
Physical re-education to improve posture and movement, thus relaxing distorting tensions.

ALKALI
A bitter, caustic or soapy substance, such as ammonia, that can be neutralized by an acid.

ALLERGY
An abnormal response by the body to some foreign substances, which may be foods.

ALLOPATHY
Treatment of disease by inducing an opposite condition; the basis of Western orthodox medicine.

AMULET
A protective charm or talisman.

ANABOLISM
That part of the metabolic process during which substances are used to build the body.

ANTIBODY
A protein produced by the body as part of the defense system when invaded by a foreign substance.

ANTISEPTIC
Prevents sepsis; destroys harmful bacteria.

ARCHETYPE
Primeval image or symbol.

ASEPTIC
Surgically sterile; absence of harmful bacteria.

ASTROLOGY
The study of planetary influences.

AUTOGENIC TRAINING
A six-step training to attain a state of passive relaxation; similar to self-hypnosis.

AUTONOMIC
Any involuntary, self-governing activity, including physical functions such as the heart beat.

BIOENERGETICS
Exercises designed to release chronic muscle tensions and the emotions associated with them.

BIRTH CHART
A circular diagram of the position of the planets at the time of birth, used in astrology.

BRAIN DEATH
The absence of electrical activity in the brain shown as a flat reading on an electroencephalogram (EEG).

CADUCEUS
Greek herald's wand, usually that of Mercury, the messenger of the gods. A symbol of healing.

CATABOLISM
That part of the metabolic process during which substances are broken down to release energy.

CATALYST
A substance that facilitates a (usually chemical) change but does not participate in it.

CHAKRAS
The seven centers of energy along the spine (Yoga).

CHARACTER ARMORING
Pattern of chronic muscular tensions that determine attitude (Reichian therapy).

CH'I or QI ENERGY
Flow of life energy in the body (Oriental).

CHIROPRACTIC
Manipulation of the joints of the vertebrae in the spine to restore normal functioning of the body.

CLINICAL DEATH
The absence of clinically detectable signs of life, such as heart beat, breathing and warmth.

CLINICAL ECOLOGIST
A physician who specializes in allergies due to chemical or environmental causes.

CLONING
Forming an organism asexually, i.e. reproducing an exact duplicate of an organism from one of its cells without any fertilization taking place.

CONTAGIOUS DISEASE
A disease that is spread by direct contact.

CONTAGIOUS MAGIC
The continued influence upon each other of things that previously have been in contact.

CRYONICS
Placing a human body in deep freeze, because of the belief that it can be thawed out, and cured to live in the future.

CYCLE
A regular sequence of recurring events.

DIASTOLIC
The blood pressure between contractions of the heart.

DIVINER
One who foretells the future through signs & portents.

DNA
Deoxyribonucleic acid, an essential part of all living cells; a protein chain that carries the genetic code.

DRUG
A substance that produces a psychotropic change in the consumer, i.e. is mind-altering.

EGO
The part of the mind that deals with reality; a person's consciousness of his or her individuality.

EIDETIC MEMORY
Remembering by seeing something exactly as if it were there in reality and can be examined.

ELECTROLYTE
A solution of a salt that conducts electricity.

ELEMENT (Ancient use of word)
Four or five active constituents of the universe including fire, earth and water, the other two varying from culture to culture: e.g. wood, metal, air, ether.

ELEMENT (Chemical use of word)
A substance that can form other substances such as sodium and chlorine, forming sodium chloride.

ENZYMES
Substances in the body that control or speeds up biological and chemical reactions in the body.
ESOTERIC
Secret knowledge available only to the initiated.
EUGENICS
Attempts at the production of perfect offspring by improving genetically inherited qualities.
FAMILIAR
A spirit, ghost or demon that obeys the shaman, medicine-man or witch who regularly calls upon it.
FELDENKRAIS EXERCISES
A series of precisely structured movements designed to re-align the skeleton correctly.
GESTALT
A perceived, organized whole, which is greater, in effect, than the sum of its parts (Psychology).
GESTURE
Communication by small movements of the body, limbs, fingers or facial features.
GINSENG
Panax ginseng is a plant that grows in China, the root of which has been used for centuries for healing and as a tonic. Other *Panax* varieties grow elsewhere.
HEALER
A person who causes healing to take place by his or her own presence or touch.
HEMOGLOBIN
Oxygen-carrying substance in red blood cells.
HIGH
Having feelings of joy, pleasure or ecstasy, caused naturally or by taking drugs (see TRIP).
HOMEOPATHY
Treatment of disease by inducing a similar condition in general or in particular.
HORMONES
Substances which stimulate the organs of the body into action and determine what kind of action.
HUMORS
Body fluids, such as bile, allied to temperament.
HYPNOSIS
An altered state of consciousness induced by the self or by another person, which reduces some inhibitions, including the sensation of pain.
HYPOCHONDRIA
Morbid anxiety about health.
HYPOTHERMIA
Lowered body temperature, usually due to extreme cold.
IATROGENIC DISEASE
A new illness caused by the diagnosis or treatment of another disease; more than just a side-effect.
IMMUNE RESPONSE
The response of the body to antigens, i.e. foreign substances that stimulate the defense system.
IMPEDANCE
The total resistance offered by the medium through which electric impulses are passing; measured in ohms.
IMPRINTING
Leaving an impression on one substance, often water, of the essence (perhaps the energy pattern) of another substance (principle of homeopathic remedies).
INFECTIOUS DISEASE
A disease spread by air, water and contact with a diseased person.
INTROVERSION
A reserved, inward, unsociable attitude of mind.
ION
An atom that is carrying a positive or negative charge due to having lost or acquired an electron.
KARMA
A person's destiny, determined by their actions in previous lives (Hinduism).
KILNER SCREEN
A double sheet of glass containing a solution of diocene, used for viewing the human aura.
KINESIOLOGY
Applied kinesiology is a form of nutritional diagnosis and monitor of treatment using measured muscle tone.
KUNDALINI
Life-force or sexual energy (Indian).
LEGEND
Historical myth rooted in a real person or event.
MACROBIOTICS
A way of life based on a diet of brown rice, grains, vegetables and little else.
MAGATAMA
Japanese word for the curved "tadpole" symbol of life. Two magatama together form a circle.
MAGIC
The art of influencing events by occult and other inexplicable means. Magic can be good, bad or amoral. See also CONTAGIOUS and SYMPATHETIC MAGIC
MANTRA
A repetitive incantation for religious purposes.
MESMERISM
Healing by magnetic forces drawn from the moon and planets. Invented and used by Austrian physician, Franz Anton Mesmer (1734–1815).
METABOLISM
Processes in living organisms using food and oxygen for body building and energy production.
MIASMAS
Infectious or noxious emanations; tendency to disease.
MOUTZA
Greek; insulting open hand gesture.
MYTH
Traditional story about a fictitious person or idea.
NATUROPATHY
Health and healing attained by using natural methods such as correct diet, fasting, cleansing and massage.
NEUROTIC
Behavior that is based on unrealistic ideas.
NEUROTRANSMITTER
Chemical substances that carry electrical impulses from one nerve cell to the next.
NUCLEIC ACIDS
The two acids, DNA and RNA, present in all living cells.

OCCULT
Secret, supernatural or mystical knowledge.
OSTEOPATHY
The diagnosis and treatment of malfunctions in the musculo-skeletal system by manipulation.
PALMISTRY
Reading personality and personal destiny in the hands, particularly using the lines on the palms.
PARASYMPATHETIC NERVOUS SYSTEM
That part of the autonomic system that is in control during relaxed states.
PHAGOCYTOSIS
Absorption of bacteria or other foreign bodies by white blood cells.
PLACEBO
A pleasant, inactive substance given in place of a drug, e.g. a sugar-pill.
POLARITY THERAPY
Reflex healing by stimulating the charge of polar opposites in the body.
PORTENT
A sign of what is to come; an omen.
POTENTIZING
Homeopathic process involving shaking or grinding during which a substance is said to leave its imprint in water, an alcohol or a powdered lactose base.
PSIONIC MEDICINE
Diagnosis by dowsing and treatment by psychic means.
PSYCHIC
Having a sixth sense or keenly intuitive skill.
PSYCHOPOMP
Shaman who helps souls transfer into the next world.
PSYCHOSIS
Severe mental illness involving the whole personality.
PSYCHOSOMATIC
Physical illness aggravated by mental stress.
PSYCHOTHERAPY
Psychological treatment by verbal intercourse.
PSYCHOTROPIC
Having a mind-altering effect.
RADIONICS
Method of diagnosis and treatment at a distance.
REFLEX HEALING
Healing by stimulating the autonomic reflex pathways, using thumb pressure or massage.
REFLEX MASSAGE
A gliding form of thumb pressure used in reflexology.
REFLEXOLOGY
Reflex healing through selected points on the feet.
REINCARNATION
Rebirth after death as a new person in a new body.
RNA
Ribonucleic acid, an essential part of all living cells. See also DNA.
ROLFING See STRUCTURAL REINTEGRATION
SHAMAN
Healer, originally in the Asian Arctic, who healed by contacting the spirits during a trance state. A person became a shaman by inheritance and suffering.
SHIATZU
Japanese form of acupuncture treatment done by a finger massage known as acupressure.
SOLAR PLEXUS
Nerve mass just behind the stomach which services most of the involuntary organs.
STRESS
Anything from outside an organism that causes erosion of its normal physiological functioning.
STRUCTURAL REINTEGRATION or **ROLFING**
A deep massage program to soften chronically tight connective tissues, allowing the skeleton to ride easily and making the whole body feel lighter.
SUBLIMATE
To purify; to re-channel; to vaporize from a solid and then return to a solid state.
SYMPATHETIC MAGIC
Things that are similar have similar magical effects.
SYMPATHETIC NERVOUS SYSTEM
That part of the autonomic system that is in command during stress.
SYNCHRONOUS
Two things occurring at the same time.
SYNDROME
The group of symptoms that are typical of a disease.
SYSTEMIC
Of a system as a whole.
SYSTOLIC
The pressure of the blood on contraction of the heart, i.e. at the heart beat.
TANKA
Buddhist religious painting designed to activate the unconscious and stimulate awareness (also the name of a Japanese poetic form).
TANTRA
An Indian religious cult.
TINCTURE
A medicinal substance finely ground and dissolved in water or alcohol.
TRACTION
Stretching the body, head to foot, to relieve the compression of the vertebrae on the spinal cord.
TRANSFERENCE
Psychological term meaning the patient has transferred his feelings for a parent, etc. to the therapist.
TRANSMUTE
Change from one form into another, for example metals into gold in alchemy.
TRIP
Name given to experiences of altered perceptions usually due to the use of drugs (see HIGH).
VIRUS
Sub-microscopic pieces of nucleic acids in a protein shell that can only grow inside living cells.
VITAMIN
A substance in food that is an accessory nutrient.
VOTIVE
An offering, sometimes consecrated, to fulfill a vow.

WET NURSING
Breast-feeding a child other than one's own.
YIN-YANG (Chinese)
Opposing forces within the total flow of life energy.
ZONE THERAPY
Reflex healing by massaging zones of the feet and hands to stimulate corresponding horizontal and vertical zones of the body.

Index

A
Ablution 98
Aborigines 69
Abrams, Dr Albert 106
Acids 139
Acoustic images 24
Acupressure 32, 38
Acupuncture 30, 32–35, 147
Additives 83
Aging process 11, 102
Ainyahita 99
Alchemy 55, 70–73
Alcohol 80, 128
Alexander technique 47
Alkalis 139
Allergies 83, 146
Allopathy 22, 153
Alternative medicine 29
Amulets 48–49, 62–63, 99
Anabolism 24
Anatomical Chinese Inch (ACI) 33, 36
Anesthetic hypnosis 112
Animal fats 82
Animal feeds 153
Animal wisdom 77
Ankh 62
Anthroposophy 24
Antibiotics 22
Anticoagulant 84–85
Aphrodisiacs 80
Apple cider vinegar 138
Archetypal patterns 102
Aromatherapy 25
Astrology 115, 148
Atkins, Dr R.G. 82
Augury 148
Auras 106, 108, 119, 142, 144
Autogenic therapy 113

B
Bach, Dr Edward 136–137
Back-walking 40
Back stretching 41
Balahi (Hindu) medicine 66–67
Baldness 126
Ball, Lawrence 24
Balneology 86
Barwa 66–67
Bates, Dr William H. 90
Baths 75, 86–87
Bee stings 88–89
Biochemics 93
Bioenergetics 23
Biorhythms 20–21, 146
Black box 106–107
Blaise, St 96, 97
Blood-letting 74, 84–85
Blood pressure 150
Bonding 44
Bone-setting 41
Bovis, Antoine 102
Brain death 17
Brompton cocktail 129
Broussais, F.J.V. 84
Budwig, J. 88

C
Cadmus 71, 73
Caduceus 63, 72–73, 91
Cannabis 128–129
Cantelupe, St Thomas 100–101
Castenada, Carlos 131
Catabolism 24
Celestial Bed 79
Celiac disease 140
Chaology 11
Chiropractic 40
Chung-Ching, Chang 15
Clairvoyance 108, 146
Clinical death 17
Cocaine 129
Cold water treatment 150
Color therapy 109, 118–119
Complementary medicine 29
Consultants 66–67
Contagious magic 19
Contraception 81
Convulsions 111
Cosmetics 123
Coventina's well 99
Creative cycle 20–21
Cupping 25

D
Degenerative diseases 11, 12
de la Warr, George 106
Deoxyribonucleic acid (DNA) 17, 91, 95
Developmental healing 12
Diagnoses 144–145, 148–149
Diet 82–83
Divestment 126–127
Dowsing 108, 109, 148–149
Drbal, Karl 102
Drown, Ruth 106
Drugs 122, 128–129
Drumming 116–117

E
Ehrlich, Paul 123
Eidetic memory 112
Electrical stimulation 26–27
Electro-convulsive therapy 111
Electroencephalograph (EEG) 17, 144
Electrolytes 93
Electro-magnetic spectrum 119
Elements 10, 36, 56, 70
Elixir of Life 72
Endorphins 26–27, 105
Essential oils 25
Eurhythmy 24
Eugenics 99
Evers, Joseph 83
Exercise 22, 94
Exorcism 12–13
Eye exercises 90
Eysenck, Prof. H.J. 114

F
Familiars 66–67
Feet 50–53
Feldenkrais exercises 47
Fertility 78–79
Finger massage 32, 52
Fliess, Dr W. 146
Flower remedies 136–137
Fly agaric 131
Folklore 13, 126–127
Folk medicine 28, 124–125
Food, importance of 77, 82–83
Footwear 27, 47
Fractals 11, 130
Fresh air 77

G
Gassner, Father 110
Gattefossé, M. 25
Genetic changes 152
Genetic engineering 91
Geomancy 148
Gestalt therapy 23
Gimble-Seilung, Max 118
Gimble, Theo 118–119
Ginseng 77, 89
Golden series 103
Graham, James 79, 87
Grape diet 88
Greatriks, Valentine 110
Great Work, the 71, 72–73
Grindrod, Dr 150
Groddeck, George 23

H
Hahnemann, Dr Samuel 123, 134
Hail chant ritual 61
Hallucinogens 130
Hand gestures 48–49
Ha'nish, Otoman Zar-Adusht 99
Health 12, 150
Heat stimulation 32
Herbalism 76–77, 120, 124–125
Hippocrates 47, 82, 88, 145, 151
Hirudin 85
Hoffer, Dr Abram 140
Hoffmann, Dr Albert 131
Holistic medicine 29
Holy water 98–99, 127
Homeopathic medicine 18, 22, 102, 109, 123, 134
Honey 88, 138
Huxley, Aldous 131
Hypnotism 112–113
Hypochondria 12
Hypothalamus 92

I
Immune deficiency 11, 153
Impotence 81
Inherited predisposition 94
Interferon 95
Intuition 108
Ion therapy 25
Iridology 145

J
Jarvis, Dr D.C. 138
Jesus of Nazareth 42
Jogging 91
Jung, Carl 11, 19
Junk foods 152

K
Kamiya, Joseph 144
Kelp 83
Kidneys 92
Kilner screen 106, 118–119
Kinesiology, applied 146
King's Evil 30, 42
Kirlian photography 144
Kondratieff, Nikolai D. 21
Kundalini 91

L
Lapp shamans 76
Lawrence, Dr George 108
Laying on of hands 19, 30
Leaf, Dr Alexander 138
Leboyer, Frédéric 45
Leechdom 132–133
Leeches 84–85
Levin, Dr Allen Scott 153
Lévi-Strauss, Claude 105
Light 90–91, 118–119
Littlejohn, John M. 40
Lorenz, Edward 11
Lourdes 96, 100, 101
Love potions 80
Lowen, Alexander 16, 23
LSD 130–131
Lydiard, Arthur 91
Lynn, R. 12

M
Mackarness, Dr R. 82
Macrobiotics 77
Magic mushrooms 131
Magnetism 79, 110–111
Maharishi Mahesh Yogi 57
Mandelbrot, Benoit 11
Manipulation 40–41
Massage 41, 43, 52
Materia Prima 71, 72
McDonagh, J.E.R. 108
McDowell, Roger 82–83
McGilvray, Isobel 24
McLuhan, Marshall 58
Melatonin 91
Memory 112
Menstruation 20, 80–81
Meridians 32, 36–37, 147
Mescaline 131
Mesmer, Franz 97, 110–111
Miasmas 108, 134
Mineral waters 86
Mistletoe 78
Moxabustion 32, 77
Mud baths 87
Multiple sclerosis 82–83
Music 117
Musoli 65
Mystical senses 108–109

N
Natural immunity 153
Natural remedies 138–139
Naturopathy 82, 99
Navaho rituals 60–61, 64–65
Navaho sand-paintings 61, 65
Ndembu medicine 64–65
Necromancy 148
Needles 33
Nerves 37
Niehans, Dr Paul 94

O
Old wives' tales 120, 126–127
Oneiromancy 148
Onions 125
Opium 121, 129
Optimism 94, 114
Oracles 142, 148–149
Orthomolecular medicine 140
Osteopathy 40
Ouser 63
Outlining 69
Owen, Dr Julia 88–89

P
Pain 26–27, 113
Paisley pattern 39
Palmer, Daniel 40
Palmistry 48
Paracelsus 110, 123
Pasteur, Louis 85
Pauling, Linus 140
Peripheral Nervous System (PNS) 17
Peters, Dr Lulu Hunt 151
Philosopher's Stone 72
Pilgrimages 100–101
Polarity therapy 51
Pollution 25, 94, 153
Posture 27, 46–47
Potencies 134–135
Precognition 108
Price, Dr W.A. 83
Priessnitz, Vincenz 150
Psionic medicine 108
Psychometry 108
Psychotherapy 23
Pulse 14, 147, 150
Pyramids 102–103
Pythagoras 10

R
Radiesthesia 146
Radionics 106–107, 146
Rae, Malcolm 102–103, 106
Reflex healing 50–51
Reflex massage 52–53
Reflexology 146
Regression 113
Reich, Wilhelm 16, 23, 97
Rein, Dr G. 118
Reiter, Professor Russel 91
Rejuvenation 90–91
Resuscitation 17
Reticuloendothelial system (RES) 94
Richards, Dr Guyon 106
Rituals 58–61, 78
Rolfing 47

S
St Anthony's Fire 130
Salvarsan 123
Sauna 86
Scapegoats 12–13
Scarab 62
Schuessler, Dr Wilhelm H. 93
Schultz, Dr Johannes 113
Sclerology 145
Seaweed 83
Secondary infections 22
Self-understanding 99
Semen 57
Serotonin 25
Sexual orgasmic cycle 21
Shackleton, Basil 88
Shamanism 54, 76, 104–105
Shiatzu 38
Shrines 100–101
Sioux rituals 60, 116
Smith, Dr R.F. 140
Soil deficiency 152
Solar breathing 153
Solomon's Seal 63
Soubirous, Bernadette 101
Sound 24, 116–117
Spagyrik therapy 147
Spas 86, 150
Sport 22
Star of David 63
Steiner, Rudolf 24, 118–119
Still, Andrew 40
Stoll, Arthur 131
Stress 23, 25, 113, 153
Structural Integration 47
Succussion 134
Sudatorium 86
Suggestion 69, 112
Sun-cults 118
Sweating 86–87
Swovoda, Dr H. 146
Sympathetic magic 18

T
Tai Chi 22
Talisman 62
Tansley, David 106
Tantra 31, 50–51
Teeth 81, 83
Telepathy 108
Temple of Health 79
Tesla, Nikola 112
Thalassotherapy 87
Thermalism 86
Tibetan medicine 77
Tinctures 18, 124
Tissue salts 93
Tituration 134
Tobacco 128
Tonics 89
Topology 19
Touch 30–31, 42–45
Traction 47
Transcutaneous Electrical Nerve Stimulation (TENS) 26
Tri-dosas 15
Twelve Healers 136–137

U
Unpredictability 11
Untouchables 42
Urine 92, 147
Urine testing 139

V
Vaccines 22, 143
Valnet, Dr 25
Vedas 56–57
Vision defects 90
Visualization 95
Vitamins 140–141
Votive offerings 98

W
Warts 114–115
Water 92–93, 150
Watson, Lyall 19
Weather 25
Weight 151
Well of the Heads 99
Wells 98–99
Westlake, Dr T.A. 102
Wine 88

Y
Yin-Yang 14–15, 32, 36, 38, 77
Yoruba herbalists 76
Yoruba rituals 58–59

Z
Zarathustra 99
Zone therapy 51